1202 Boulevard
Galveston (?)

HANDBOOK OF
ORTHOPAEDIC SURGERY

HANDBOOK OF
ORTHOPAEDIC SURGERY

By

ALFRED RIVES SHANDS, Jr., B.A., M.D.

Medical Director of the Alfred I. duPont Institute of the Nemours Foundation,
Wilmington, Delaware; Visiting Professor of Orthopaedic Surgery,
University of Pennsylvania School of Medicine,
Philadelphia, Pennsylvania

In Collaboration With

RICHARD BEVERLY RANEY, B.A., M.D.

Professor of Surgery in Orthopaedic Surgery, University of North Carolina,
Chapel Hill, North Carolina; Lecturer in Orthopaedics,
Duke University School of Medicine,
Durham, North Carolina

Illustrated by
JACK BONACKER WILSON AND OTHERS

Fourth Edition

St. Louis
The C. V. Mosby Company
1952

Press of
The C. V. Mosby Company
St. Louis

TO

WILLIAM STEVENSON BAER

1872-1931

PREFACE TO FOURTH EDITION

In the preparation of this fourth edition, the heads of the departments of orthopaedic surgery in the medical schools of the United States have been consulted. They were asked to express their opinions concerning the Handbook and particularly how it was thought the publication could be improved for the teaching of medical students. Out of the replies to this inquiry came many helpful suggestions which the author has carefully considered and deeply appreciates. The most pertinent suggestion was that the roentgenograms should be reproduced as roentgenograms and not as drawings. In the revision this has been accomplished almost completely. Many suggested that there should be more elaboration and detail in the presentation of the entities and that chapters should be added on surgical and plaster technics. This has not been done as the book would be increased in size to an extent that it would be no longer in the Handbook class of publications which the author does not think advisable. However, there have been ten short sections added on Arachnodactyly, Vitamin Disturbances and Skeletal Changes, Gargoylism, Morquio's Disease, Fibrous Dysplasia, Brucellosis, Gout, Herniation of the Fascial Fat in the Low Back, The Foot of the Normal Child, and Radiohumeral Subluxation in Children. The text has been brought up to date and the bibliography has been revised to March 1, 1952.

More attention has been paid to illustrations than in any of the previous revisions of the original text. There are one hundred six new illustrations as follows: seventy-nine new roentgenograms, twenty new drawings, two retouched drawings, two replacements of drawings from the first edition, and three copies of drawings from other publications; forty of the illustrations of the third edition have been deleted, most of which were drawings from roentgenograms.

The author wishes to express his thanks to the Radiology and Orthopaedic Departments of the University of Pennsylvania Hospital of Philadelphia, of the Duke Hospital of Durham, N. C., and of the Watts Hospital of Durham, N. C., who have contributed so generously of their roentgenographic material for illustrations; to the artists, Mr. Carl W.

3

Brill of Philadelphia and Mr. Don Alvarado of Baltimore, who have furnished the new drawings; to Mr. Nelson Sanborn, Jr., who has labored long and hard to obtain just the right prints of the roentgenograms; and to my secretary, Miss E. Ann Thomas, who has so satisfactorily typed, checked, and rechecked all of the printed and illustrative material. To the group of residents at the Alfred I. duPont Institute, Colonel Knox Dunlap, Medical Corps, United States Army, Lieutenant Commander Alvis B. Dickson, Medical Corps, United States Navy, Major Lucius C. Hollister, Jr., Medical Corps, United States Air Force, Dr. J. Stuart Gaul, Jr., and Commander Harold A. Streit, Medical Corps, United States Navy, who have prepared so much of the original material for the new sections, searched hard and long for just the right roentgenograms, and helped revise the bibliography, my especial thanks goes. Lastly, to Dr. R. B. Raney, my collaborator since the first edition, I wish to express my deepest appreciation for all he has done working oftentimes under most difficult conditions in a distant state.

A. R. SHANDS, JR., M.D.

Wilmington, Delaware

PREFACE TO FIRST EDITION

The purpose of this book is to present for the consideration of the medical student and the general practitioner the fundamental facts and principles of orthopaedic surgery as concisely as possible and yet in sufficient detail to convey a well-rounded knowledge of the subject.

An attempt has been made to present, not the views of one man or of one school, but the consensus of opinion as recorded in the orthopaedic textbooks and in the more recent orthopaedic literature, criticized and tempered with the experience and thought of twenty-four teachers of orthopaedic surgery and allied subjects representing eighteen different medical schools. It was believed to be unfair to ask any one man or group of men to criticize the whole text. To obviate the labor which this would necessarily impose upon a few individuals, various sections of manuscript were sent to these authorities for their criticism. This has been productive of most helpful suggestions for the betterment of the text. Each chapter has been reviewed by more than one authority. When there were conflicting opinions, the author has reserved the right to choose the subject matter which he thinks most suitable. Because of limitation of space certain important parts of orthopaedic teaching have been omitted; among these are the subjects of fresh fractures, plaster technic, and orthopaedic apparatus, as well as certain forms of treatment which in the past have been widely used but which are not generally accepted today. On the other hand, it may appear to some readers that too much material has been included for an elementary textbook. In the bibliography are grouped most of the outstanding American and English articles on the various orthopaedic subjects, and the reader who is desirous of gaining further knowledge will find these an excellent source of detailed and authoritative information.

Illustrations which are clear and to the point are used. Those taken from textbooks and journals have been redrawn. The majority of the illustrations are original pen and ink drawings, many of which were made from specimens provided by the author's collections of pathologic bones. No photographs or roentgenograms have been reproduced directly; all have been redrawn to emphasize their characteristic features. The drawings of operative technic have been chosen to illustrate certain principles of orthopaedic surgery. A great many surgical procedures which are described in the text have not been illustrated because of limitation of space.

The subject matter of the text has been divided into twenty-four chapters in accordance with a report of the Committee on Undergraduate Instruction in Orthopaedic Surgery of the American Orthopaedic Association, which in 1934 called attention to the fact that in several of the leading medical schools approximately twenty-four class periods of an hour's duration are profitably employed for undergraduate orthopaedic instruction. Sixteen of the chapters are arranged upon the basis of pathology; seven chapters are arranged according to anatomical region, and include disease entities which do not fall readily into the pathology grouping. It is realized that this arrangement is imperfect; nevertheless it has seemed to the author that such an organization of the subject matter provides an approach to completeness, at the same time reducing unnecessary repetition to a minimum.

While the value of a historical background is appreciated, it is believed that the student should not be confused with the names of too many individuals. Experience in teaching has shown that it is advisable to emphasize the principle of diagnosis and treatment rather than the identity of the originator; therefore, first importance has been given to the description of orthopaedic entities, and individual credit for their original presentation has in most cases been acknowledged as a secondary consideration.

The first chapter on chronic arthritis (Chapter X) has been taken from the *Arthritic Primer*, prepared by the American Committee for the Study and Control of Rheumatism. This Primer treats most ably the entire subject of chronic arthritis and presents the mature opinion of authorities who are most interested in this subject and best qualified to discuss it. The chapter on the low back (Chapter XIX) is a modification of Dr. Steindler's presentation of this subject in his text, *Diseases and Deformities of the Spine and Thorax*.

Most sincere appreciation is expressed to the following for their invaluable criticisms of various sections of the text: Dr. Lloyd T. Aycock, Boston, Mass.; Dr. G. E. Bennett, Baltimore, Md.; Dr. Willis C. Campbell, Memphis, Tenn.; Dr. W. B. Carrell, Dallas, Texas; Dr. F. A. Chandler, Chicago, Ill.; Dr. H. Earle Conwell, Birmingham, Ala.; Dr. R. S. Crisvell, Durham, N. C.; Dr. A. H. Freiberg, Cincinnati, Ohio; Dr. J. A. Freiberg, Cincinnati, Ohio; Dr. R. V. Funsten, University, Va.; Dr. Ralph K. Ghormley, Rochester, Minn.; Dr. A. Bruce Gill, Philadelphia, Pa.; Dr. R. W. Johnson, Jr., Baltimore, Md.; Dr. J. Albert Key, St. Louis, Mo.; Dr. Richard Kovacs, New York, N. Y.; Dr. Arthur Krida, New York, N. Y.; Dr. Arthur T. Legg, Boston, Mass.; Dr. Leo Mayer, New York, N. Y.; Dr. J. R. Moore, Philadelphia, Pa.; Dr. J. J. Morton, Rochester, N. Y.; Dr. I. W. Nachlas, Baltimore, Md.; Dr. Robert B. Osgood, Boston, Mass.; Dr. W. M. Phelps, Baltimore, Md.; Dr. Robert D. Schrock, Omaha, Neb.; Dr. R. Plato Schwartz, Rochester, N. Y.; Dr. Arthur Steindler, Iowa City, Iowa; Dr. John C. Wilson, Los Angeles, Calif.; and Dr. Philip D. Wilson, New York, N. Y.

Appreciation is expressed to Dr. W. M. Roberts, of the North Carolina Orthopaedic Hospital, and to Dr. O. L. Miller, of Charlotte, for the use of their case records and roentgenograms. Sincere thanks are extended to Dr. D. C. Hetherington for his criticism of construction and syntax. Appreciation is expressed also to the Radiological Division of Duke Hospital and to various members of the staff who have offered many helpful suggestions in their special fields of work. We also feel indebted to the following who have so kindly made suggestions regarding certain of the drawings: Dr. Toufick Nicola and Dr. Isadore Zadek, of New York; Dr. Irvine M. Flinn, Jr., of Wilmington, Del.; Dr. I. W. Nachlas, Dr. G. E. Bennett and Dr. R. E. Lenhard, of Baltimore; and Dr. J. Warren White, of Greenville, S. C.

Without the splendid work of the artists the value of the book would be greatly impaired. The author feels deeply indebted to Mr. Jack Bonacker Wilson, who has done a major part of the illustrative work, to Mr. Elon Clark, and to Mrs. E. M. Collins, who drew many of the preliminary sketches, and to Miss Elizabeth Brödel, whose illustrations of arthritic spines have proved most useful. For valuable stenographic aid appreciation is expressed to Mrs. Lucille Lyon and to Miss Henrietta Fagan and her associates.

It is hoped that this short textbook will assist in the teaching of orthopaedic surgery, and that it may find a permanent place of usefulness in this special field of medicine.

A. R. Shands, Jr., M.D.

Durham, N. C.

CONTENTS

CHAPTER I

CHAPTER II

CHAPTER III

CHAPTER IV

CHAPTER V

CHAPTER VI

CHAPTER VII

CHAPTER VIII

CHAPTER IX

CHAPTER X

CHAPTER XI

CHAPTER XII

CHAPTER XIII

CHAPTER XIV

HANDBOOK OF
ORTHOPAEDIC SURGERY

HANDBOOK OF ORTHOPAEDIC SURGERY

CHAPTER I

INTRODUCTION

The development of orthopaedic surgery as a specialized division of medical practice has been a long and gradual process. It was early recognized that the problems peculiar to this field of work should be grouped together as one subject for study and that these problems are best handled by individuals especially trained and experienced in their diagnosis and treatment. This principle can be observed in the works accredited to Hippocrates in the fifth century B.C., which contain many excellent descriptions of affections of the bones and joints. The first work devoted exclusively to the subject of orthopaedics, Andry's *L'Orthopédie,* was published in 1741. It provided an occasion for the frank separation of orthopaedics as a specialized branch of medical science. With the accelerated development of surgical technic one hundred years later, orthopaedic surgery finally became separated from the general field of surgery and established as a specialty. With the introduction of anesthesia and asepsis, rapid progress was made in the development of surgery of the bones and joints. Operations could be performed successfully which in earlier years had been impossible because of the extreme suffering of the patients and the severe infection which often followed the opening of joints and the exposure of bones. The developments in the technics of anesthesia in the last decade, during which period the specialty of anesthesiology has become established more firmly in medical practice, have made it possible for still further advancement in the surgical treatment of bone and joint conditions to be made. The development and widespread use of roentgenography in visualizing bone and joint lesions increased greatly the accuracy of diagnosis and perfection of surgical technic. With the advent of modern industrial machinery, the automobile, and the airplane, the incidence of traumatic orthopaedic problems rapidly increased. The care of large numbers of men crippled by injuries during the first and second World Wars was an additional influence leading toward an increased development of orthopaedic surgery. In recent decades attention has been called to the importance of the care and treatment of the crippled child, and, as a result, there have been instituted extensive state and national programs for this work. Still more recently, similar programs for rehabilitation of the crippled adult have been inaugurated.

In all definitions of orthopaedic surgery emphasis is placed equally upon the prevention and the correction of deformity and disability. Certain phases of orthopaedics can be interpreted as representing a mechanical aspect of preventive medicine; for example, the deformity which might follow a crippling disease can often be prevented by the orthopaedic measures of braces, splints, traction, or other mechanical devices. This conception of prevention dates back to the original orthopaedic textbook, written by Nicholas Andry of the University of Paris, which includes a summary of certain previous publications on related subjects. The term "orthopaedic" has been adopted from the title of Andry's work; he originated it by combining the two Greek words "orthos," straight, and "pais," a child. Andry stated that the purpose of his book was "to teach the different methods of preventing and correcting the deformities of children." From this definition has been expanded the modern interpretation of orthopaedic surgery as applying not only to children but to patients of all ages.

The subject matter of orthopaedic surgery includes the deformities and diseases of the bones and joints and of their related structures, namely, the muscles, tendons, ligaments, and nerves. Of the many definitions of orthopaedic surgery, one accepted by the American Orthopaedic Association is most descriptive: "Orthopaedic surgery shall be considered to be that branch of surgery, the purposes of which are to prevent and correct deformity and to preserve and improve the function of the bones and joints and motor apparatus when function is threatened or impaired by defects, lesions, or diseases." The American Board of Orthopaedic Surgery has adopted the following shorter definition: "Orthopaedic surgery is that branch of surgery especially concerned with the preservation and restoration of the functions of the skeletal system, its articulations, and associated structures."

In this textbook of orthopaedic surgery the various entities which are etiologically related have, insofar as possible, been placed together. Affections which cannot be satisfactorily classified in this manner have been grouped under the heading of the anatomic region involved. It is hoped that this arrangement will enable the physician and student unfamiliar with orthopaedic surgery to obtain a clearer understanding of relationships between its different entities. It is anticipated that this type of approach, rather than one which presents a series of unrelated pathologic conditions, will give the reader a broader and clearer insight into the problems of orthopaedics.

General Considerations of Bone and Joint Affections

Embryology, Anatomy, and Physiology.—Bone is derived from the mesenchyme or primitive connective tissue. In its development it passes first through either a membranous or a cartilaginous phase. In the membranous phase there is a gradual replacement of the primitive connective tissue by osteoid tissue. The osteoid tissue then becomes mineralized and the fully differentiated bone results. Only a few of the flat bones of the skull have this type of development. In the cartilaginous or endochondral type of development the mesenchymal tissue is transformed into hyaline cartilage. The interstitial tissue of this cartilage is replaced by osteoid tissue, and the hyaline matrix is gradually replaced by mineral deposits to form bone. The long bones, spine, scapulae, ribs, sternum, and pelvis undergo this type of development.

Grossly, bones are of three shapes: flat, irregular, and long. Except for the Haversian systems contained in the compact portion of long bones, all bone is histologically similar. The flat and the irregular bones consist of an inner and an outer plate of compact bone, between which is situated a cancellous or spongy portion. Each long bone is composed of, from within outward, an elongated medullary canal; a fine layer of connective tissue called the endosteum; the cancellous or spongy portion at either end, which in children is the epiphysis; the compact layers with their numerous Haversian systems, which form the diaphysis or shaft; and the outer fibrous covering called the periosteum. The periosteum is firmly bound to the compact layer of bone, or cortex, by anchoring fibers called Sharpey's fibers.

Bone formation in the diaphyses, from primary centers of ossification, is well developed by the time of birth. Ossification of the epiphyses, which proceeds from secondary centers, is a much slower process. At birth, ossification centers are not usually visible roentgenographically in any epiphyses except those of the lower end of the femurs. Thereafter, ossification appears in the various epiphyses in orderly chronological sequence. Between epiphysis and diaphysis is the epiphyseal cartilaginous plate, which is silhouetted in roentgenograms as the epiphyseal line. Long bones increase in length by growth at the epiphyseal plates; their shafts thicken by appositional growth beneath the periosteum. As local skeletal maturity is reached, the thinned epiphyseal plate is replaced by fusion between diaphysis and epiphysis. Certain of the vertebral epiphyses are last to fuse, doing so at about twenty-five years of age.

The Haversian systems of compact bone can be considered as long, patent columns, irregularly parallel to the long axis of the shaft of the bone. The central space of the column is known as the Haversian canal; surrounding it are concentric layers of calcified intercellular substance, called lamellae. Within the lamellae are spaces called lacunae, occupied by the bone cells or osteocytes. The lacunae are connected with one another and with the Haversian canal by tiny irregular channels, termed canaliculi, which contain the processes of the osteocytes. From the Haversian canals arise the Volkmann's canals, which are broad, irregular channels perpendicularly placed; they transmit the vascular supply from the periosteum to the Haversian systems and thence to the medullary canal.

The bone receives its nourishment from blood circulating through the nutrient arteries and the periosteal vessels. The nutrient arteries of the long bones enter the shafts obliquely and send branches to the ends of the diaphysis where they form an abundant capillary bed close to the epiphyseal line. Vessels from the nutrient arteries supply also the marrow and the endosteum. The periosteum is supplied from the outside, and from its dense arterial network numerous small vessels pass into minute orifices in the compact bone and run through the Haversian canals. Other vessels pass from the periosteum through orifices in the compact bone to supply its spongy portion. The epiphysis is nourished by branches of the anastomotic vessels surrounding the joint. Lymphatic vessels are present in the periosteum and have been traced into the bone substance. Nerves are distributed freely to the periosteum and accompany the nutrient arteries into the interior of the bone.

A joint is formed by contact between the articular surfaces of two or more bones, surrounded by a fibrous capsule and held in place by ligaments and muscles. The cancellous ends of the long bones are covered by a thin layer of compact bone and a layer of hyaline cartilage. The cartilage contains no blood vessels but is nourished through the arteries of the subjacent bone, the joint fluid, and the small vessels in the region of the attachment of the synovial membrane. For articular cartilage to maintain its normal state, it is necessary that the joint function normally.

The lining of the joint cavity is a delicate serous membrane, called the synovial membrane, which in the embryo covers the articular cartilage but which disappears from the cartilaginous surfaces when growth and joint motion take place. This membrane secretes a clear, light yellow, viscid liquid called the synovial fluid, which acts as a joint lubricant. Nerve fibers are not present in articular cartilage but are contained in the capsule and the synovial membrane and there mediate the pain of joint reactions.

The synovial membrane is surrounded by a strong fibrous capsule. Flexible but inelastic ligaments thicken and reinforce the capsule, and in turn are partly covered by muscles and muscle attachments. In addition, certain joints, such as the knee and jaw, possess intra-articular fibrocartilages which decrease shock, facilitate joint motion, and provide increased stability. Fibrocartilaginous disks between the bodies of adjacent vertebrae perform a similar function. The motion in joints is brought about by muscle activity. In order to function properly, a joint requires normal tone, strength, and synergism in the muscles by which it is moved.

About the joints are bursae, which are closed sacs lined by specialized connective tissue and containing synovial fluid. Bursae are usually found over bony prominences, especially where a muscle or tendon moves over a projection of bone. The function of bursae is to facilitate gliding movements by diminishing friction.

Etiology.—The following are the most common etiologic factors leading to pathologic changes in bones and joints.

1. *Congenital Deformities.*—These anomalies of prenatal development may be primary or secondary. Primary abnormalities, which are the more common, arise from defects in the fertilized ovum and irregularities in its development during the first month of embryonic life. Secondary congenital defects develop in a previously normal fetus as the result of extra-embryonic influences exerted during intrauterine life. Dietary factors, vitamin deficiencies, and virus infections of the embryo may also cause these deformities.

2. *Trauma.*—This may be acute, as a sudden blow or wrench, or chronic, as the stress on the knee joint which may accompany flatfoot.

3. *Infection.*—Pathogenic organisms may enter the bone or joint through the blood stream, directly through a lacerating wound, or by direct extension from a neighboring focus. Their presence may or may not result in the formation of pyogenic arthritis or an osteomyelitis.

4. *Metabolic Disorders.*—Numerous changes take place in and about the bones and joints as a result of disturbances of metabolism. Gout, occasioned by a disturbance of purine metabolism, is an outstanding example.

5. *Endocrine Disorders.*—Extensive changes in the bones may take place as a result of endocrine gland abnormalities. A notable example is the absorption of bone salts and development of bone cysts associated with the excessive production of parathormone in hyperparathyroidism.

6. *Tumors.*—Malignant bone tumors are the most important neoplasms encountered in orthopaedic patients.

7. *Circulatory Disorders.*—Disturbances which decrease the blood supply of certain epiphyses are believed to cause profound changes in these growing areas. Lesions of this type have been termed aseptic or avascular necrosis. Changes sometimes observed in the head of the femur, tarsal scaphoid, distal end of the second metatarsal, semilunar, and certain other bones are examples of aseptic necrosis.

8. *Neurologic Disorders.*—This is a large and varied group constituting approximately one-third of all orthopaedic affections. If the lesion is located (1) in the brain, it may produce a type of cerebral palsy; (2) in the spinal cord, infantile paralysis, muscular atrophy, or neuropathic disorders of the bones or joints; and (3) in the peripheral nerves, obstetric paralysis or other forms of localized paralysis.

9. *Psychologic Disorders.*—Neuromuscular manifestations of hysteria and other abnormal psychosomatic conditions often simulate primary orthopaedic affections. Orthopaedic conditions may be aggravated by psychologic disorders.

Physical Diagnosis.—Every student of orthopaedic surgery must gain an accurate understanding of the physical diagnosis of orthopaedic affections. Such knowledge is best acquired by a careful study of each patient. A number of points in the history and examination are worthy of emphasis.

1. *History.*—The age, sex, occupation, racial background, and economic status of the patient should be recorded. Careful analysis of the

presenting complaint should then be made. It is necessary to determine whether the complaint concerns a new symptom or the recurrence of an old one. Accurate appreciation of the time and manner of onset should be gained. It is important to determine whether the onset was (1) gradual or sudden, (2) associated with an injury or strain, and (3) accompanied by constitutional symptoms such as chills, fever, and malaise. A gradual onset may indicate a static disability such as that which may accompany arch strain; sudden onset of disability suggests acute trauma, and if accompanied by febrile symptoms, a bone or joint infection.

In analysis of the character and type of *pain*, determination of the following points is important: (1) the severity of the pain, and whether it is aching or sharp, (2) whether the pain is becoming progressively worse or is diminishing, (3) whether it is less severe in the morning after rest and worse at night, (4) whether activity and cold or damp weather increase its severity, (5) whether radiation of the pain occurs and in what course, and (6) whether pain is present also in other parts of the body. The extent of disability produced by the pain should be ascertained, as well as the character and result of previous treatment. Pain, although always an important symptom, is variable and must be analyzed, as far as possible, with full appreciation of the patient's psychic stability and tolerance of discomfort. Sharp pain may indicate bone injury with muscle spasm or a purulent exudate under pressure within a closed cavity; increasing pain may indicate a progression of this infectious process; pain which becomes worse with activity during the day usually indicates joint strain; pain worse in bad weather and felt in more than one part of the body may be associated with chronic arthritis; and radiating pain frequently accompanies a rupture of an intervertebral disk.

If *deformity* is present, the following points should be ascertained: (1) the patient's conception of the character of the deformity, (2) when and by whom it was first noted, (3) whether its onset was associated with known injury or disease, (4) whether the deformity appears to be increasing, and (5) the degree of disability which the patient experiences. Deformity, unless immediately associated with trauma, is seldom recognized first by the patient. Lateral curvature of the spine, for example, is usually first called to the attention of the child's parents by a dressmaker.

If there has been *paralysis*, one should note: (1) the time and mode of onset, (2) the distribution and degree of paralysis, (3) the improvement or increase of symptoms, (4) the presence of sensory disturbance, (5) the presence of trophic changes, and (6) the presence of disturbance in the control of bladder or bowel.

When the past history is reviewed, careful attention should be given to evidence of foci of infection, as well as to the other subjects usually investigated in the taking of a routine history. Attention should be paid to whether there have been previous orthopaedic disabilities, such as a short leg; a limp when growing up, which might indicate a coxa plana or mild slipping of the upper femoral epiphysis; sprains, fractures, or dislocations; and whether the patient has had a venereal disease, a chest complaint which might indicate pulmonary tuberculosis, abscessed teeth, or a series of boils or furuncles. It is essential to be always on the lookout for misleading subjective exaggeration of the symptoms and for malingering. The family history is of significance particularly from the viewpoint of tuberculosis, hemophilia, malignancy, and congenital anomalies.

2. *Examination.*—Whenever possible a complete physical examination should be done, in addition to careful study of the local area. This is particularly important in conditions marked by low back pain, since the possibility of referred pain must be considered. A complete physical examination is also indicated in the search for foci of infection and for visceral neoplasms which may have metastasized to bone. In order to obtain the confidence of the patient, which is so important, especially in children, the examiner should proceed gently. In addition to the routine physical examination, careful observation of the patient both standing and walking should be made, since abnormalities of posture and gait are extremely important. It should also be noted whether the patient is of slender or stocky build and what the muscle development is, i.e., whether the muscles are overdeveloped, normal, or underdeveloped. Poor posture might be setting the stage for backache and long arch disturbances. Overdevelopment of the muscles in a child may indicate a pseudohypertrophic muscular dystrophy.

Often a diagnosis can be made on the gait alone, such as the duck waddle associated with a congenitally dislocated hip and the sway to one side which is associated with a gluteus medius paralysis in infantile paralysis.

Careful inspection of the affected region should be made, and any dissimilarity as compared with a corresponding normal area should be noted.   Any redness or swelling, and any atrophy or other deformity should be noted. Muscular atrophy is frequently a valuable confirmatory sign of disuse and local disability. Following inspection, careful palpation of the affected region should be done in an attempt to determine the presence of increased local heat, tenderness, crepitation, changes in consistency, or abnormal masses.

Both active and passive motion of the joint or joints should be observed carefully (Figs. 1, 2, and 3).   It is important to compare the range of motion of the pathologic joint with that of the corresponding normal joint.   The range of motion should be measured with a *goniometer* wherever possible (Fig. 4); if such an instrument is not available, an approximate estimation of the range of joint motion should be made. This estimation should be expressed always in degrees and entered in the clinical record. The presence of muscle spasm and of crepitus should be noted when the examination of joint motion is made. Any joint which has a normal range of smooth, painless, active motion can be presumed to be free of any advanced lesion. It is often desirable to measure the length of the extremities and their circumference at corresponding levels. Such measurements of the lower extremities approach accuracy only when made with the patient lying relaxed on a table with his pelvis level. About the hip it may be useful to determine the relationship of the greater trochanter to *Nélaton's line* (the line from anterior superior iliac spine to tuberosity of the ischium) (Fig. 5) and to note the length of *Bryant's line* (the distance between lines projected perpendicular to the long axis of the body at the anterior superior spine and at the greater trochanter) (Fig. 5). Displacement of the tip of the greater trochanter above Nélaton's line and shortening of Bryant's line indicate a lesion of the head or neck of the femur. One should become acquainted with conventional methods of expressing deformity and the degree of limitation of motion. The following will serve as an example. In deformities of the hip, routine examination sometimes fails to demonstrate the degree of hip flexion in the presence of hyperextension of the lumbar spine (Fig. 6). In such cases the examiner should flex the patient's normal hip fully on the abdomen. This procedure will flatten the lumbar spine against the examining table, and an accurate determination of the amount of flexion contracture of the affected hip can then be made.   At times it is difficult to ascertain abnormal limitation of motion of the spine.   There is great variation in the flexibility of the spinal column in different individuals. Abnormal limitation of motion is

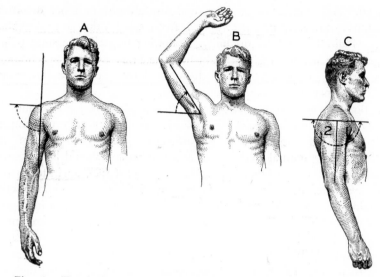

Fig. 1.—Terminology of shoulder motion.   Arrows indicate direction of *A,* abduction; *B,* elevation; *C,* flexion (*1*) and extension (*2*).   (After Cave and Roberts.)

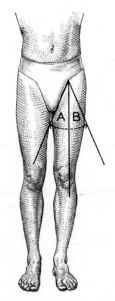

Fig. 2.—Terminology of hip motion.   *A,* Adduction; *B,* abduction.   (After Cave and Roberts.)

usually present when there is tenderness and evidence of muscle spasm; stiffness of long standing may be present in the absence of pain, tenderness, and spasm. Occasionally auscultation of joints, especially in the case of the knee, is helpful in determining whether crepitation is present.

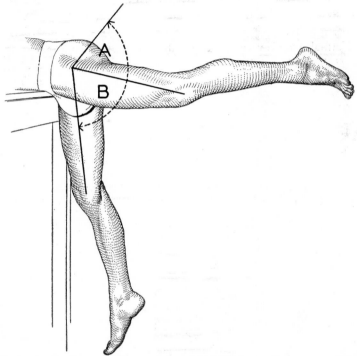

Fig. 3.—Terminology of hip motion. Arrows indicate direction of *A,* hyperextension; *B,* flexion. (After Cave and Roberts.)

A careful neurologic examination is necessary when a neuromuscular disturbance is suspected. The type and distribution of motor paralysis should be determined, the character of the reflexes should be recorded, any change in sensation should be charted, and the presence of atrophy should be noted. In cases of paralysis it is most important to estimate the power of each muscle or muscle group. Muscle testing should be done with great care, and the findings should be recorded in detail. It is convenient to use the following scale, which was introduced by Lovett and published in 1932 by Legg:

Gone—no contraction felt.

Trace—muscle can be felt to tighten, but cannot produce movement.

Poor—produces movement with gravity eliminated, but cannot function against gravity.

Fair—can raise part against gravity.

Good—can raise part against outside resistance as well as against gravity.

Normal—can overcome a greater amount of resistance than a "good" muscle.

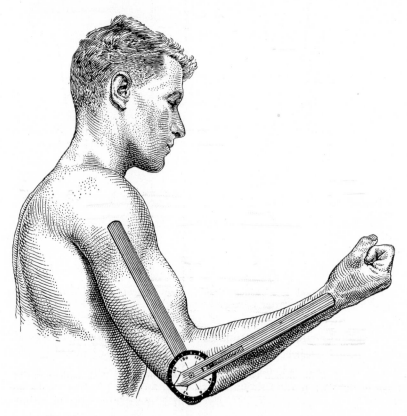

Fig. 4.—Goniometer for measuring the range of joint motion.

Congenital abnormalities should be recorded. Static deformities should be noted, as well as abnormalities of posture, and especially those which may be associated with unequal lengths of the legs, flat feet, or knock-knees. As a rule these postural abnormalities are outstanding and can be determined without difficulty.

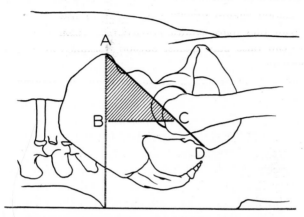

Fig. 5.—Bryant's triangle, *ABC*. Bryant's line, *BC*. Nélaton's line, *AD*. *A*, Anterior superior iliac spine; *B*, intersection of vertical line through anterior superior spine with horizontal line through greater trochanter; *C*, greater trochanter; *D*, tuberosity of ischium.

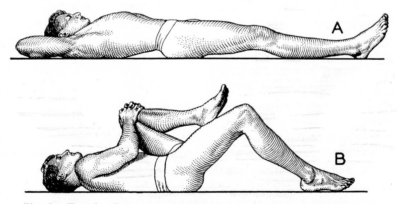

Fig. 6.—Test for flexion contracture of right hip. *A*, With patient supine, flexion of right hip is concealed by arching of lumbar spine; *B*, with normal hip held in extreme flexion to flatten the lumbar lordosis, flexion contracture of right hip is evident.

Roentgenographic examination of the bones and joints is frequently necessary to clarify or confirm the clinical diagnosis. The roentgen findings may include bone atrophy or hypertrophy, erosion or increased calcification, change in bone relationships, change in joint contour, or change in the soft tissues. In interpreting roentgenograms the student or practitioner should not rely on the roentgenologist's report but should himself examine and interpret every film in the light of the clinical findings. Comparison of roentgenograms of the involved structure with films of the opposite, normal side is often essential, particularly in children because of the normal variations incident to growth. Certain cases may require, in addition to routine roentgenograms, films made in oblique positions, stereoscopic films, or laminagrams.

The clinical examination of the patient should be supplemented, when indicated, by laboratory studies of the blood, urine, synovial fluid, spinal fluid, aspirates, or other material, which often reveal facts essential to the diagnosis and treatment. Microscopic examination of pathologic tissue is especially indicated when the presence of tuberculosis or of malignancy is suspected. Joint cultures and inoculation of guinea pigs with joint fluid are often essential in establishing the presence of tuberculosis. Often the intracutaneous tuberculin test is of considerable diagnostic value.

Treatment.—Orthopaedic treatment may be divided into nonoperative and operative types. Nonoperative treatment comprises such procedures as rest and support, secured by strapping, braces, splints, traction, and plaster casts; physical therapy, including the use of heat, massage, ultraviolet light, and selected exercises; occupational therapy, and medical treatment, such as the administration of drugs and the prescription of diets. Operative treatment may be classified as closed or open. The closed operations consist of manipulative procedures, such as the reduction of dislocations and fractures, the stretching of contractures, and osteoclasis. The most frequently performed open operations are tenotomy, osteotomy, arthrotomy, arthrodesis, and open reduction for fracture. Tendon and muscle transplantation, nerve transplantation or resection, bone grafting, and arthroplasty are indicated less frequently. The object of all operative treatment is to improve function. Operation should never be performed at the risk of decreasing function, lessening needed stability, or leading to pain.

The treatment of orthopaedic patients frequently requires consultation with one or more of the following specialists: internist, general surgeon, pediatrist, neurologist, neurosurgeon, psychiatrist, urologist, gynecologist, otolaryngologist, ophthalmologist, roentgenologist, physiatrist, dentist, and others; if obtained, the consultants' advice should be carefully weighed with the orthopaedic findings before the final decision concerning treatment is made. The orthopaedic surgeon who fails to obtain these related opinions when indicated may be embarrassed by finding, after months of unsuccessful treatment, that the diagnosis is not primarily orthopaedic.

Lesions of the bones and joints and allied structures often require a longer time for healing than do those of other tissues of the body; hence the convalescence of the average orthopaedic patient is notably slow. Because of the long period often necessary for treatment, the patient may become disheartened, lose morale, and develop a mental state which may act as a psychologic barrier to a normal convalescence. To offset this, patience and optimism are required of the physician, and a well-rounded program of medical rehabilitation should be started early. This program should include intelligently planned physical and mental activities. Too quick a recovery cannot be expected and should not be promised. Because of the slowness of the improvement often encountered in orthopaedic patients, they, as a group, are likely to change from doctor to doctor and from one form of treatment to another, and ultimately to find themselves in the hands of the unethical practitioner or the cultist. For the best understanding between the patient and the doctor, a frank and honest statement should be made by the doctor to the patient, or the family, or both, explaining in detail as much as is known about the cause of the complaint, the treatment, and the prognosis. Consultation with other physicians should be encouraged if the diagnosis is uncertain or the results of treatment are slow.

When injury or disease is followed by a permanent disability, the economic and social adjustment of the physically handicapped person often presents a serious problem. Vocational rehabilitation of the crippled adult should be started early. The physician should do all in his power to show the patient how much he can accomplish in spite of his handicap, and how he can make the best of his abilities with disregard, as far as possible, of his disabilities. By so doing the physician can help the patient make the best of his misfortune.

NOTE.—Any student or practitioner who is further interested in the subjects presented in these chapters should make use of the bibliography for more extended reading. The bibliography is by no means exhaustive; an attempt has been made, however, to select as references the most authoritative orthopaedic textbooks and the most recent informative articles written in English.

CHAPTER II

CONGENITAL DEFORMITIES

Congenital deformities are abnormalities of development present at birth. They are frequently observed in all orthopaedic clinics, and it is the belief of the author that they have increased in frequency in the last decade. There are many different types of anomaly and numerous minor variations which may involve any bone or joint structure. Congenital deformities therefore vary in significance from very minor abnormalities, such as webbing of the toes, to serious and disabling defects, such as absence of the major portion of an extremity.

Current conceptions of the causation of congenital deformities are hypothetical rather than proved. A defect of a particular part of the early germ plasm may be responsible. In some instances this is hereditary, being a result of the inheritance of the defect of an ancestor. It is possible that anomalies are produced when weakened or dying ova are fertilized. External influences acting upon the developing fetus, such as excessive pressure from abnormal position in the uterus, may account for some deformities. In recent years there has been clinical evidence to show that virus infections, such as measles, contracted in the first twelve weeks of pregnancy, may lead to deformities in the embryo. Experiments on laboratory animals have shown that congenital deformities can be produced by dietary and vitamin deficiencies and the injection of certain drugs and hormones. In experiments recently reported, typical congenital anomalies appeared in 85 per cent of chickens hatched after injection of insulin into the yolk in the first few days of embryonic development; the normal expectancy of congenital malformations in chickens is from .25 to 1.00 per cent.

Largely because of their uncertain etiology, congenital deformities are not preventable, but it is likely that improved care of the health, diet, and vitamin intake of the expectant mother may lessen their incidence. Treatment should in most instances be started quite early in infancy, before abnormal changes in the affected tissues become more advanced and fixed by increasing age and trauma and before they lead to deforming secondary changes in adjacent structures. The effectiveness of treatment in reducing disability and disfigurement varies widely with the type of anomaly and with the promptness with which the treatment is instituted.

The two most common and important congenital anomalies are clubfoot and dislocation of the hip. Congenital dislocations are considered in Chapter III. In the present chapter, congenital clubfoot and a number of other congenital deformities are described. Several additional types of congenital anomaly, including cervical rib, torticollis, and lumbosacral variations, are discussed in subsequent chapters which deal with the individual region affected.

Congenital Talipes

The term *talipes* is used in connection with many foot deformities, whether congenital or acquired. It is derived from the Latin *talus,* meaning ankle, and *pes,* meaning foot, and was originally used to designate a deformity of the foot which caused the patient to walk on the ankle. Deformities of the foot and ankle are conventionally described according to the position of the foot. The four cardinal positions are (1) *equinus,* or plantar flexion, (2) *calcaneus,* or dorsiflexion, (3) *varus,* or inversion, and (4) *valgus,* or eversion. Of the congenital deformities of the foot, the combination of equinus and varus is the most common, and that of calcaneus and valgus next. The equinovarus foot has a clublike appearance, and is the classical type of congenital clubfoot.

Congenital Talipes Equinovarus (Congenital Clubfoot)

Etiology.—An hereditary factor is often concerned in the etiology of clubfoot, its presence being observed in from 5 to 22 per cent of the cases in reported series. The most widely accepted hypotheses of the pathogenesis of clubfoot are the following:

1. Arrested or anomalous development of this particular part of the germ plasm may be the cause. This theory receives indirect support from the statistical fact that from 4 to 12 per cent of the patients with congenital clubfoot have other congenital anomalies as well.

2. At about the third month of intrauterine life the foot occupies normally an equinovarus position. As the fetus develops, inward rotation of the leg normally takes place, and the foot gradually assumes its adult position by the seventh month. If inward rotation fails to occur, however,

the foot remains in an equinovarus position, and the child is born with a clubfoot. By some embryologists, however, this hypothesis is not accepted.

3. Recent investigations of pathologic changes in the soft tissues in congenital clubfoot have shown abnormalities in the relative maturity and length of the muscles, as well as variations in their tendon insertions. These findings suggest that muscle imbalance may play a considerable part in the causation of congenital clubfoot.

Incidence.—Congenital talipes equinovarus forms 75 per cent of all congenital abnormalities of the foot. It is found to occur about once in each 1,000 births. It is more common in some parts of the country than in others, and is particularly frequent in the South. It is twice as common in boys as in girls. The statistics of most clinics have shown that it is observed in a single foot more frequently than in both, but a few reports have shown the reverse. Occasionally there is talipes equinovarus on one side and talipes calcaneovalgus on the other. Clubfoot occurs relatively more often in multiple pregnancies than in single pregnancies.

Pathology.—All degrees of talipes equinovarus, from a very mild deformity to one in which the toes touch the medial side of the lower leg, are found. The Achilles tendon is always shortened. The anterior and posterior tibial tendons are contracted in proportion to the degree of varus deformity. In some cases degenerative changes in the fibers of certain muscles and anomalous insertions of tendons in the foot have been demonstrated.

The most marked bony changes occur in the astragalus and os calcis. The astragalus may be wedge shaped, with only its posterior surface apposed to the tibia. The neck is elongated, depressed, and deflected medially, and the head is flattened. A small portion of the scaphoid bone articulates with the inner border of the head of the astragalus. The os calcis points downward and is tilted in such fashion that its medial tuberosity approaches the tibial malleolus. The anterior extremity of the os calcis is pointed medially and follows the direction of the neck of the astragalus. The os calcis lies more nearly under the astragalus than normally. The distal portions of the tibia and fibula usually show slight inward rotation; this deformity of the tibia is called *tibial torsion.* Structural changes are found in all other bones of the foot but are less extreme in degree.

In older patients proliferative bone changes due to weight-bearing take place about the edges of the articulating surfaces. The articular cartilage undergoes atrophy. New bone is practically always formed around the greatly thickened and broadened proximal end of the fifth metatarsal bone. A large bursa forms over the weight-bearing surface on the lateral portion of the dorsum of the foot and may contain a semi-solid gelatinous material (Fig. 7). In the older cases genu valgum is frequently associated.

Clinical Picture.—The heel is drawn up, the entire foot below the astragalus is inverted, and the anterior half of the foot is adducted. The medial border of the foot is concave, the lateral is convex, and there is a transverse crease across the sole at the level of the mediotarsal joint. When the infant starts to walk, he suffers a tremendous handicap because of his inability to bear weight normally. The muscles of the leg quickly become fatigued and show marked atrophy. Pain is experienced only in the adult patient in whom arthritic changes have developed.

Unilateral clubfoot causes a marked limp. The patient with bilateral clubfoot deformity exhibits a typical gait called the "reel walk," in which considerable wobbling from side to side takes place.

In extreme talipes equinovarus the weight is borne upon a bursa which rapidly develops over the cuboid and proximal end of the fifth metatarsal bone when the child begins to walk. This pad acts to absorb shock in the same manner as does the heel cushion of the normal foot (Fig. 7).

Diagnosis.—In infants the diagnosis of congenital clubfoot is made with ease, but in older children and adults it is sometimes difficult to exclude paralysis as a cause of the deformity. Clubfoot is seen frequently in association with paralytic changes in the lower extremities in spina bifida. Often the first sign of the peroneal type of progressive muscular atrophy is the development of talipes equinovarus. Occasionally in progressive muscular dystrophy the foot has a similar appearance. Old injury of the lower tibial epiphysis, osteomyelitis, and fracture in the region of the ankle joint are other causes of equinovarus deformity.

Prognosis.—When treatment is begun within the first six months of life there is an excellent chance that the deformity may be completely corrected by nonoperative procedures. The course of treatment is usually long, however, requiring several years, and, according to Kite, from 10 to 15 per cent of the cases tend later to relapse and require a second period of treatment. In the patient who is treated late, i.e., after the first year, the prognosis for a normally functioning foot is poor. In untreated cases the deformity usually increases until the patient walks upon the lateral portion of the dorsum of the foot, and the disability becomes greater as the patient grows older (Fig. 7).

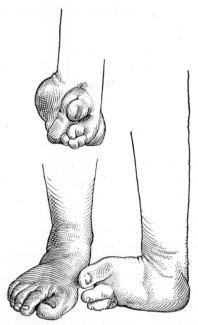

Fig. 7.—Left talipes equinovarus of extreme degree. Note large bursa on weight-bearing portion of foot.

Treatment.—Treatment should be started as soon as the deformity is recognized. If treatment is begun immediately after birth, the problem of correcting the deformity is simple as contrasted with the difficulty encountered in older children.

The treatment is divided into three stages: (1) correction of the deformity, (2) maintenance of correction until normal muscle balance has been regained, and (3) observation for several years in order to forestall any recurrence of the deformity.

It is most important that the first stage of treatment be continued until a position of marked overcorrection has been reached. Anything short of this constitutes inadequate treatment. The position of dorsiflexion and eversion of the foot and abduction of the forefoot is the goal of every form of treatment.

It is generally agreed that the functional result is far better if the final position can be obtained without the trauma of forceful manipulation and without radical surgery, either of which may be followed by bone changes and stiffness of the joints of the foot. Simple lengthening of the Achilles tendon and posterior capsulotomy of the ankle joint, however, usually produce no unfavorable effects.

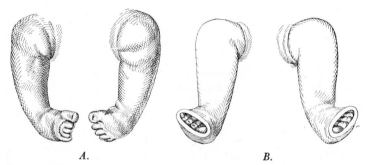

A.   B.

Fig. 8.—Bilateral talipes equinovarus in infant. *A,* Before correction; *B,* undergoing correction in plaster casts.

The ease with which correction may be obtained and the choice of method in *the first stage of treatment* vary according to the age of the patient. In young infants a series of plaster casts, applied without manipulation other than holding the foot in a position of as much correction as can be obtained without the use of force, is usually effective (Fig. 8). The cast should be changed at intervals of from three to fourteen days. The successive casts provide an opportunity for the tight structures on the medial side of the foot to stretch and for the lax structures on the lateral side of the foot to contract. In this way a gradual correction of the deformity is obtained without the application of excessive force. The casts should be padded, particularly over bony prominences, and should extend above the flexed knee to allow effective correction of the rotation deformity. It is often convenient to use the technic of wedging the cast instead of changing the entire cast. A wedge of plaster is taken out over that aspect of the foot toward which correction is desired, the sides of the wedge are brought together, and plaster is applied in circular fashion over the closed-in wedge. The adduction deformity should be corrected first; this phase of the treatment must be continued until the scaphoid bone is brought directly in front of the head of the astragalus. Next, the inversion deformity is corrected; care must be taken to continue this until there is no inversion of the os calcis. As suggested by Kite, complete correction of the astragalus-os calcis relationship may be verified by a roentgenogram showing anterior divergence of their long axes. Finally, the plantar flexion or equinus is corrected by gradually increased dorsiflexion of the ankle. Attempts to correct simultaneously all three elements of the deformity may produce a misshapen, "rocker-bottom" foot. Correction of the equinus may be hastened by (1) lengthening the Achilles tendon, and (2) posterior capsulotomy of the ankle joint. The final cast is often left on for a period of four to eight weeks to allow thorough accommodation to the new position. It may be necessary for many months to use a splint at night which holds the foot in the corrected position.

An alternative method of correcting the deformity of congenital clubfoot is the use of the Denis Browne splint. The popularity of this method has steadily increased in the last decade. This splint consists of two padded metal plates which are securely fastened with adhesive tape to the infant's feet and which are then connected by a crossbar. The stretching of contracted structures is accelerated by the infant's kicking. The foot plates can be so rotated outward on the crossbar that progressive correction of the adduction and later of the equinus may be obtained. For good results this treatment also must be continued for a long period, until wide overcorrection of each element of the deformity has been secured. The results of this treatment, in many instances are excellent, but it is not considered by the author to be so satisfactory as the use of wedged casts. In the second stage of treatment the Denis Browne splint may also be applied by means of the shoes and used to maintain the correction of clubfeet, after full correction has been obtained either by wedged casts or by the use of Denis Browne splint applied with adhesive plaster (Fig. 9).

During *the second stage of treatment* measures are taken to maintain the correction and to encourage the development of normal muscle balance. After the deformity has been overcorrected by either method, a special clubfoot shoe to hold the corrected position should be used. Many braces have been designed for this purpose, but because of the tendency of the foot to slip in the shoe to which the brace is attached, they have not been very effective. The clubfoot shoe has a lateral deviation of its anterior half and a slight raise (⅛ to ¼ inch) of its entire

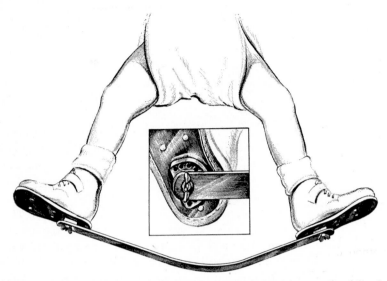

Fig. 9.—Denis Browne splint being used to maintain the correction following the first stage treatment of clubfoot. Note the external rotation of the legs and the dorsiflexion of the ankles. The mechanism of the attachment of crossbar to foot plate, shown in the insert, allows changing of the relationship of the bar to the plate. When the splint is used in this way, it may be worn either as a night and day splint or only as a night splint.

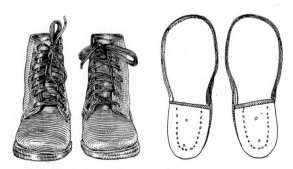

Fig. 10.—Clubfoot shoes. Note the turning out of the shoes and outer wedge of the sole. This wedge has a tendency to roll the foot into pronation and to maintain the correction of the varus deformity.

lateral border (Fig. 10). When special clubfoot shoes cannot be obtained, ordinary shoes can be altered to aid in preventing a recurrence of the deformity. It is often helpful also to extend the outer border of the sole and heel of the shoe ¼ inch laterally. Corrective night shoes and splints are also useful. Walking should be encouraged in order to strengthen the weakened muscles. If the patient is old enough to cooperate in muscle training, exercises should be given to strengthen the muscles of abduction, eversion, and dorsiflexion of the foot and ankle. Such muscle re-education is an extremely important factor in obtaining a permanent cure.

In certain of the more difficult cases, casts alone may prove inadequate for correcting the deformity in a reasonable length of time. This is particularly true in older children. In such cases it may be necessary to hasten the correction by the use of forceful manipulation under anesthesia. The adduction deformity is first corrected by gradually forced abduction of the foot, usually over a padded block of wood. Then the inversion of the os calcis is corrected, and finally the plantar flexion. After the adduction and varus have been corrected and while the patient is still under anesthesia, the Achilles tendon may be lengthened. This is followed by the application of a plaster cast which extends above the knee. It may be necessary to perform two or more forceful manipulations before a position of satisfactory overcorrection can be obtained. After such manipulation it is best not to immobilize the foot too long because of danger of the formation of adhesions. In some of the more resistant cases it may be necessary also (1) to divide the medial ligaments of the mediotarsal and subastragalar joints, (2) to strip the plantar fascia from the os calcis, and (3) to perform a posterior capsulotomy of the ankle joint. Section of the resistant soft tissue structures is more favored in Europe, especially in England, than in America.

For the adult or for the older child with a clubfoot which cannot be corrected by these conservative means, operation upon the bones is justified. A *wedge osteotomy,* the base of the wedge being on the dorsal and lateral aspect of the foot, is most frequently done. As much bone as is necessary to correct the deformity completely is removed from the region of the mediotarsal joint. At the same time the subastragalar joint is usually fused.

The third stage of treatment consists of prolonged observation, until the child has reached adolescence or in the case of older patients for at least several years. During this period any tendency toward recurrence of the deformity should be promptly and thoroughly treated. A recurrent deformity is often more difficult to treat than the original clubfoot. Lateral transplantation of the anterior tibial tendon, as advocated by Garceau, is often helpful in preventing a recurrence of the varus and adduction deformity.

Other Forms of Congenital Talipes

In comparison with talipes equinovarus, other forms of congenital talipes are less common and form less difficult therapeutic problems.

Talipes Calcaneovalgus.—This type of congenital deformity of the foot, characterized by eversion of the foot, increased dorsiflexion of the ankle, and apparent lengthening of the Achilles tendon, is second to congenital equinovarus in frequency. It is often of mild degree and, unlike congenital equinovarus, is not fixed but can be easily overcorrected by stretching. It is most noticeable immediately after birth. As the child begins to use his muscles and kick his legs, the condition becomes less marked and often seems to disappear completely. When the infant later begins to stand, however, persistent changes in the affected foot or feet may be evidenced by excessive pronation.

If the deformity does not respond to passive stretching, wedged casts may be applied in the same manner described for clubfoot. It is sometimes best to use a Denis Browne splint to hold the feet in the equinovarus position for a number of months. This should be followed by a night splint to maintain overcorrection, while each morning and night the foot may be gently manipulated. Every foot which has shown an early calcaneovalgus deformity should be fitted with a strong shoe with a ⅛ inch raise of its medial border when the infant begins to stand and walk; usually the shoe modification should be continued for several years. Seldom do the contracted structures have to be sectioned. This type of foot deformity is often unnecessarily alarming to the parents of the infant.

Talipes Valgus.—At times a valgus deformity is seen without accompanying calcaneus and lengthening of the Achilles tendon. The treatment is identical with that described above for talipes calcaneovalgus.

Talipes Calcaneus.—This deformity may be associated with hyperextension of the knee. It is thought by some observers that talipes calcaneus is due to extreme flexion of the thighs on the abdomen in utero. The type of treatment outlined for talipes calcaneovalgus is indicated.

Talipes Varus.—Talipes varus is usually an incomplete form of congenital equinovarus deformity. The treatment is the same as that described for talipes equinovarus. Talipes varus sometimes has the appearance of a relapsed equinovarus deformity.

Talipes Equinus.—This congenital deformity is about half as common as talipes varus. In the older child it is often necessary to lengthen the Achilles tendon and to perform a posterior capsulotomy of the ankle joint before the equinus can be fully corrected. Operation should be followed by a plaster cast for from four to six weeks.

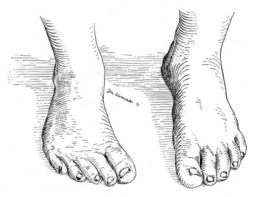

Fig. 11.—Metatarsus varus of the right foot. Note the turning in of the fore-foot and of the toes.

Metatarsus Varus.—This deformity consists of adduction of the forefoot at the tarsometatarsal joints; in some cases inversion of the forefoot is present also (Fig. 11). It sometimes has been called "skewfoot." Many observers, among them Kite, report that the incidence of this deformity is increasing. It may involve one or both feet; when unilateral it is sometimes associated with clubfoot of the opposite extremity. At times it may be a residual deformity associated with an old congenital talipes equinovarus. Metatarsus varus may also be of acquired type, when it is usually combined with valgus deformity of the posterior portion of the foot. In early childhood the deformity may sometimes be corrected by gentle manipulation and casts, after which special shoes with outswung toes should be prescribed. In older children forcible correction under anesthesia may be necessary. In the more difficult cases arthrodesis of the medial metatarso-cuneiform joints and resection of a portion of the lateral three metatarsal bones are sometimes indicated.

Clubhand

Clubhand is a rare congenital malformation usually associated with complete or partial absence of one of the bones of the forearm (Figs. 12*A* and 12*B*); it is sometimes hereditary and may be bilateral. The hand may be in a flexed, extended, adducted, or abducted position. Of these the most common type is abduction or radial deviation of the hand, associated with defective development or complete absence of the radius. The thumb is usually very small or completely absent. In this type of deformity the ulna is practically always bowed with its concavity directed laterally. Despite the deformity, the hand is ordinarily quite useful. It has been observed that clubhand with radial deviation is often associated with the presence of a cervical rib. In some instances the radial nerve or the artery cannot be demonstrated.

Treatment.—An attempt to improve the deformity by manipulation or wedged casts may be made, especially in the early years. These procedures must be followed by a brace or splint to maintain the corrected position. Several operative procedures for correction of the deformity of the hand have been devised. If the radius is absent, the following operations are to be considered: (1) a bone graft may be placed to reach from the ulna to the lateral portion of the carpus, (2) the distal end of the ulna may be split and the end of its lateral portion transposed to the carpus, (3) a bone graft may be taken from the ulna and laid in the position of the radius, and (4) the end of the ulna may be beveled anteriorly and posteriorly and inserted into a longitudinal split made in the carpus. The latter operation is the choice of the author. If the ulna is defective, analogous types of operation upon the radius may be considered. The results of these operations are not always satisfactory, especially if they are performed when the patient is too young and the bones are small.

Congenital Defects of Individual Bones

Congenital partial absence of one of the bones of the extremities is seen more frequently than total absence. Defects in the bones of the

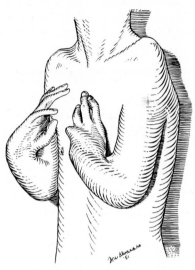

Fig. 12A.—Bilateral clubhand in a girl ten years of age. Note the turning in of the hands, the very short forearms, and the webbing between the arm and forearm.

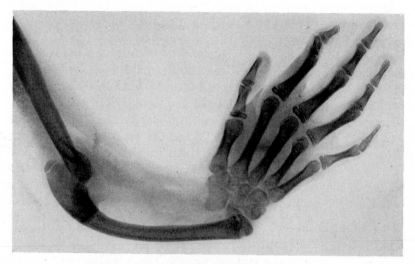

Fig. 12B.—Roentgenogram of clubhand of patient in Fig. 12A. Note the turning in of the hand, the complete absence of the radius, the dislocation of the lower end of the ulna, and the posterior bowing of the shaft of the ulna.

upper extremity are more often bilateral than those occurring in the lower extremity. These bone defects are often associated with other congenital abnormalities. In many instances they form a most difficult therapeutic problem.

Humerus.—An isolated defect of the humerus is very rare.

Radius.—Partial absence of the radius is observed more often than complete absence, the upper end being most often missing. Clubhand is nearly always associated with this deformity. In 40 per cent of the cases of clubhand associated with a defect of the radius, the condition is bilateral.

Ulna.—Defects of the ulna are not so common as those of the radius. Clubhand associated with deficiency of the ulna exhibits a bowing of the forearm with its concavity directed medially.

Femur.—Underdevelopment or partial absence of the femur, especially of the upper third, of which several varieties have been described, is much more common than complete absence. Partial absence of the femur is often associated with complete absence of the patella and with anomalies of the pelvis on the affected side.

Tibia.—Absence of the tibia is rare. The limb exhibits a characteristic deformity. The thigh is rotated externally and adducted, the knee is flexed, and the upper end of the fibula is displaced laterally and backward from the femur. The fibula is bowed with its concavity directed medially, and the foot is in a varus or equinovarus position. In some cases operations have been performed to correct the deformity of the foot, and at the same time the fibula has been fused to the femur. The end-results, however, have not always been satisfactory.

Fibula.—Congenital absence of the fibula is more common than that of any other long bone. Total absence is observed more frequently than partial absence (Figs. 13A and 13B). The tibia is usually bowed anteriorly, and the foot is short, occupies an equinovalgus position, and may show deformities of the toes. The whole lower extremity is short. The treatment of absence of the fibula is to correct the deformity of the foot and to straighten the curvature of the tibia by osteotomy performed above the site of maximum bowing. There need be no fear of nonunion after osteotomy; this is in contrast to osteotomy in congenital pseudarthrosis of the tibia, with which absence of the fibula may be confused. Absence of the fibula may be associated with congenital abnormalities of the arterio-venous system of the leg. Occasionally following surgery to correct the deformity, a circulatory block may occur; this complication demands early recognition and immediate treatment. Extension shoes and braces may be indicated to equalize leg length.

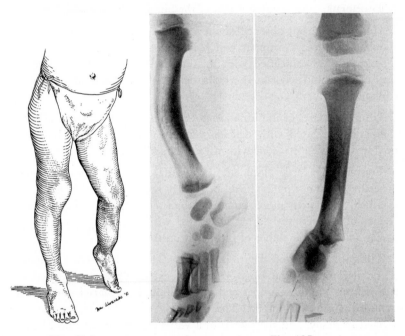

Fig. 13*A*.

Fig. 13*B*.

Fig. 13*A*.—Congenital absence of the fibula in a boy four years of age. Note the short left lower extremity, the anterior bowing of the leg, and the equinus deformity of the foot.

Fig. 13*B*.—Lateral and anteroposterior roentgenograms of patient in Fig. 13*A*, showing congenital absence of the fibula. Note the complete absence of the fibula, the anterior bowing of the thick, short tibia, and the lateral displacement of the foot with marked valgus deformity in the anteroposterior roentgenogram.

Patella.—The development of the patella may be delayed or imperfect, or the bone may be completely absent. Occasionally, an ossification center in the upper and lateral segment fails to fuse with the remainder of the bone, producing a *bipartite patella*. This condition is usually bilateral and ordinarily causes no symptoms. Partial or complete absence of the patella is usually associated with underdevelopment of the quadriceps tendon and occasionally with congenital dislocation of the knee. Clubfoot, dislocation of the hip, and other congenital anomalies are sometimes associated. Deformity and weakness of the knee depend more upon the associated anomalies than upon the defect of the patella. Massage and exercises are indicated in an effort to strengthen the quadriceps muscle, and occasionally the wearing of a brace to prevent strain of the quadriceps is advisable.

Congenital Radio-Ulnar Synostosis

Congenital radio-ulnar synostosis is an infrequent congenital anomaly which is usually bilateral. The synostosis occurs as a rule at the proximal end of the radius and ulna (Fig. 14). Occasionally there is only a small bridge of connecting bone. There is practically always a fibrous union between the bones in the lower third of the forearm. The head of the radius is sometimes dislocated. Occasionally there is fusion of the radius, ulna, and humerus, with absence of the elbow joint. The forearm may be fixed in a position of pronation or midway between pronation and supination. Extension of the elbow is limited. As the patient learns to compensate for his loss of forearm rotation by increased use of the shoulder, however, the disability is slight.

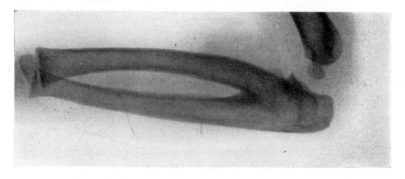

Fig. 14.—Roentgenogram showing congenital synostosis of the radius and ulna. Note the bony fusion between their upper ends.

Treatment.—The whole upper end of the radius may be resected, or only the bone between the radius and ulna, and the space so formed may be filled with fat, muscle, or fascia. Rarely, however, do these operative procedures meet with success. The disappointing postoperative results have been ascribed to the persistence of fibrous bands between the bones in the distal part of the forearm and to the congenital absence of muscles controlling rotation of the forearm.

Congenital Contractures

Congenital contractures may involve any of the joints. When present at the ankle or the wrist, they produce the conditions of clubfoot or clubhand, respectively. They are usually associated with other congenital malformations.

In the hand the contractures most commonly cause a flexion deformity of the little finger and are frequently bilateral. Congenital contracture of the elbow is usually associated with a flexion deformity of the wrist. The shoulder often suffers a limitation of abduction. Congenital hip flexion contracture is rare; it may be associated with flexion of the knee. When the knee is flexed, there may be redundant skin in the popliteal space. It is thought that these contractures of the knee and of the hip may be due to a long-continued position of flexion in utero.

Treatment.—The treatment of all of these contractures is essentially the same. It consists of (1) gradual manipulation into the corrected position, (2) exercises to develop the weak muscles, usually the extensors, and (3) the use of a retention splint. Occasionally it may be desirable to incise the tight skin and underlying resistant bands; it may be necessary to graft skin over resulting denuded areas.

Congenital Abnormalities of Fingers and Toes

Syndactyly (Webbed Fingers or Toes).—Syndactyly (Fig. 15) occurs twice as often in boys as in girls, and more often in the hand than in the foot. In the hand the fingers on the ulnar side are more often affected than those on the radial side, and the thumb is seldom involved. The union between the affected parts may consist only of skin and connective tissue or may include bone. Webbing is sometimes associated with polydactyly, and both of these conditions may be hereditary. Syndactyly is often associated with multiple congenital deformities of the hands and feet.

Separation of the involved fingers or toes is accomplished by dividing the soft tissues and bony structures and should be done between the second and the sixth year. A great many different plastic procedures have been devised, most of which are followed by satisfactory results.

Macrodactyly.—Macrodactyly is an overdevelopment of one or more fingers or toes (Fig. 15). It is due presumably to an abnormal growth capacity of the germ plasm forming this part. In some cases lesions of local nerve trunks have been found. The usual treatment is amputation, but occasionally a plastic operation to effect a reduction in size is preferable.

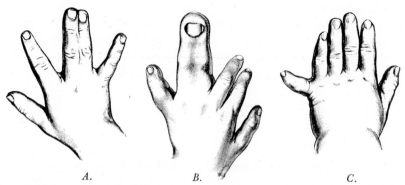

Fig. 15.—Congenital deformities of the hand, showing (*A*) syndactyly, (*B*) macrodactyly, and (*C*) polydactyly.

Polydactyly.—Supernumerary digits are found in the hand and foot with about equal frequency (Fig. 15). The condition is often bilateral and may be combined with syndactyly. Amputation of the extra finger or toe is indicated.

Cleft Hand and Cleft Foot.—This anomaly consists of a cleft or division in the middle of the hand or foot which results in the formation of large digits or parts. It is spoken of as the "lobster claw" hand or foot and is sometimes associated with polydactyly. These hands and feet are unsightly but often function satisfactorily. No operative procedure should be considered if the hand or foot is useful and painless. Operations are undertaken more often for cosmetic effect than for improvement of function.

Arachnodactyly (Marfan's Syndrome)

This unusual congenital and sometimes hereditary condition, which occurs in tall and slender individuals, is characterized by thin fingers and toes with elongated phalanges, metacarpals, and metatarsals. It is sometimes spoken of as "spider fingers and toes." It is thought by some to be due to a dysfunction of the anterior portion of the pituitary gland. In approximately 80 per cent of the cases, there is an asymmetry of the skull. About half of the patients have eye deformities with dislocation of the lens, and approximately a third have a congenital heart lesion. There are marked atrophy and weakness of all muscles, and hypermobility of joints due to laxity of the ligaments. There may be a coxa vara and a lateral curvature of the spine which increases as the child grows older. In some respects, arachnodactyly is similar to amyotonia congenita. Arachnodactyly is to be differentiated from the Ehlers-Danlos syndrome, which also is characterized by hypermobility of the joints, but includes increased elasticity of the skin and fragility of the walls of the blood vessels.

Treatment.—There is no specific therapy. Individual deformities or disabilities should be treated as indicated.

Intrauterine Amputations and Constrictions

Intrauterine amputations (Fig. 16) have been thought to be due to constriction in utero, but the publications of Streeter have shown that in most instances they are primary congenital changes due to abnormal constitution of the germ plasm. Often there is a deep circular constriction about the arm or leg without actual amputation. The constriction may occur in any portion of the arm or leg. Beyond it the distal portion of the extremity may be enlarged.

Treatment.—When the presence of a deep indented band is associated with disturbance of the distal circulation, it may be necessary to dissect out the band and to approximate the edges of the uninvolved subcutaneous tissue and skin. Occasionally it may be desirable to complete the amputation which began in utero.

Asymmetrical Development (Congenital Total Hemihypertrophy, Hemimacrosomia)

In the normal individual there are often slight differences between the development of the two lateral halves of the body. This condition, however, is sometimes severe and of congenital origin. It has been stated that it is caused by an increased blood supply to one side of the body, resulting from a primary developmental abnormality of the circulatory system. It has also been said to be the result of an asymmetrical growth capacity of the germ plasm. Neurofibromatosis may occasionally produce a similar appearance. Hemihypertrophy may at times resemble a unilateral elephantiasis, the redundant tissue being of fibrous and fatty nature. The increase in size usually ceases at the end of the growth period, but the disproportion constitutes a permanent deformity. Sometimes one extremity only is involved. Occasionally an arteriovenous fistula may be the cause. Treatment is not uniformly effective, but cosmetic operative procedures, such as shortening of the longer leg, are indicated in selected cases.

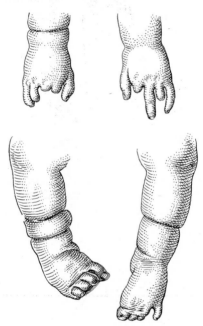

Fig. 16.—Multiple congenital deformities. Note constrictions, complete and partial absence of several fingers and toes, and band across toes of left foot.

Arthrogryposis Multiplex Congenita (Amyoplasia Congenita)

Arthrogryposis multiplex congenita is an incomplete congenital fibrous ankylosis of many or all of the joints except those of the spine and jaw, and is usually symmetrical. The spine may show a lateral curvature. It is thought to be due to a primary aplasia or failure of muscle development early in embryonic life. The joints appear enlarged, and the periarticular tissues show contractures and fail to develop normally. In contour the extremities may resemble stuffed sausages. (Fig. 17.)

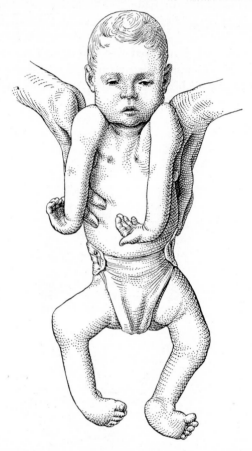

Fig. 17.—Arthrogryposis multiplex congenita. The cylindrical contours of the arms, extended elbows, contracted knees, clubhands, and clubfeet are characteristic.

The typical patient shows internal rotation of the arms and flexion contractures of the wrists. The elbows and knees have a fusiform appearance and may be hyperextended. The hips may be flexed. The thighs are rotated outward and the tibias twisted on the femurs. The patellae are sometimes absent. There are usually associated clubfeet and sometimes clubhands. Numerous other congenital anomalies, such as syndactyly and polydactyly, may be present.

Treatment.—Because of the muscle deficiency the treatment is unsatisfactory and the deformities often recur. The feet are in general more amenable to treatment than the hands. Gentle manipulations performed several times a day may be helpful. Elastic splinting for the hands, traction for the hips and knees, and corrective casts for the feet are indicated in selected cases. The position of the arms and legs may be improved with tenotomies and myotomies; arthroplasties of the joints may be done in older patients. Following these procedures physical therapy should be diligently carried out for a long period of time.

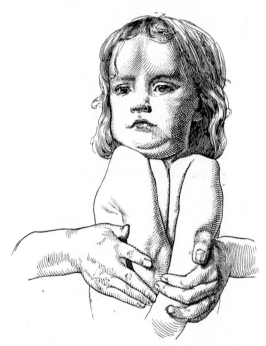

Fig. 18.—Cleidocranial dysostosis. Partial approximation of the shoulders is made possible by absence of clavicles. Note typical depression in middle of forehead. (From clinical material of Dr. E. A. Park.)

Cleidocranial Dysostosis

Cleidocranial dysostosis (Fig. 18) is a partial or complete absence of both clavicles together with changes in the skull. It is rare and is of hereditary origin in about half of the cases. The sexes are affected with equal frequency.

Pathology.—The characteristic changes are partial or complete absence of both clavicles and an exaggerated development of the transverse diameter of the cranium with delayed ossification of the fontanels. The muscles which are attached to the clavicle and chest always develop in an anomalous manner. Often other congenital malformations are associated, such as coxa vara and imperfect pubic ossification and spinal segmentation.

Clinical Picture.—Usually the patient is brought to the physician because it has been found adventitiously that there is something wrong with one or both shoulders. A defect of the clavicle is demonstrable clinically. Because of the extreme relaxation of the shoulder girdle the patient can often bring the tips of the shoulders together below the chin.

Treatment.—As a rule there is little disability and no treatment is indicated. If the patient complains of pain, however, one or both ends of the clavicles, if present, should be removed.

Congenital Elevation of the Scapula (Sprengel's Deformity, Congenital High Scapula)

In this congenital malformation and malposition, the scapula is elevated from 1 to 4 inches above its normal position, and its inferior angle is rotated medially (Fig. 19). The deformity may be present on one or both sides. It is often associated with other congenital anomalies, and particularly with defective development of the cervical vertebrae.

Etiology.—Failure of the scapula to descend below the high position which it occupies in the embryo has been postulated as the cause of this deformity. Other observers, however, have believed that it is due to faulty position of the fetus in utero. It is thought by some to be related to congenital synostosis of the cervical spine.

Pathology.—The scapula is shortened in its vertical diameter. The upper part bends forward and hooks over the clavicle. The cervical muscles are shortened on the affected side and are changed in direction. In 25 per cent of the cases there is union between one of the lower cervical vertebrae and the scapula; such union may consist of bone, cartilage, or fibrous tissue. When a bony connection is present, it extends from the transverse process of one of the cervical vertebrae to the scapula. Such an osseous bridge is spoken of as an *omovertebral bone.*

Clinical Picture.—Asymmetry of the shoulder is often the first evidence of abnormality. In most of the cases abduction of the shoulder is markedly restricted. In 10 per cent of the cases torticollis is present, together with lateral curvature of the spine. In bilateral cases the neck appears shortened.

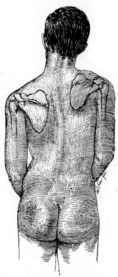

Fig. 19.—Sprengel's deformity. Note elevated right shoulder and scapula.

Diagnosis.—The diagnosis is made from the physical signs and the roentgenogram. Congenital elevation of the scapula must be differentiated from paralysis of the serratus anterior and the trapezius muscles and from obstetrical paralysis.

Prognosis.—Without operation no improvement of the deformity is to be anticipated. Operative correction is sometimes followed, however, by recurrence.

Treatment.—Postural training, exercise of the shoulder, and manipulation may increase the joint function. In cases in which motion is markedly limited and the deformity is unsightly, operative measures may be indicated. If an omovertebral bone is present, it should be carefully resected.

Subperiosteal transplantation of the scapula, within its muscular envelope, downward to the desired level, and its anchorage to one of the ribs by fascia or wire, as described by Schrock, is the most satisfactory operative procedure. To be effective, operation must be performed in childhood.

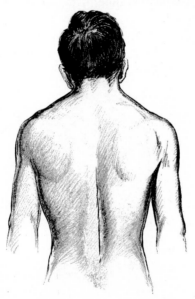

Fig. 20.—Klippel-Feil syndrome. Note the broad thick neck and the webbing of the sides of the neck from the head to the shoulders. This is sometimes spoken of as web-neck or pterygium colli.

Congenital Synostosis of the Cervical Spine (Klippel-Feil Syndrome)

Congenital synostosis of the cervical spine is a rare malformation resulting from an arrest of development. The outstanding pathologic change is fusion of all or of only the lower cervical vertebrae into one homogeneous mass of bone. The posterior portion of some or all of the laminal arches is not developed, resulting in spina bifida which usually involves the lower cervical vertebrae and one or two of the upper dorsal vertebrae. A cervical rib, crowding of the upper ribs, and congenital anomalies in other parts of the body are often associated. Roentgenograms show the anomalies of the cervical spine, including the clefts in its vertebral arches.

Clinical Picture.—Abnormal shortness of the neck is the most noticeable feature, sometimes causing the head to seem to rest directly on the trunk (Fig. 20). There is painless restriction of neck motion in all directions. Flexion and extension of the cervical spine, which may take place wholly at the joints between occiput and atlas, are better preserved than is lateral motion. The head and neck may be held in an oblique position which simulates that of congenital torticollis. Occasionally the trapezius muscles stretch winglike from the mastoid processes to the shoulders, suggesting the term of pterygium colli or web-neck.

Treatment.—As a rule, no treatment is indicated. In early childhood a neck brace is occasionally helpful. Attempts to increase mobility by manipulation have proved harmful.

CHAPTER III

CONGENITAL DEFORMITIES (CONTINUED)

Congenital Dislocation of the Hip

In 1826 Dupuytren first described accurately the pathologic changes which occur in congenital dislocation of the hip, but not until 1888 did Paci suggest reduction of the dislocation as a means of treatment. Until this time such deformities of the hip had been considered incurable. The suggestions made by Paci were first popularized in 1895 by Lorenz. It is now generally agreed that if a congenitally dislocated hip can be reduced early, and if the corrected position can be maintained for an adequate period of time by means of a plaster cast or brace, a stable joint with satisfactory function will often result.

Defective development of the acetabulum with or without dislocation is termed *dysplasia* of the hip. This condition, which is apparent roentgenographically, has an hereditary background. If slight in degree it causes no symptoms and may disappear spontaneously; if more severe it may produce disability of the hip in adult years or may be associated with congenital subluxation or frank dislocation.

Incidence.—Congenital dislocation of the hip, in contrast to that of other joints, is not a rare deformity. It is observed far more frequently in some sections of the United States, particularly in the northeastern states, than in others. It is found with especial frequency in the Latin races, especially in Italy and France. Among Negroes it is very seldom observed. It is approximately six times as common in girls as in boys. Congenital dislocation of the hip is more often unilateral than bilateral. In unilateral cases the left hip is affected more often than the right.

Etiology.—There are various hypotheses to explain the origin of the dislocation. (1) It may result from a primary developmental defect causing imperfect formation of the posterosuperior margin of the acetabulum in utero, or acetabular dysplasia. (2) It may be due to a position of excessive flexion and adduction in an abnormal uterus, causing a stretching and lengthening of the ligaments of the hip joint. This relaxation of the capsule may allow the head of the femur to become subluxated at birth and later to become completely dislocated from the acetabulum. (3) The dislocation may be due to an injury which has taken place in utero.

In some instances congenital dislocation of the hip is of hereditary origin. One large Italian clinic has noted an hereditary influence in 13 per cent of 1,900 cases.

Pathology.—The pathologic changes are characteristic and vary definitely with age. The changes are minimal in the early case and increase with the duration of the dislocation. There is often a shallow acetabulum with an oblique superior and posterior surface. Later the acetabulum becomes triangular or oval in shape and may be filled with fat and fibrous tissue. The head of the femur is nearly always displaced upward and backward upon the ilium. Anterior dislocation is rare, and some observers question whether there can ever be a primary anterior dislocation. When the epiphysis of the femoral head appears, it is smaller than that of a normal hip; this is believed to be due to decreased functional stimulation. The head of the femur becomes flattened and later mushroom-shaped. The neck of the femur is short and thick, and may show an increase in the angle with the shaft (coxa valga) (Fig. 28). The whole upper portion of the femur usually develops a structural alteration as a result of which the neck or shaft and neck undergo torsion, assuming a more anterior position in relation to the lower end of the femur (antetorsion or anteversion). The capsule over the head, which on weight-bearing acts as a suspensory ligament, becomes elongated, thick, and fibrous; it may become constricted in the middle and assume an hourglass shape. The ligamentum teres may be extremely thin, ribbonlike, and atrophic, and may even be absent; in some cases, however, it is broad and thick. The muscles about the joint, especially the adductor group, become shortened and contracted.

With continued weight-bearing a shallow secondary acetabulum may develop on the wing of the ilium. The pelvis is underdeveloped on the affected side, and a postural deviation of the lumbar spine toward this side takes place. Forward tilting of the pelvis and increase of the lumbar lordosis develop to a slight degree in unilateral dislocation and to a much greater degree in bilateral dislocation.

Clinical Picture.—It may be difficult to recognize dislocation of the hip in early infancy. In a unilateral case the mother may notice that the affected hip is prominent laterally and that the extremity is short (Fig. 21). By placing the child on his back on the examining table and then flexing both of the child's hips and knees to a right angle, the examiner can see that on the affected side the knee is lower than on the normal side (Fig. 22). Then by abducting the flexed hip as far as possible, the examiner will note restriction of motion due to adductor tight-

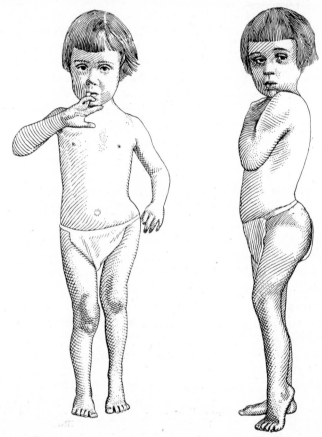

Fig. 21.—Congenital dislocation of left hip. Note shortening of left leg, prominence of left hip, and increased lumbar lordosis.

ness on the side of the dislocation or subluxation. If the extended thigh is first pushed toward the patient's head and then pulled distally, the greater trochanter and head of the femur can be felt to move up and down in the buttock. This is commonly called "telescoping" or "piston mobility." The instability may sometimes be recognized more easily by testing with the hip and knee flexed to 90 degrees. There are usually asymmetric skin folds in the thigh, and the trochanter is more prominent than normal. Instability of the hip on weight-bearing delays the child in learning to stand and walk and causes a characteristic limp. In young children there are no other complaints. Function is usually good. In older children fatigue may be present on exertion and pain may develop after activity, yet at times, even in adult patients, there is no complaint of pain.

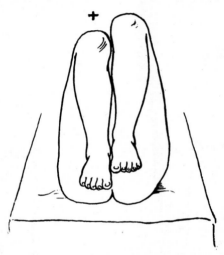

Fig. 22.—Knee test for congenital dislocation of hip. The hips and knees are flexed with patient on a hard table. When the test is positive, the knee is lower on the side of the dislocation than on the normal side. (From Hass: Congenital Dislocation of the Hips, Charles C. Thomas, Publisher, 1951.)

In bilateral dislocation the gait is especially characteristic; the patient, because of the instability of the joints, sways from side to side, exhibiting a "duck waddle" gait. This gait is also present in less marked degree in unilateral dislocation. In bilateral dislocation the perineum is wide, the buttocks are broad, and the transverse gluteal folds are obliterated. The normal lordosis of the lumbar spine is increased and there is marked protrusion of the abdomen. In both unilateral and bilateral cases the greater trochanter is prominent and appears above Nélaton's line (the line from anterior superior iliac spine to tuberosity of the ischium) (Fig. 5). When the patient stands, bearing his weight on the affected hip, the pelvis is tilted downward on the normal side (positive Trendelenburg's sign) instead of tilting upward as it would if the hip possessed normal stability (Fig. 23). The femoral head can usually be felt outside of the acetabulum. The range of abduction and of external rotation may

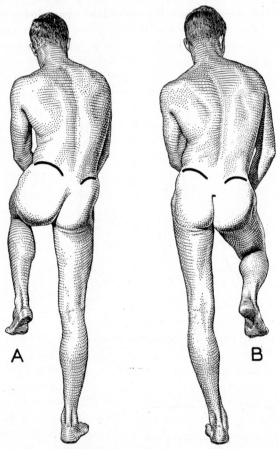

Fig. 23.—The Trendelenburg test in instability of the left hip. *A*, Negative test—when entire weight is borne on normal leg, opposite side of pelvis is elevated to maintain balance. *B*, Positive test—when entire weight is borne on abnormal leg, elevation of opposite side of pelvis cannot be accomplished because of instability of the hip.

be decreased. In older persons a definite flexion deformity of the hip can be demonstrated upon flattening the lumbar spine on the examining table.

Diagnosis.—In the infant it may be impossible to make a diagnosis with certainty until roentgenograms of the hip have been examined. These should be taken first with the knees together and the patellae pointing forward and second with the hips in maximum abduction and internal rotation. If Shenton's line is disrupted (Fig. 24A), the diagnosis is strongly suggested. Outstanding roentgenographic findings in older children are increased displacement of the femur, continued underdevelopment of the femoral head, and obliquity of the acetabular roof. Aside from the roentgenogram, the diagnosis depends upon eliciting the signs above described, particularly the palpation of the femoral head in an abnormal position. Because of the waddling gait of patients with either unilateral or bilateral congenital dislocation of the hip, the diagnosis may be confused with that of coxa vara, excessive lumbar lordosis, rickets with muscular hypotonia, tuberculosis of the lumbar spine, infantile paralysis with weakness of the gluteus medius, and early progressive muscular dystrophy, in each of which conditions the gait is somewhat similar.

Treatment.—Treatment should be begun as soon as the condition is recognized. The earlier the treatment is started the better will be the ultimate result.

It has been shown that in young babies abduction of the hip tends to stimulate the development of the acetabulum. Putti has demonstrated that an effective method of treating hip dislocations in the first year of life is to apply a triangular abduction splint. Many modifications of this splint have been devised; they include firm pillows for maintaining wide abduction of the hips, casts with turnbuckles for gradually increasing abduction, and shoe splints with adjustable spreader attachments. In recent years the abduction pillow splint of Frejka has become popular (Fig. 25). This holds the legs in moderate abduction and the patient is encouraged to stand with the splint applied. Before application of the splint, a period of from one to several weeks of skin traction in increasing abduction will accommodate the hips to this position and often will effect reduction with a minimum of trauma.

When the dislocation has been first recognized at the age of about one year, it is treated by closed reduction under anesthesia. The most favorable period for the closed method terminates, however, at the age of three years. Statistics show that in children under the age of six years satisfactory results follow closed reduction in from 40 to 60 per cent of the cases, while in cases in which treatment is undertaken prior to three years of

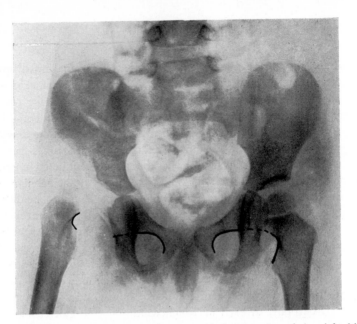

Fig. 24A.—Roentgenogram showing congenital dislocation of the right hip in a two and one-half year old girl. Note the upward and outward displacement of the head of the right femur, the increased obliquity of the superior portion of the acetabulum, and the small, underdeveloped capital epiphysis. The right obturator-coxofemoral line (Shenton's line) is disrupted.

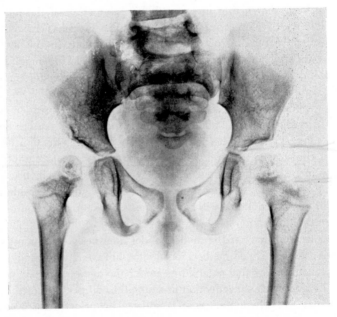

Fig. 24B.—Same patient as Fig. 24A, thirteen months following closed reduction of right hip dislocation. Note the continued increased obliquity of the acetabulum, the continued underdevelopment of the epiphysis, and the atrophy of the shaft of the femur. The head of the femur is now in the acetabulum.

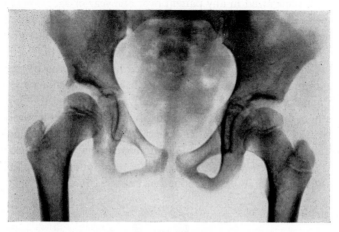

Fig. 24C.—Same patient as Fig. 24A, five and one-half years after closed reduction of right hip dislocation. Patient now nine years of age. Note the head of the right femur has almost the same appearance as the left. The right acetabulum has deepened but still is not so well developed as the left.

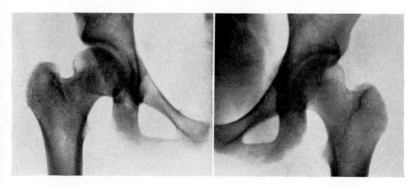

Fig. 24D.—Same patient as Fig. 24A, eleven years after closed reduction of right hip dislocation. Patient now fourteen years of age. Note well-rounded, smooth head of femur. The acetabulum is almost as well developed as that on the left, but the head and neck of the right femur are not quite so large as those on the left.

age, 60 to 80 per cent of satisfactory results may be anticipated. Some orthopaedic surgeons, however, advocate open reduction as soon as the condition is recognized in any patient over one year of age; others recommend open reduction in the younger child only when the closed reduction is unsuccessful. Advocates of immediate open operation contend that no damage is done to the head of the femur by operation but that with closed reduction the femoral head is often injured by the trauma of manipulation, and that such damage may later lead to osteochondritis of the capital femoral epiphysis and degenerative changes in the hip joint. The author believes that the method of choice depends entirely upon characteristics peculiar to the individual case and that no single rule can be followed; he considers the optimum treatment to be closed reduction at the age of one year; the earlier use of an abduction splint, however, may make manipulative reduction unnecessary.

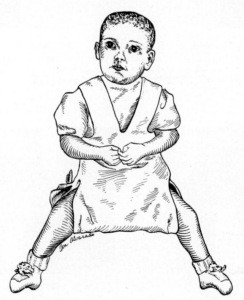

Fig. 25.—Abduction pillow splint (Frejka). Used for treatment of early congenital dislocation of hip. (After Hart.)

Crego has shown that skeletal traction may be of great value as a preliminary to either open or closed reduction. Before open reduction, traction reduces the time of operation, obviates radical division of resistant soft parts, and minimizes trauma at the time of placement of

the head into the acetabulum. To be effective, the traction must pull
the head of the femur down below the level of the center of the
acetabulum and hold it in this position for a week or ten days before
either closed or open reduction is attempted. At times the reduction
may be accomplished by skeletal traction alone; in this case, the hip
should be in wide abduction and internal rotation.

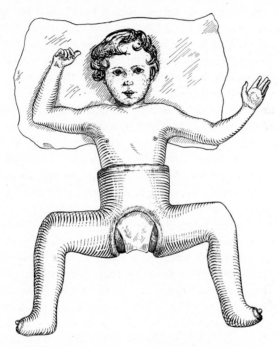

Fig. 26.—Bilateral hip spica cast applied in the "frog-leg" position of 90
degrees of abduction, 90 degrees of external rotation, and 90 degrees of flexion
(reduction attitude).

In the closed reduction, emphasis must be placed upon gentleness.
In the original "Lorenz bloodless reduction" there was actually a tremendous amount of trauma and hemorrhage. In the technic of
the closed reduction some orthopaedic surgeons recommend, after anes-
thetization, a gentle, thorough stretching of the muscles and ligaments by
carrying out flexion, extension, abduction, and adduction before attempting to reduce the dislocation. Reduction should be effected in this
manner: first flex the hip and the knee to 90 degrees, externally rotating
the hip slightly, and then gradually abduct the hip in the flexed position

as upward pressure is exerted on the head and greater trochanter of the femur. When the hip is brought into 90 degrees of abduction, the head of the femur will lie in the acetabulum if reduction is successful. During a successful manipulation, the head of the femur can be felt to slip over the acetabular rim. Occasionally a myotomy of the contracted adductor muscles will facilitate reduction. If the dislocation is reduced, the head of the femur will slip out with a click when the abduction of the limb is lessened. In both bilateral and unilateral cases both hips should be immobilized in the frog-leg position of 90 degrees of flexion, 90 degrees external rotation, and 90 degrees of abduction (Fig. 26). Usually a plaster cast is applied to maintain this position; sometimes, however, a splint is employed.

There is a difference of opinion as to how long a reduced congenital dislocation of the hip should be kept in a plaster cast and as to the position in which such fixation should be maintained. The author believes that immobilization should usually be continued for nine months. Originally it was recommended that the frog-leg position should be maintained during practically the whole of the period of immobilization. More recent experience, however, has shown that a better functional result is obtained by converting relatively soon this reduction attitude (Fig. 26) to one more nearly approximating a functional attitude (Fig. 27), and that the change of position is attended by little risk of redislocation. The change may be made from three to four months after closed reduction. The functional attitude is one of extension, moderate abduction, and internal rotation (Fig. 27). The proper degree of internal rotation depends upon the degree of anteversion of the femoral neck, or antetorsion of the femur. Following either closed or open reduction, correction of the antetorsion may be accomplished by supracondylar osteoclasis or osteotomy with outward rotation of the lower femoral fragment adequate to correct the deformity. In the growing child, especially under three years of age, however, much of the excessive antetorsion will undergo spontaneous correction and an osteoclasis or osteotomy is rarely necessary.

When an open reduction has been done, the period of postoperative immobilization is as a rule not less than three months. After operation, the extremity is usually immobilized in plaster in the functional attitude of extension, abduction, and internal rotation (Fig. 27). Following the removal of plaster or splint, after either a closed or an open reduction, the patient should receive physical therapy to strengthen muscles and loosen contracted joints. This may include pool therapy.

With weight-bearing it may be advisable to keep the hips or limbs in moderate abduction by a brace which includes the pelvis. For a year or more following the removal of the plaster cast, it is frequently desirable for the patient to use a night splint which maintains the hips in wide abduction by means of a long bar between the shoes.

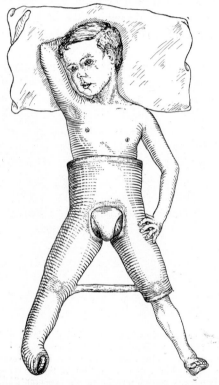

Fig. 27.—Bilateral hip spica cast applied with affected right hip in extension, abduction, and internal rotation (functional attitude). This position is commonly used to maintain correction after open reduction of congenital dislocation of the hip.

Gill and others have shown that disability from subluxation or redislocation of the hip frequently develops years after an apparently successful closed or open reduction. Patients with reduced dislocations should be kept under observation for many years; roentgenograms should be taken at long intervals, and no patient should be discharged as cured until the roentgenographic appearance of the acetabulum and femoral head has become normal. The development of symptoms due to upward subluxation, and failure of the upper lip of the acetabulum to develop satisfactorily as shown by roentgen examination, are indications for surgical reconstruction of the acetabular roof or a shelf operation (Fig. 28).

Colonna has reported successful results following an arthroplastic procedure performed in children between three and eight years of age. This consists of enlarging or deepening the acetabulum and placing in it the head of the femur after covering the head with the elongated capsule.

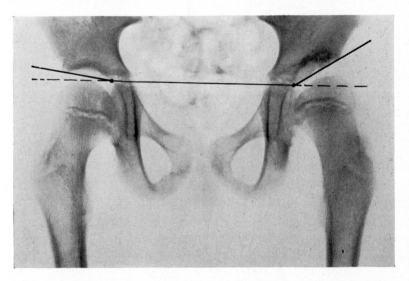

Fig. 28.—Roentgenogram showing congenital dysplasia of left hip in six-year-old boy. Note the irregular ossification and the increased obliquity of the superior portion of the acetabulum. The acetabular angle is 30 degrees on the left and 10 degrees on the right. The superior portion of the acetabulum does not cover the head of the femur as completely as in the normal right hip. The capital epiphysis has the so-called "jockey cap" appearance. Note the bilateral coxa valga (155 degrees). This case is a congenital dislocation of the left hip, four years after closed reduction.

The treatment of dislocation of the hip in children over ten years of age and in adults forms a different and more difficult problem. It has been found that reduction is usually impracticable because of the shape of the head of the femur, the acetabular changes, the thickened and contracted capsule, and the extensive shortening of the muscles. Three operative procedures which provide increased stability and at the same time preserve a useful amount of motion are most commonly used: (1) the shelf operation, (2) subtrochanteric osteotomy, and (3) the bifurcation operation.

1. The shelf operation consists of improving the acetabular socket by constructing a ledge of bone over the head of the femur after it has been pulled down as far as possible. This may be done by turning down a bone flap from the ilium and reinforcing the back of this ledge with a triangular piece of bone from the iliac crest, as shown in Fig. 29, or with bone chips, or by inserting tibial grafts into the ilium over the head of the femur. If the head is in the acetabulum, the shelf of bone should be created at the superior acetabular margin and should constitute an extension of the roof of the acetabulum over the head of the femur. This type of operation is frequently advised by Gill for an acetabular dysplasia (Fig. 28) following the reduction of a congenital dislocation.

2. The subtrochanteric osteotomy of Schanz may at times be advisable. This operation permits the femur to be placed in abduction with its large upper portion lying against the pelvis in such fashion as to provide greatly increased stability; it also allows the femur to be shifted anteriorly and hyperextended, which decreases the pelvic tilt and the strain on the lumbar spine. The blade plate recently described by Blount may be used for internal fixation following this osteotomy.

3. The bifurcation operation of Lorenz is sometimes indicated in the older cases when marked adduction and flexion are present. In this operation an oblique osteotomy of the femur is performed below the level of the lesser trochanter. The proximal end of the lower fragment is placed in the old acetabulum. The upper fragment is then allowed to unite with the lower fragment in its new position.

In the older cases marked by instability, stiffness, and pain, an arthrodesis of the hip may be advisable for relief of the symptoms.

In the older untreated cases, a high cork sole under the shortened leg will sometimes relieve the strain. When back pain due to this strain is present, a corset or snugly fitting back brace should be applied.

Prognosis.—In congenital dislocation of the hip, the prognosis for good joint function is excellent if treatment is started before the third year of age and if late redislocation or subluxation is prevented. In older patients good results are much less certain. Circulatory changes in the femoral head sometimes lead to local deformity and impairment of function. The patient with an incomplete reduction is likely to complain of weakness and early fatigue, and later in life of pain on weight-bearing. Secondary hypertrophic bone changes which gradually develop in the hip region and the lumbar spine may cause considerable pain of a chronic type. A completely unreduced dislocation causes deformity, limping, and hip and low back discomfort which increases as the patient grows older.

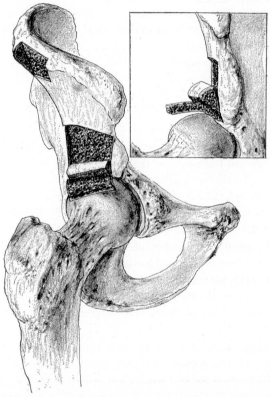

Fig. 29.—Shelf operation for late unreduced congenital dislocation of the hip. A procedure of this type may be used when it is impossible to effect reduction or difficult to maintain reduction because of shallowness of the acetabulum. A shelf of bone is turned down from the ilium and held in place by a triangular wedge of bone taken from the iliac crest.

Summary.—Congenital dislocation of the hip is found more often in girls than in boys, more often in one hip than in both, and more often in the Latin races. No wholly satisfactory hypothesis has been advanced to explain the pathogenesis. The saucer-shaped acetabulum, mushroom-shaped head, anteverted femoral neck, and hourglass capsule are the most characteristic pathologic features. The shortened extremity, positive Trendelenburg test, protruding abdomen, duck waddle gait, and sway-back are the most important physical signs. Treatment should be started as soon as the condition is recognized. Abduction splinting is advocated in early infancy, closed reduction up to three years of age, and open reduction after this. The shelf operation to provide stability is the most satisfactory procedure in the older untreated cases and in late cases of subluxation. Congenital dislocation of the hip is no longer a hopeless and incurable condition.

Congenital Dislocation of Other Joints

These entities, in sharp contrast to congenital dislocation of the hip, are rare. In many instances they are more correctly considered subluxations or relaxations of the joint ligaments than true dislocations.

KNEE

Two types of congenital luxation are encountered. One is a hyper-extension of the knee or congenital genu recurvatum; this is more common than true dislocation. The second type exhibits an actual posterior displacement of the condyles of the femur on the head of the tibia, constituting an anterior dislocation of the knee joint. The most plausible explanation for the origin of these conditions is an abnormal position of the knee in utero, because when the deformity is corrected the knee develops normally.

Clinical Picture.—In true congenital dislocation of the knee the leg may be brought to a straight line but will not flex beyond this point, because of contracture of the quadriceps muscle and the patellar ligament. Often the patella is absent, or it may be very small. There is usually a wrinkling of the skin over the patella, and there may be an associated varus or valgus deformity of the knee. Lateral instability is often present.

Treatment.—As soon as dislocation of the knee is recognized, an attempt should be made to correct the displacement. This can be done usually either by gentle manipulation of the joint and stretching the quadriceps tendon or by wedged casts. Massage of the anterior muscles may relax them and facilitate the manipulation. After reduction the knee should be kept in a flexed position by means of a posterior splint. This position should be maintained until the flexors of the knee are strong enough to prevent a recurrence of the deformity. It is sometimes necessary to lengthen the quadriceps tendon, and occasionally the iliotibial band must be released, before satisfactory reduction can be obtained.

PATELLA

Congenital dislocation of the patella rarely occurs. It may be bilateral and is usually associated with a genu recurvatum and genu valgum. The patella is usually displaced laterally. An attempt should be made to replace the patella, and a dressing should be applied to maintain the corrected position. If the correction cannot be held, an operative procedure such as that described for recurrent dislocation of the patella (page 462) is indicated when the child has become older.

ANKLE

Occasionally with defective development of the tibia or fibula there exists from birth an inward or outward dislocation of the ankle joint. Volkmann has described a congenital dislocation of the ankle in which a partial defect of the bones of the leg produces an obliquity of the ankle joint and causes the foot, which in itself is normal, to assume an abnormal position, usually that of valgus. In congenital absence of the fibula a lateral displacement of the ankle may occur.

Treatment.—Very little can be done in the early period of life. In later years it may be necessary to carry out an osteotomy for correction of the deformity.

SHOULDER

Congenital dislocation of the shoulder is extremely rare. The dislocation may occur in utero. The head of the humerus usually lies beneath the spine of the scapula with the arm in a position of abduction and internal rotation. The condition may be associated with other congenital malformations. True congenital dislocation of the shoulder must be differentiated from dislocation caused by trauma at birth and from subluxation secondary to obstetric paralysis.

Treatment.—Manipulative reposition of the head of the humerus should be done as early as possible. If the result is unsatisfactory, it may be necessary to carry out later an arthrodesis of the shoulder joint.

ELBOW

Congenital dislocation of the elbow is also a rare condition. Partial luxation of the head of the radius sometimes occurs. If the radial head is displaced posteriorly, extension of the elbow is usually limited. It is necessary to remove the head of the radius in order to put the elbow in a corrected position. If the ulna and radius are dislocated posteriorly on the humerus, flexion is usually restricted. Congenital dislocation of the elbow is often associated with an elongation of the upper third of the radius or with a radio-ulnar synostosis.

WRIST

Congenital dislocation of the wrist is most often associated with club-hand and defective development of the bones of the forearm. Posterior luxation of the lower end of the ulna is spoken of as *Madelung's deformity* (Fig. 190) (page 535). This is an acquired deformity but is believed by some orthopaedic surgeons to develop on the basis of an underlying congenital abnormality which may result in a growth defect in the lower end of the radius.

CHAPTER IV

AFFECTIONS OF GROWING BONE

Introduction: The Functional Adaptations of Bone.—By its physical properties of strength, resilience, and lightness, bone is admirably adapted to its function as the supporting framework of the body. Bone is not on this account to be regarded as an inert structural material, however, since it is an actively living tissue and like other tissues is constantly undergoing the simultaneous processes of tissue destruction and regeneration. With this continuous breaking down and rebuilding is associated an adaptive remodeling of the bones in response to the functional demands, including muscle tension, which are placed upon them. This far-reaching principle, stated by Julius Wolff in 1868, has become known as *Wolff's law:* "Every change in the form and the function of bones, or in their function alone, is followed by certain definite changes in their internal architecture, and equally definite changes in their external conformation, in accordance with mathematical laws."

Increased functional demands cause the physicochemical processes of bone regeneration to outdistance those of resorption, and a condition of *bone hypertrophy* results. The thick, heavy bones of athletes and laborers, as contrasted with the lighter bones of sedentary individuals, are illustrative of bone hypertrophy. Of greater clinical concern, however, is the converse process of *bone atrophy,* which results from a predominance of the catabolic and resorptive processes over those of regeneration.

Bone atrophy, in accordance with Wolff's law, may be caused by disuse. The bone atrophy which constantly develops during therapeutic immobilization of an extremity is a classical example. The cortical bone becomes thinned, the medullary cavity widened, slight narrowing of the shaft occurs, and generalized porosity and loss of weight may become very marked. These bone changes represent merely a quantitative variation, however, since the chemical composition undergoes no demonstrable alteration, the breaking strength in relation to weight is normal, and the power of repair after fracture is unimpaired. Extreme bone atrophy is of particular importance when involving the growing bones of childhood, since atrophic bones grow slowly and may never attain full size.

Bone atrophy appears in roentgenograms as a loss of density of the bone shadow as compared with that of the soft tissues. Narrowing of the cortex and attenuation of the bony trabeculae are frequently pronounced. It must be remembered that roentgenographic density is simply an index of the total lime salt content of the bones and gives no information regarding the pathologic changes which may be taking place in their organic constituents. Little is known of the chemistry or physiology of this organic part of the bone, or of what part the proteins and carbohydrates play in bone formation and metabolism. It is believed by the author that research in this field, which is greatly needed, may lead to an understanding and explanation of many of the unusual bone conditions about which there is so little information at this time.

Since the bony skeleton is not an inert mechanical structure but a living and continually changing tissue, it is like other tissues subject to characteristic metabolic and nutritional disorders. These diseases are alike in producing widespread skeletal changes but vary markedly in etiology. Some, such as *rickets* and *scurvy,* are of dietetic origin; others, as *cretinism* and *acromegaly,* are the result of endocrine disturbances; while several, for example, *osteogenesis imperfecta* and *osteitis deformans,* may be grouped together as of unknown etiology. In the past few decades much has been accomplished toward defining the causation of bone diseases; thus the rôle of the parathyroid glands in producing the extensive bone changes of *hyperparathyroidism* is a comparatively recent discovery. Such advances suggest that the causation of other members of this group of diseases will eventually be learned and that with discovery of the etiologic factors will come improvement in our methods of prevention and treatment.

In age incidence, as in etiology, the members of this group of bone diseases vary widely. In age of onset they range from embryonic life, as in the case of *achondroplasia,* to old age, as in *senile osteomalacia.* It is convenient to divide these disorders arbitrarily into two groups: (1) *affections of growing bone,* which are considered in the present chapter, and (2) *affections of adult bone,* which will be discussed in Chapter V.

Skeletal Changes Associated With Vitamin Disturbances

In recent years much attention has been paid to the bone and joint changes and the imbalance in calcification associated with both the lack and the excess of vitamins in the body. The part which vitamin A plays in calcification has received especial consideration. Many previously un-explained bone conditions in the growing child are being interpreted in the light of new knowledge. Some forms of hypervitaminoses have been due to the mother's thinking that if one tablespoonful of cod liver oil or a few drops of cod liver oil concentrate will help her child, a larger dose will help more. This is particularly true of the administration of large doses of vitamins A and D. An excess of vitamin B, C, or E has no known harmful effect. The following is a brief summary of the effect of vitamins A, B, C, D, and E on the skeletal system.

1. **Vitamin A.**—This has a specific effect on the osteoblasts, osteo-clasts, and epiphyseal chondroblasts of growing bone. It determines the pattern of bone growth. Thick, short bones will result from either a lack or an excess of the vitamin. Hypervitaminosis A will cause an elevation of the periosteum followed by subperiosteal calcification similar to that seen in scurvy. This appears usually after six months of age with exces-sive administration and is associated with pain in the extremities and irri-tability. It may be confused, not only with scurvy, but also with *infantile cortical hyperostosis (Caffey's disease)*, which is usually accompanied by swelling of the jaw and occurs in the infant from one to four months of age, and *progressive diaphyseal dysplasia (Engelmann's disease)*, which is extremely rare, occurs in the older child and young adult and is asso-ciated with a waddling gait and muscular weakness.

2. **Vitamin B.**—A lack of vitamin B_2 or riboflavin in early preg-nancy, i.e., in the first to the twelfth week, is thought to be an etiologic factor in the formation of congenital anomalies. This has been proved experimentally. Nicotinic acid is thought by some observers to stimulate callus formation and the consolidation of fractures by means of its ability to activate phosphatase. Experimentally it has been shown that lack of the B complex causes thinning of the epiphyseal cartilage plates and cessa-tion of growth.

3. **Vitamin C.**—This vitamin promotes the formation of collagen and maintains the intercellular substance. A deficiency causes the activity of the osteoblasts and chondroblasts to cease, resulting in resorption and rarefaction of bone. The fibrous periosteum may be elevated by sub-periosteal hemorrhages. There is a marked widening of the epiphyseal cartilages. Scurvy, which is caused by this deficiency, is discussed as an entity on page 89.

4. **Vitamin D.**—The principal physiologic action of this vitamin is regulation of the calcium and phosphorus in the blood. It regulates also the deposition of these salts in the osteoid matrix or protein framework of bone which has been laid down by the osteoblasts. The organic salts of calcium and phosphorus in the blood stream are changed by vitamin D into the inorganic salts, which are deposited in the osteoid tissue. A deficiency of this vitamin produces rickets in the young and osteomalacia in adults. If the osteoid matrix is not laid down by the osteoblasts, so that there is no framework in which calcium and phosphorus salts may be deposited, an osteoporosis will result. In the young with defective calcification there is a compensatory hypertrophy of the epiphyseal cartilage which results in thickening and irregularity of the epiphyseal plates.

An excess of vitamin D will cause a high blood calcium level. Often metastatic calcification will take place in periarticular structures, bursae, and tendon sheaths. In the kidneys this process may lead to the formation of stones.

5. **Vitamin E.**—Less is known about this vitamin than about the others. The lack of vitamin E may be a cause of certain neuromuscular disorders such as pseudohypertrophic muscular dystrophy and may be a factor in producing the typical concentric bone atrophy observed in these conditions.

Rickets

Rickets is a constitutional disease of infancy and childhood caused by a disturbance of nutrition and evidenced by bony deformities which may be striking in degree and widespread in distribution. The orthopaedic problems of rickets are always secondary to the pediatric ones.

Etiology.—Underlying the rachitic syndrome is a disorder of calcium metabolism, the exact mechanism of which remains obscure despite enlightening results of dietetic investigations made in recent years. Three factors are generally considered to be important in the prevention of rickets; viz., the antirachitic vitamin D, adequate amounts of calcium and phosphorus in the diet, and sunlight or artificial ultra-violet irradiation.

Pathology.—The chief characteristic of the pathologic changes is subnormal calcification and a relative increase of osteoid tissue throughout the skeleton. This results in an increased plasticity of the bones which allows them to undergo changes in shape and to become deformed by gravitational and physiologic stresses which would be withstood by bony structures of normal strength. At the epiphyseal lines ossification is delayed and disordered, and the epiphyseal cartilages become thickened and abnormally vascularized. Involvement becomes most marked in epiphyses at which growth is most rapid.

In active rickets, characteristic blood chemistry findings include a normal calcium content, decreased phosphorus, and increased phosphatase.

Roentgenographic Picture.—These bone changes cause the roentgenographic appearance of a rachitic joint to undergo a cycle of typical alterations as the disease pursues its course.

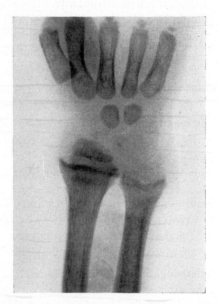

Fig. 30.—Healed rickets in patient three and one-half years of age. Note the irregular cup-shaped metaphyses with spotty, fuzzy calcification at the epiphyseal lines.

In the early stages the end of the diaphysis is widened and concave, and presents an irregular and indistinct margin. The epiphyseal line is broad. The epiphysis itself is obscurely outlined and contains one or more indistinct areas of ossification; as growth proceeds it assumes a vaguely mottled appearance. The shaft may show periosteal thickening and occasionally a fracture line.

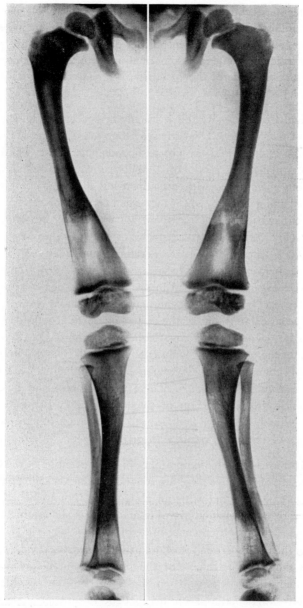

Fig. 31.—Healed rickets in patient six years of age. Note broadening of epiphyseal cartilage disks with genu valgum, distortion of tibiae and lower ends of femurs, and bilateral coxa vara.

In later stages the end of the diaphysis loses most of its concavity but remains unmistakably widened. The epiphysis becomes more distinct in outline and more homogeneous in density. The shaft shows an increased calcium content. Abnormal curvature, with thickening of the cortex on the side of the concavity, is a characteristic finding (Figs. 30 and 31.)

Clinical Picture.—Rickets is usually first recognizable near the end of the first year of life. The early symptoms are of pediatric rather than orthopaedic interest, and are not pathognomonic. They consist chiefly of an abnormal restlessness and irritability; a catarrhal inflammation of the mucous membranes with accompanying diarrhea, constipation, or bronchitis; and a tendency toward excessive perspiration.

The clinical picture of the more advanced case, however, is characteristic (Fig. 32). The typical rachitic patient has a pale skin, flabby subcutaneous tissue, and poorly developed musculature. The joints, because of changes in the epiphyses, are slightly enlarged. The liver and spleen are likely to be increased in size, and the abdomen is prominent. The thorax may be of grossly abnormal shape and may show the *rachitic rosary*, due to enlargement of the costochondral junctions, or *Harrison's groove*, a transverse sulcus across the lower portion of the chest, thought to be due to the pull of the diaphragm. The skull is large and because of its decalcification exhibits a delicate crepitation on palpation, a condition which is known as *craniotabes*. There is noticeable delay in closure of the fontanels, in development of the teeth, and in acquisition of the ability to stand. Bowleg, knock-knee, coxa vara, scoliosis, and other deformities of the bones occur with great frequency in rickets.

Treatment.—Of chief importance in the prevention of rickets and in the treatment of its active stage are adequate dietary calcium, phosphorus, and vitamin D, together with an abundance of sunshine and general hygienic care. An ample intake of vitamin D must be assured by supplementary medication with a concentrate of cod liver oil.

When the disease is established and still in its active stage, orthopaedic measures should be added. For the prevention of deformity, weight-bearing and sitting with the legs crossed should be avoided. It is occasionally advisable to keep the patient recumbent upon a frame. Slight degrees of deformity in the relatively plastic bones of infants may sometimes be corrected gradually bv closed methods. The use of wedged casts is sometimes effective in correcting bowing of the long bones. A well-padded and closely fitting cast applied to the deformed extremity is later cut for wedging, and thereafter at intervals of one or two weeks

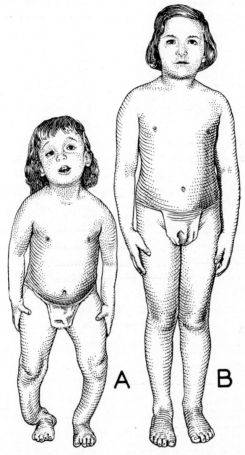

Fig. 32.—*A*, Rachitic dwarf, aged eight years. The prominent forehead, sagging abdominal musculature, and lateral and anterior bowing of the legs are characteristic. *B*, Normal child of same age. (From clinical material of Dr. E. A. Park.)

gentle manipulation is carried out without anesthesia, the successive corrections being maintained by additional plaster applied to the original cast. Frequent inspection must be made to guard against ulcers or circulatory impairment caused by the pressure of the cast.

Osteoclasis, or fracture without operative exposure, has been used frequently in the past for the correction of deformity of the long bones in infants and young children, but is now less often employed. This procedure is most useful either in active rickets while the bone is still plastic, or after it has become so from disuse atrophy accompanying immobilization. Osteoclasis may then be performed manually with little danger of injuring the soft tissues, after which the extremity is immobilized in a corrected or slightly overcorrected position by means of a plaster cast until healing of the fracture is well advanced.

Osteotomy, or operative section of the bone, is the procedure of choice in most instances of severe rachitic bowing and particularly in the late cases. Osteotomy is a quick, simple, and accurate procedure requiring only a small incision and obviating contusion of the soft tissues. The exact level and degree of the desired correction should be determined preoperatively from analysis of the roentgenograms. During operation caution must be observed not to injure the vessels or nerves with the osteotome. Following closure a well-padded plaster cast is applied with the extremity in a slightly overcorrected position. It is sometimes advantageous to do an incomplete osteotomy and to follow it after three weeks by osteoclasis, as described by Moore. Immobilization is continued for from six to twelve weeks or until there is a satisfactory union as indicated by adequate callus shown in the roentgenogram and by absence of mobility at the site of osteotomy. Gradual return to weight-bearing is then carried out under observation.

Vitamin-Resistant Rickets

In some infants and young children, active rickets fail to respond to ordinary doses of vitamin D. These patients do not have a disease of the kidneys or alimentary tract but are thought to have a congenital or acquired resistance to vitamin D. The typical deformities of rickets may develop. Vitamin-resistant rickets may be treated successfully by the administration of massive daily doses of vitamin D, i.e., doses of from 150,000 to 1,500,000 units. The dosage should be great enough to maintain a one-plus or two-plus Sulkowitch urine reaction. Over-dosage of vitamin D, manifested by nausea, weight loss, and hematuria due to hypercalcemia, must be avoided. The orthopaedic correction of the deformities is the same as that described for rickets (Fig. 33).

Adolescent Rickets

A condition characterized by the appearance in late childhood of symptoms and deformities of rachitic type, usually limited to one or two bones, has been called *late* or *adolescent rickets*. The same fundamental pathologic changes are found as in infantile rickets, but there are fewer epiphyseal changes and more decalcification. There is a delay in the calcification of the epiphyseal plates as shown in the roentgenograms, and occasionally there may be an associated epiphyseal separation, especially of the capital femoral epiphysis. The orthopaedic treatment consists principally of correction of deformity of the long bones by means of osteotomy.

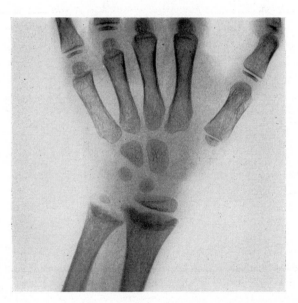

Fig. 33.—Vitamin-resistant rickets in child six years of age. Note the cup-shaped metaphyses and the irregularities at the epiphyseal lines of the radius and ulna.

Genu Varum (Bowleg)

Deforming curvature of the legs, most frequently found in association with rickets, occurs so commonly as to merit consideration as an entity. The most frequent of these deformities is *genu varum*, or *bowleg*, in

which the major convexity of the limb is disposed laterally (Fig. 34).
Curvature in which the major convexity lies anteriorly is occasionally
seen and is called *anterior bowleg.*

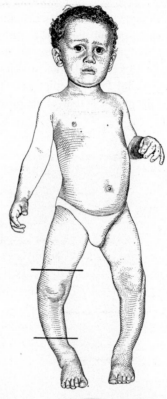

Fig. 34.—Bilateral bowleg (genu varum) resulting from rickets. The sites of
osteotomy for correction of the deformity of right tibia and femur are indicated.

Etiology and Pathology.—The curvature is usually due to the
gradual bending of pathologically softened bone under the influence of
weight-bearing or of postural stresses. Normal bone possesses sufficient
strength to resist these forces; hence healthy children never acquire bowleg from walking. Bowleg in infancy and childhood is therefore suggestive
of rickets. Bowleg may be due to an unknown change in the upper tibial
epiphysis, in which growth does not take place normally on the medial
side of the epiphyseal plate. This is an epiphyseal dysplasia sometimes

termed *tibia vara*. Rarely the healed fractures of osteogenesis imperfecta may lead to similar deformities; in differential diagnosis the roentgenograms are of value. The *saber shin* of congenital syphilis is differentiated from anterior bowleg by collateral clinical evidence of syphilis, a positive complement fixation reaction, and the roentgenographic findings. In adults bowleg may occur from the changes of osteitis deformans, osteomalacia, hyperparathyroidism, malunited fracture, and destructive disease of the knee joint.

The curvature may be present in only one leg or in both. It may involve the tibia alone, the tibia and femur equally, or rarely the femur alone; sometimes it is the result of a lateral yielding at the knee joint while the shafts of femur and tibia remain straight. As the three-cornered column of the tibial shaft bends, torsion necessarily takes place, and the lower end of the tibia becomes internally rotated. Anterior bowleg may exist independently or in association with the lateral form.

Clinical Picture.—Bowleg is present if the extended knees are separated when the medial malleoli of the ankles are approximated. Measurements of the space between the knees, other elements of the position being unchanged, provide a ready clinical estimation of the degree of deformity and of its progress. Because of the outward bowing at the knee and the inward rotation at the ankle, the child tends to walk with the feet widely separated and the toes turned in; this may lead to considerable lateral shift of the body weight with each step and thus to a waddling type of gait.

Treatment.—The stage at which the patient is first seen influences the treatment. Antirachitic dietetic and hygienic measures should always be instituted when any degree of active rickets remains. In such early cases weight-bearing should be discouraged, and gentle corrective manipulation, carried out several times daily, may help to render more strenuous measures unnecessary. Braces will sometimes prevent increase of the bowing and will aid in its correction. In the majority of cases, however, the deformity is best corrected by *osteotomy* (see page 84). As a rule, osteotomy should not be done before the age of three years.

Genu Valgum (Knock-Knee)

In genu valgum, or knock-knee, there is an abnormal curvature of the leg with the apex of the convexity disposed medially at the level of the knee (Fig. 35). Knock-knee may occur in one or both legs; it may be present in one leg while a bowleg deformity exists in the other; or elements of knock-knee and bowleg may be present at different levels of the same extremity.

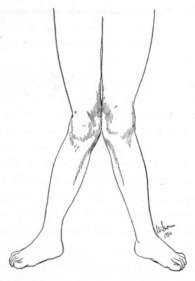

Fig. 35.—Knock-knees (genu valgum) due to rickets. The external torsion of the tibias and the pronation of the feet are common secondary deformities.

Etiology and Pathology.—Normally the medial femoral condyle is slightly longer than the lateral, thus maintaining the horizontal plane of the knee joint despite the obliquity of the femur. The axis of weight-bearing at the knee, however, passes lateral to the center of the joint, so that the lateral condyle bears more weight than the medial. With the bone-softening changes of rickets, a gradual depression of the lateral tibial condyle is therefore likely to occur, leading to various degrees of valgus deformity. With increasing knock-knee, external rotation of the tibia takes place from the pull of the lateral hamstring muscles. The foot usually develops marked pronation; in occasional cases, however, compensatory adduction of the anterior part of the foot occurs and leads to a position of varus. Knock-knee is sometimes due not to obliquity of the joint line but rather to curvature of the tibial or femoral shaft.

Rickets is the most important cause of genu valgum in children. Nonrachitic children, when standing, sometimes show a knock-knee deformity which is not the result of bony changes in the tibia or the femur but is associated with eversion of the foot and exaggerated by relaxation of the collateral ligaments of the knee joint. In other cases genu valgum of slow development may be due to an impairment of bone growth in the lateral half of the epiphyseal plate as a result of trauma or infection. Genu valgum may also occur in advanced tuberculosis of the knee, in severe poliomyelitic paralysis, and after "bumper fractures" of the tibia with uncorrected depression of the lateral condyle.

Clinical Picture.—As in bowleg, the diagnosis of knock-knee deformity is made on inspection of the extended knee. On flexion the valgus deformity of rachitic knock-knee disappears, since the posterior portion of the femoral condyles is not deformed, and in this position an abnormal length of the anterior portion of the medial femoral condyle, as compared with the lateral, may be evident. The child, as viewed from the front, may stand with the knees overlapping. The gait is altered by an internal rotation of the leg and foot to prevent the knees from striking each other while passing, and by an increased lateral sway of the body to carry its weight to a position directly over the foot.

Treatment.—When deformity of the knee is associated with active rickets, dietetic and hygienic treatment of the underlying disease is essential. In such early stages and in slight degrees of knock-knee, conservative treatment, consisting of a limitation of walking, elevation of the medial side of the shoe, and corrective manipulation carried out several times daily, may prove entirely adequate. As in the treatment of bowleg, braces sometimes are effective.

In later cases *osteotomy* (see page 84) is the procedure of choice. The level of section, determined after roentgenographic analysis of the deformity, is usually in the supracondylar region of the femur, but at times high tibial osteotomy is preferable. In older patients the removal of a small wedge of bone may be necessary. Care must be taken to overcorrect slightly the valgus deformity. The external rotation, estimated from the position of the foot with respect to the patella, must also be carefully corrected.

Scurvy

Scurvy is an acquired constitutional disease caused by an abnormality of nutrition and manifesting itself chiefly by signs related to the bones.

Etiology and Pathology.—The cause of scurvy is a dietary lack of the antiscorbutic vitamin C. This vitamin occurs in largest amount in the citrus fruits, unboiled milk, and fresh vegetables.

The pathologic changes involve an alteration in certain intercellular materials throughout the tissues, resulting particularly in subperiosteal and submucous hemorrhages.

Clinical Picture.—Like rickets, scurvy usually makes its clinical appearance in infants between six and eighteen months of age. Adult cases caused by the same dietary deficiency, however, have in the past been common among sailors and others whose diets have been abnormally restricted, and sporadic cases of scurvy in adults are still occasionally seen.

The scorbutic infant is poorly nourished and irritable and experiences extreme pain on motion of the joints and on slightest pressure over the affected bones. In well-marked cases the subperiosteal hemorrhage (Fig. 36) causes a palpable thickening of the bone. This thickening may be visible in the roentgenograms but often does not appear until calcification has taken place following dietetic treatment. In extreme cases there may be loosening of the epiphyses from the shafts, resulting in an obvious crepitation on clinical examination. Slipping of an epiphysis, followed by a deformity with subsequent growth, is a rare complication. In adult cases, and in infantile scurvy when the teeth have already appeared, the gums are likely to be swollen, spongy, and hemorrhagic.

Treatment and Prognosis.—The treatment of scurvy is primarily of pediatric nature, and consists chiefly of the administration of ascorbic acid and adequate amounts of foods, such as orange juice, which contain relatively large quantities of vitamin C. Clinical improvement is usually rapid, and the prognosis for complete cure is excellent. The orthopaedic treatment of scurvy is largely of symptomatic type. During the acute stage, complete recumbency is indicated for protection of the affected bones, and occasionally simple splints are useful to relieve pain and minimize further subperiosteal hemorrhage. During the stage of recovery, heat, massage, and exercise are useful in accelerating the healing process and in restoring function to the affected extremities.

Cretinism

Cretinism is a form of dwarfism caused by hypofunction of the thyroid gland. The condition manifests itself usually in the second six months of life. In sporadic cases no pathologic changes in the thyroid gland of the mother are demonstrable, and here the etiology is obscure. On the other hand, cases of endemic type occur frequently in goitrous regions and may be ascribed to a lack of iodine in the mother. In such instances the fetus may develop as a cretin in utero.

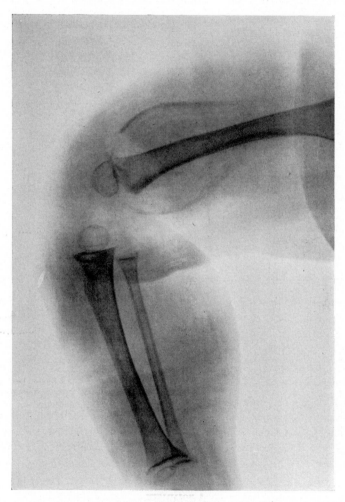

Fig. 36.—Roentgenogram of lower extremity of infant six months of age, showing changes due to scurvy. Note calcification in large subperiosteal hemorrhage in the thigh, and increased calcification and cupping on the metaphyseal side of the epiphyseal lines of the tibia and fibula.

The cretin (Fig. 37) must be carefully differentiated from the rachitic (Fig. 32*A*) and the achondroplastic (Fig. 38) dwarfs. The cretin has a large tongue which often protrudes between his thickened lips, a flattened nose with sunken bridge, puffy eyelids, and a dry skin. The facial expression is characteristically stupid and usually the mental development is obviously impaired. Ossification of the epiphyses is irregular and

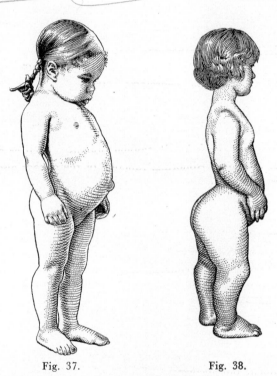

Fig. 37.   Fig. 38.

Fig. 37.—Cretinoid dwarf, aged eight years. The facies is characteristic. The sagging abdominal musculature and flattened feet are evidences of muscular hypotonicity. Note umbilical hernia. (From clinical material of Dr. E. A. Park.)

Fig. 38.—Achondroplastic dwarf, aged sixteen years. The trident hand, shortness of the extremities, large head, and increased lumbar lordosis are characteristic. (From clinical material of Dr. E. A. Park.)

delayed. Since the kidneys are unable to excrete phosphate in normal amounts, it accumulates in the blood serum. Although the epiphyseal cartilages may remain ununited for twenty or thirty years, growth of the long bones ceases, and the arms and legs remain short and stumpy.

The roentenograms show transverse bony shadows at the ends of the diaphyses.

Cretinism may be treated by the administration of thyroid preparations.

Gigantism

Gigantism is a condition in which skeletal overgrowth results from a pathologically increased activity of the anterior portion of the pituitary gland during youth. It is thus of orthopaedic interest in demonstrating clearly a close relationship between skeletal development and endocrine function. Subjective symptoms are slight or absent. The treatment of these cases belongs to the neurologic rather than to the orthopaedic surgeon.

It is probable that the pituitary gland, with its major influence on the growth processes, is to be considered in the etiology of a number of rare and obscure disorders of the developing organism, such as symmetrical dwarfism, or *ateleiosis.* Abnormal function of the gonads also can cause disturbances of growth.

Renal Dwarfism (Renal Rickets)

Renal dwarfism is a rare disease of childhood characterized by the coexistence of skeletal changes and a chronic interstitial nephritis. In the past two decades this syndrome has been established, chiefly through the work of British investigators, as a definite disease entity. Failure to recognized the entity may be followed by disastrous results, since the renal insufficiency makes general anesthesia and operation extremely dangerous.

Pathology.—The nephritis is evidenced by a low urinary specific gravity, frequent but inconstant albuminuria, a diminished urea clearance, and an increase of the nonprotein nitrogen of the blood. Postmortem examinations in these cases have consistently shown an advanced bilateral interstitial nephritis. The bones exhibit a replacement of red marrow by fat, and microscopically there are marked changes in the ossification at the epiphyseal plates. The roentgenographic changes also occur characteristically at the epiphyses and consist of a widening of the epiphyseal lines and a broadening of the diaphyses, as in rickets, but usually to a lesser extent and without the characteristic rachitic cupping (Fig. 39). The epiphyses themselves are not markedly altered but may appear fragmented. Epiphyseal separation is common. Deformities of the shafts of the bones, so characteristic of rickets, do not occur in renal dwarfism.

Clinical Picture.—The clinical course is marked by gradually developing dwarfism, which is usually not evident until about the fifth year, by thirst and polyuria beginning insidiously during childhood and later accompanied by drowsiness, vomiting, and headaches, and by bone deformities appearing near the age of puberty and simulating those of late rickets. The advanced stage of renal dwarfism is marked by the development of uremia.

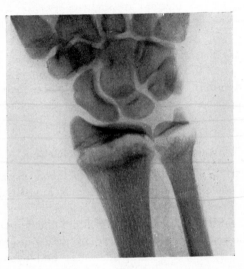

Fig. 39.—Renal rickets. Note broad epiphyseal bands of radius and ulna, the normal appearance of the epiphyses, and the areas of irregular absorption in the metaphyses.

Prognosis and Treatment.—The disease is almost always fatal, no effective therapy being known. Vitamin D not only does not help but may do harm. From an orthopaedic point of view the chief importance in recognizing renal dwarfism lies in appreciation of the futility and risk of attempting operative correction of the deformities. A brace to prevent the increase of deformity is sometimes indicated.

Dwarfism Associated With Other Types of Visceral Disease

Dwarfism and skeletal deformities of various types are occasionally seen in infancy and childhood in association with advanced visceral disease, such as cirrhosis of the liver, disorders of the pancreas, and celiac disease. Characteristic bone changes, consisting of thickening of the cranial bones and widespread osteoporosis, are frequently observed in severe and long-continued hemolytic anemias.

In such cases the primary visceral disorder is usually severe and the prognosis for survival grave. The major therapeutic consideration is treatment of the underlying visceral disease, while orthopaedic measures for the prevention or correction of specific deformities may occasionally be indicated.

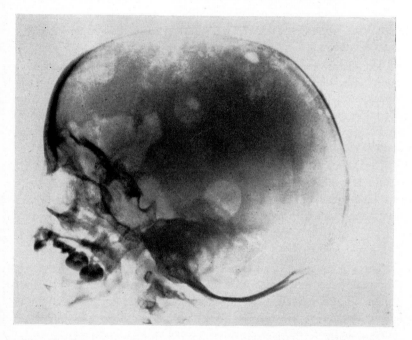

Fig. 40.—Lateral roentgenogram showing xanthomatosis of the skull. Note the irregular punched-out areas which are the sites of the invasion of the bone by the deposits of the xanthoma cells.

Xanthomatosis

(Christian's Syndrome, Schüller-Christian Disease, Lipoid Granulomatosis)

Christian's syndrome is a rare metabolic disorder characterized by bone defects which render its differential diagnosis from other bone diseases important. The disorder is essentially a disturbance of lipoid metabolism similar to that of Gaucher's and of Niemann-Pick's diseases. However, some observers regard it as a reticulo-endotheliosis in which the lipoid material is found at one stage of the disease and eosinophils at another stage. It causes a storage of lipoid substances in bone, most characteristically in the skull (Fig. 40). These deposits consist microscopically of large numbers of reticulo-endothelial cells showing lipoid infiltration. These cells have a foamy cytoplasm and are called *xanthoma cells*. The deposits are most common in the skull but occasionally are found in other bones and give rise to characteristic defects which are visible on roentgenographic examination. They may occur also in the tendons or tendon sheaths. In well-marked cases these changes may be quite extensive.

The disease usually makes its clinical appearance in childhood. Commonly associated factors, dependent upon the localization of the lipoid deposit, are diabetes insipidus, gingivitis, and exophthalmos. Dwarfism and infantilism are sometimes present, and the patient may be jaundiced. Studies of the blood chemistry have shown that lipemia is not a constant finding.

Treatment by means of a low-fat diet and the administration of insulin is indicated, and symptomatic improvement may be induced by shrinking the lipoid deposits by means of roentgen therapy. In spite of treatment, cases with extensive involvement of the bones are often fatal.

Gargoylism (Lipochondro-Osteodystrophy)

This is a congenital and familial syndrome of children, associated with abnormal bone development with widespread deposition of lipid or protein in the various tissues of the body. It is usually fatal in the second decade of life because of heart failure from lipid infiltration.

Gargoylism is characterized by marked shortening of the trunk and neck, a dorsal kyphosis, protruding abdomen, and enlargement of the liver and spleen (hepatosplenomegaly). The facial features are coarse and somewhat repulsive. There are a misshapen, enlarged skull, prominent forehead, widely spaced eyes, prominent supraorbital ridges, "saddlenose," thick tongue, and prognathism. The corneas are clouded by multiple deep opacities. There are usually short arms, impaired joint mobility, and flexion deformities of the joints, especially of the fingers, which are thickened. Because of cerebral infiltration of the lipid substance a mental deficiency develops. Characteristic roentgenographic changes include abnormalities in development of the cranial bones, abnormal vertebral contours, widening of the medial ends of the clavicles and underdevelopment of their lateral ends, and tapering of the distal phalanges. There is no known treatment.

Eosinophilic Granuloma

This is a benign inflammatory lesion of bone occurring almost exclusively in children and young adults and much more common in males than in females. Its etiology is unknown. It involves both long and flat bones and may be solitary or multiple. The lesion most often is discovered accidentally by roentgen examination. However, the signs and symptoms of local swelling, tenderness, redness, heat, and pain, with some limitation of function, may call attention to the lesion.

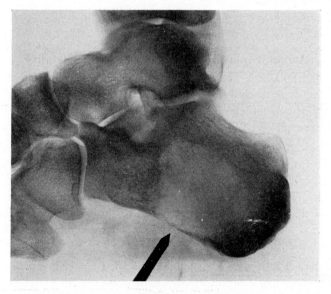

Fig. 41.—Lateral roentgenogram showing eosinophilic granuloma of os calcis. Note large circumscribed area of decalcification in central portion of the os calcis.

The roentgenographic picture is usually a circumscribed area of bone destruction from one to four centimeters in diameter with a sharply punched-out appearance (Fig. 41). Upon gross pathologic examination the early lesion may have the appearance of soft hemorrhagic granulation tissue; upon microscopic examination there are found numbers of large mononuclear histiocytes which are phagocytic, and collections of eosinophils from which the disease derives its name. Multinuclear giant cells are often present. In the later stages the eosinophils disappear and the histiocytes become foamy and assume the appearance of xanthoma cells. The pathologic tissue is eventually transformed into bone.

Differential Diagnosis.—Eosinophilic granuloma may be confused with xanthomatosis, osteoid osteoma, osteomyelitis, Ewing's sarcoma, osteogenic sarcoma, multiple myeloma, bone cyst, benign giant cell tumor, syphilis, tuberculosis, and other conditions. Some authorities consider it to be a benign variant of xanthomatosis.

Treatment and Prognosis.—Without treatment the lesions may undergo spontaneous healing in from a few months to a year. Excision or curettage, and packing of the cavity with small bone grafts when indicated, usually result in complete cure. Roentgen therapy also may be curative.

Achondroplasia (Chondrodystrophia Foetalis)

Achondroplasia is a condition of abnormal osteogenesis which produces the typical congenital dwarf of literature and drama. The discovery of a complete achondroplastic skeleton of the early Egyptian period has established this as one of the oldest of known diseases.

Pathology and Etiology.—Essentials in the pathologic process, which begins early in intrauterine life, are disordered chondrification and ossification of the ends of the long bones and premature union of the epiphyses. These changes sometimes can be seen in roentgenograms before birth. The bones of membranous origin develop normally. The condition is always congenital and is sometimes definitely inherited. Its etiology has not been established.

Clinical Picture.—The condition is first noticed usually in the growing child when the disproportion between length of trunk and of limbs becomes evident. The arms and legs appear short and thickened in contrast to the normally developing torso. The clinical appearance of the achondroplastic dwarf is characteristic and usually permits of a ready diagnosis (Fig. 38). The facial expression resulting from high and broad forehead, flattened nose with depressed bridge, and prominent lower jaw is typical. The hands are short and broad with fingers of almost equal length which tend to spread in a radial manner and have occasioned the term "main en trident." Although growth of the trunk is of essentially normal extent, pathologic anteroposterior and lateral spinal curvatures of secondary nature are common. Bowing of the femurs and tibias is a frequent finding. Mental development is usually unimpaired, as are the sexual characteristics, although in both respects exceptions occur.

Diagnosis.—Differential diagnosis is difficult only in infancy, when rickets and cretinism are to be considered. The usual normal mentality of the achondroplastic patient forms an obvious contrast with the impaired mental development of the cretin. The roentgenograms, however, are of greatest value in differentiating sharply the short, broad, normally dense shafts and prematurely uniting epiphyses of achondroplasia (Fig. 42) from the decalcified bones and poorly ossified epiphyses of rickets, and from the broad transverse metaphyseal condensations of cretinism.

Treatment.—No successful treatment of achondroplasia is known. Occasionally, especial attention is required for the prevention or correction of specific deformities. The prognosis for length of life is good.

Dyschondroplasia (Diaphyseal or Metaphyseal Aclasis, Hereditary Multiple Cartilaginous Exostoses, Ollier's Disease

Dyschondroplasia is an infrequent congenital and sometimes inherited skeletal affection of obscure etiology characterized by disorderly cartilaginous development and irregular ossification at the ends of the long bones (Figs. 43A and 43B). Two clinical types of the condition are noteworthy. In one the deforming overgrowths are of extremely irregular shape and are confined to one extremity or to one side of the body. In the other there are multiple and often roughly symmetrical osteocartilaginous tumors which individually are identical with the benign bone tumor known as osteochondroma. There are various gradations between these two types, and in both, as a rule, secondary bone deformity and dwarfed skeletal growth occur.

Pathology.—The site of the pathologic process is the metaphysis, where disorderly overgrowth of cartilage and abnormal and incomplete ossification take place. The bones of purely membranous origin are not usually involved. The changes become most marked where growth in length is greatest, that is, at the shoulders and wrists and about the knees. Multiple tumors often take the form of narrow elongated pyra-

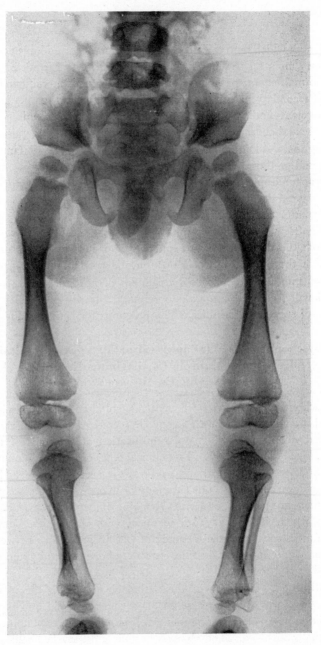

Fig. 42.—Roentgenogram showing changes due to achondroplasia in three-year-old boy. Note the short, thick femurs, tibias, and fibulas, the valgus of the hips, and the slight varus of the knees.

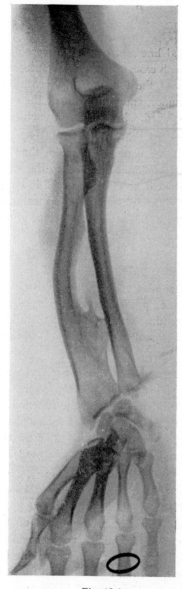

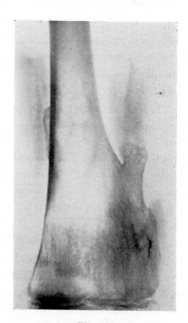

Fig. 43A.   Fig. 43B.

Fig. 43A.—Roentgenogram showing multiple congenital exostoses in a woman twenty-eight years of age. Note the exostosis at the lower end of the radius, which encroaches on the interosseous space, the exostosis at the upper end of the radius with enlargement of the bicipital tuberosity, and the outward bowing of the shaft of the radius.

Fig. 43B.—Roentgenogram showing multiple congenital exostoses in nine-year-old boy. Note the broadening of the metaphysis and the exostosis above the adductor tubercle of the femur. This patient is the son of patient in Fig. 43A.

mids with osseous base at the epiphyseal line and cartilage-covered tip directed obliquely along the shaft. In such cases symmetrical deformities are likely to occur at analogous levels of the limbs. An adventitious bursa may form over the tip of such a tumor, and with maturity the cartilaginous tip may become completely ossified. Malignant degeneration is rare.

Clinical Picture.—The disease is more common in males than in females. The presence of hard painless swellings attached to the ends of the long bones, or to the scapula or pelvis, is usually noticed in early childhood. In less marked cases such tumors make their appearance only at puberty. Patients with lesions of the more severe type show retarded general skeletal development, associated with which there may be secondary deformities, such as curvature of the bones of the forearm or fusion of the lower end of the tibia and fibula.

Roentgenographic Picture.—The roentgenograms of dyschondroplasia are, as a rule, pathognomonic, presenting large irregularly expanded diaphyseal masses with only thin sheets of cortical bone, or multiple bony outgrowths at the metaphyseal regions (Figs. 43A and 43B).

Treatment and Prognosis.—Treatment is chiefly concerned with the surgical removal of discrete tumors which by local pressure on tendon or nerve are causing pain or are interfering with the function of an adjacent joint. After ossification of the epiphyses has taken place, no further increase in deformity is likely to occur, and operative correction of outstanding deformities may be indicated. The prognosis for length of life is excellent.

Morquio's Disease (Osteochondrodystrophy)

This is a congenital condition, and approximately one-third of the reported cases have a familial history. It is usually not recognized until the child begins to walk, at which time a waddling gait is noted. There are characteristic changes in the spine and centers of ossification, especially in the capital femoral epiphyses. The femoral heads become enlarged and irregular, and there results a limitation of external rotation of the hips. The spine is stiff and usually presents a sharp kyphosis at the dorso-lumbar junction which may be confused with the gibbus of a tuberculous spine. There may be a compensatory lumbar lordosis. There is gross deformity in the bodies of the vertebrae at the dorso-lumbar junction, the front half of the vertebrae at times appearing to be missing. The neck and trunk are short in contrast to limbs of normal length. The phalanges and metacarpal bones may be stubby and the ulna and fibula short. The intelligence is usually normal.

The only treatment is that which may be indicated to correct deformities.

Fragilitas Ossium (Osteogenesis Imperfecta, Idiopathic Osteopsathyrosis, Brittle Bones, Lobstein's Disease)

Fragilitas ossium is a rare congenital and often inherited skeletal disease in which the occurrence of multiple fractures is rendered inevitable by extreme fragility of the bones. Fractures may be evident in the skeleton of the newborn infant. In roentgenograms the bones often show a generalized thinning of the cortex (Fig. 44). The fractures are usually subperiosteal.

Etiology.—The cause of the excessive bone fragility is not known. It has been ascribed by some observers to an endocrine disturbance. Abnormal numerical or functional characteristics of the osteoblasts have been described, as well as other disturbances leading to an alteration of the process of ossification of the developing bone.

Clinical Picture.—Broad lines may be drawn clinically between certain types of this disease. There is a severe form, to which the term *osteogenesis imperfecta* is restricted by some clinicians, in which the disease is obvious at birth from the occurrence of multiple fractures and definite shortening of the extremities as compared with the trunk. In these infants the prognosis for survival is poor. A less severe form of the disease, to which the term *idiopathic osteopsathyrosis* is sometimes applied, is characterized by the occurrence of fractures only in early or late childhood. It is probable that a third group of cases, patients who show perhaps two or three successive fractures after episodes of only moderate trauma, represent a milder form of the disease.

In many of the patients with fragilitas ossium a very definite China blue coloration of the sclerae will be noted. This color has been attributed to a decreased opacity of the sclerae which permits the pigmentation of the deeper coats to show through. The combination of bone fragility and blue sclerae is an inherited dominant characteristic. Many of these patients also show hypermobility of the joints and deafness, and all are of short stature.

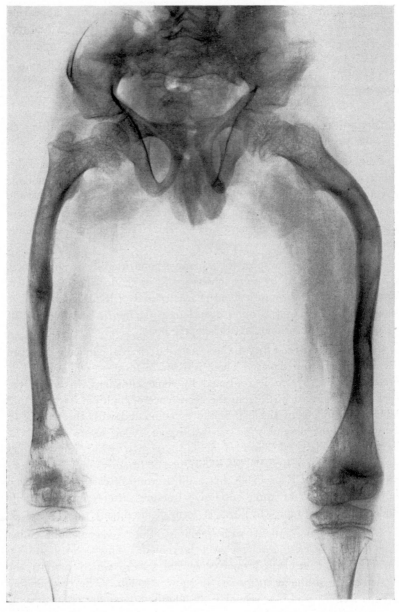

Fig. 44.—Roentgenogram showing osteogenesis imperfecta or fragile bones in a boy ten years of age. Note the distortion of femurs and pelvis with irregular calcification and thinning of the cortices. The right femur has been fractured twice and the left four times. This type of pelvis is called heart-shaped.

Treatment and Prognosis.—Since the underlying etiology is unknown, treatment is empirical and, in general, unsatisfactory. Reduction and immobilization after fracture are carried out as usual. Prophylactic measures to reduce the likelihood of trauma are indicated so far as practicable. It seems advisable to place these patients upon a diet rich in calcium, phosphorus, and vitamins and to give them an abundance of heliotherapy. Thymus extracts have been thought by some observers to be of benefit. Various hormones have been used without success.

The prognosis for union of these fractures is excellent. It is a matter of clinical experience that the fragility of the bone does not entail a loss of its capacity to unite after fracture; however, union frequently is slow. On the other hand, union may be accomplished by exuberant callus formation. With repeated fractures of various bones, it is not surprising that extensive deformities may ultimately develop. In the more severe cases deformities also result from bending of the shafts of the bones because of their plasticity. After the age of puberty is passed, the prognosis for disappearance of the abnormal fragility is good.

Osteosclerosis

Under this term may be grouped a number of interesting but rare and little known skeletal diseases characterized by an abnormal increase in calcium content of the bone. This increase of calcium gives to the affected bones a characteristic dense roentgenographic appearance, in which the cortex is greatly thickened and the medullary canal may be obliterated. The bone changes do not as a rule cause symptoms and are often discovered as an incidental finding on roentgen examination. The etiology of these diseases is quite unknown although the sporadic association of various factors in individual cases has led to a variety of hypotheses. These affections are sometimes hereditary or familial. Excessive amounts of fluorine in drinking water may cause bone changes of this type. Symptomatic treatment is occasionally indicated.

OSTEOPETROSIS (ALBERS-SCHÖNBERG DISEASE, MARBLE BONES)

The areas of increased bone density in this disease are widespread, often including pelvis, vertebrae, skull, and extremities. The affected bones show thickening of the cortex and narrowing or loss of the normal medullary canal, with fibrosis of the bone marrow. Transverse pathologic fractures may occur; they ordinarily heal without incident. Hydrocephalus, blindness, enlargement of spleen and liver, and secondary anemia may be associated.

OSTEOPOIKILOSIS (OSTEOPATHIA CONDENSANS DISSEMINATA, SPOTTED BONES)

Under this term have been described cases in which the areas of condensation are small and scattered, giving to the affected bones a spotted appearance in roentgenograms. The condensed areas consist of thickened trabeculae in the spongiosa. The metaphyseal and epiphyseal regions are most often involved. The roentgenographic picture of osteopoikilosis may be confused with the demineralization and spotted appearance of Sudeck's atrophy. Symptoms are slight or absent, and discovery of the lesions may be entirely fortuitous.

MELORHEOSTOSIS

As its name implies, this disease is a "flowing" hyperostosis of the bones of one extremity. It is slightly more common in males than females and begins in childhood, although it may be found at any age. It is characterized roentgenographically by an increased density and enlargement of the cortical bone which is limited to a single side of the bones. In advanced cases there may be associated periarticular deposits of calcium, which may cause pain and stiffness of the joints. The condition is quite rare, only approximately forty cases having been reported in the literature prior to 1949.

Myositis Ossificans Progressiva

While not primarily a disease of the skeleton, myositis ossificans progressiva is conveniently considered here because in its advanced stage it is characterized by a transformation of muscles and fasciae into immobile structures of bony consistency. The disease is rare and its etiology is unknown. An interesting hypothesis of the pathogenesis is that the mesenchymal cells do not possess the normal property of tissue differentiation, and hence progress ultimately to widespread development of bone. It is four times as common in the male as in the female.

Clinical Picture.—The disease begins in childhood. Malalignment of the great toes is frequently an associated finding. As a rule the muscles of the neck or back are first involved by the process of calcification, and although there may be remissions, one group of muscles after another gradually becomes stiffened. Ultimately the patient becomes bedridden, and as a rule death ensues from intercurrent infection.

Diagnosis and Treatment.—The diagnosis presents difficulty only in the early stage of the disease, when muscle biopsy may be helpful. At the present time no effective treatment is known.

CHAPTER V

AFFECTIONS OF ADULT BONE

Osteitis Deformans

Osteitis deformans was first described by Sir James Paget in 1876 and is often called *Paget's disease*. It is a chronic skeletal disease of middle and late life, beginning insidiously and characterized by progressive structural changes and typical deformities occurring in the long bones, spine, pelvis, and cranium.

Etiology.—The causative agent is unknown. Attempts to establish heredity or infection as the etiologic factor have failed through lack of proof. An endocrine basis has been suspected, and some observers believe that hypersecretion of the parathyroid glands may play a part. The incidence is equal in men and women.

Pathology.—The outstanding skeletal changes are a gradually developing thickening and bowing of the shafts of the long bones, particularly the tibias and the femurs, and a generalized thickening of the entire cranium (Fig. 45). Frequently, osteitis deformans affects only a single bone. In the early stages the bones lose much of their ability to withstand normal stresses, and an increase in their degree of curvature results. In the spine, which is very frequently involved, there is often a collapse of one or more of the vertebral bodies, which results in a kyphosis. In later stages more bony matrix is laid down, which slowly calcifies, producing finally a thick, hard osseous structure. The surface of the involved long bones is of characteristic unevenness and is furrowed by the periosteal vessels. Section discloses a thickened cortical layer which has lost its dense character and sharp outline and encroaches upon the marrow cavity. The marrow cavity itself may be entirely filled with spongy tissue and may contain small scattered cystic areas filled with gelatinous material. Microscopically the bone marrow may be largely replaced by a vascular fibrous tissue, in which irregular areas of osteoid tissue of abnormal and mosaic appearance are present. The serum alkaline phosphatase may be greatly increased, particularly in early stages of the disease and in patients with multiple bone involvement. The serum calcium and phosphorus are usually within normal limits.

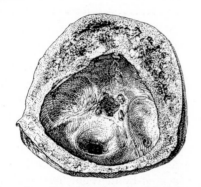

Fig. 45.—Horizontal section of skull in osteitis deformans, showing extreme thickening and other changes. (From clinical material of Dr. George W. Wagoner.)

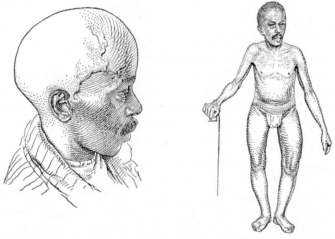

Fig. 46.—Osteitis deformans. Note massive cranium with enlargement of superficial veins, bowing of the lower extremities, and decreased height. (From clinical material of Dr. George W. Wagoner.)

Clinical Picture.—The patient suffering from osteitis deformans in its moderately advanced stage presents a characteristic clinical appearance (Fig. 46). The head appears massive and too large for the body, while the face itself is relatively small. The head may be drooped forward, and a long dorsal kyphosis may be present. The chest is likely to be barrel-shaped, the lumbar spine flexed, and the legs bowed outward and forward. This posture gives to the arms an exaggerated length, which has been compared to that of an anthropoid ape. There are no mental changes other than those of advancing age. Clinical diagnosis in well-established cases presents little difficulty.

At the onset of the disease, however, the symptoms are not characteristic. In many cases the findings are incidental to an examination for complaints unrelated to the bony framework. The patient may complain of chronic aching or discomfort in the legs, simulating chronic arthritic pains, may be affected with stiffness or clumsiness, may suffer chiefly from backache, or may simply have noticed that he is becoming bowlegged, that his back is stooped, or that his head is becoming larger as evidenced by the tight fit of his hat.

Roentgenographic Picture.—Roentgenograms are of diagnostic value, as the changes of osteitis deformans are characteristic. The contour of the bone is altered by an increase of its normal curvature. The cortex is enlarged sometimes to as much as four or five times its normal thickness and presents a blurred, fluffy appearance, the medulla is narrowed, and there is a loss of the normal definitive line between cortex and medulla. In all cases of suspected osteitis deformans, roentgenograms of the skull should be made, since its appearance is pathognomonic. The bones of the cranium are greatly thickened, with obliteration of the sutures and vascular channels, indistinct outlines, and uneven density which produce a cotton-wool appearance.

Diagnosis.—The characteristic deformities and roentgenographic changes of osteitis deformans are usually adequate to insure its recognition. In the differential diagnosis, syphilis, hyperparathyroidism, metastasis from carcinoma of the prostate, and osteomalacia must usually be considered. Diagnosis of the localized form of osteitis deformans, in which only a single bone is involved, sometimes presents difficulty. In such cases biopsy is occasionally desirable in order to exclude primary tumor, metastatic tumor, or the sclerosing osteitis of Garré.

Treatment and Prognosis.—At the present time the treatment of osteitis deformans is of symptomatic type. Salicylates and barbiturates are useful for the relief of pain. In the more active cases braces may be indicated for the prevention of deformity, and very occasionally a deformity which has already become established should be corrected by osteotomy or a similar operative procedure.

The prognosis for length of life is good. Pathologic fracture is the most common complication. It occurs most often in the femur. There is no prolongation of the healing time except in late stages of the disease, and the treatment is that of the uncomplicated fracture. A more serious complication, occurring in from 2 to 15 per cent of the series of reported cases, is the development of malignancy. The commonest type is osteogenic sarcoma. Most of the patients who develop this die within two years of diagnosis. Compression of the spinal cord by the thickened vertebrae is a rare complication.

Hyperparathyroidism (Generalized Osteitis Fibrosa Cystica, Von Recklinghausen's Disease of Bone)

It has been customary in the past to include under the designation osteitis fibrosa cystica two fairly common forms of skeletal disease which are characterized by cyst formation within bone. These two types comprise a local and a generalized form. *Localized osteitis fibrosa cystica* is typified by the solitary bone cyst which occurs in childhood and is not accompanied by demonstrable changes in blood chemistry or endocrine organs. This entity is further considered in Chapter XV under the subject of bone tumors, to which its roentgenographic characteristics give it a close relationship. The skeletal changes of *generalized osteitis fibrosa cystica* are commonly associated with a disorder of the parathyroid glands and a hypersecretion of parathormone. For this disease entity the term *hyperparathyroidism* is therefore preferable to the older, less informative designations.

Etiology.—The connection between hyperparathyroidism and skeletal changes was first brought out by the repeated finding, at postmortem examination, of parathyroid tumors associated with fibrocystic skeletal changes. Such changes can be produced in animals by the repeated injection of parathormone. The parathyroid lesion is of hyperplastic or adenomatous type. It is probably not primary but may correspond to the thyroid hyperplasia of toxic goiter; in some cases it seems to be definitely secondary to chronic renal disease. It occurs more often in men than women and at any age.

Blood Chemistry.—The serum calcium is consistently elevated, the serum phosphorus decreased, and the blood phosphatase increased. The excretion of calcium in the urine is also increased.

Pathology.—The essential feature of the bone changes is a gradual decalcification and consequent conversion of bone into connective tissue. Macroscopically this tissue presents a picture of disordered arrangement with numerous areas of softening and of hemorrhage. Cysts of irregular size and distribution often occur as the result of local degenerative changes; such cysts may have fibrous walls and may contain a grumous, serosanguineous fluid. Bone destruction is manifested microscopically by thin and disappearing lamellae, about which may be grouped numerous osteoclasts; in some places the appearance may be such as to suggest benign giant cell tumor. Other areas may show new bone formation with abundant osteoid tissue, immature bone cells, and osteoblasts. The gradual decalcification of cortical bone results in a loss of strength which may lead to curvature, compression, or spontaneous fracture.

Secondary changes in the kidneys are sometimes marked. The increased urinary excretion of calcium and phosphorus not infrequently leads to the formation of renal calculi. In other cases chronic nephritis and renal insufficiency are said to result from the precipitation of calcium phosphate within the parenchyma of the kidney.

Clinical Picture.—The symptoms are extremely diverse, depending upon the site of major involvement in the individual case, and a number of more or less well-defined clinical types have been described. General lassitude and muscular hypotonia due directly to the hypercalcemia may be the presenting symptoms. Gastrointestinal complaints are common. Skeletal involvement may be evidenced first by deep-seated pain and tenderness, the local swelling of an area of bone expansion, or the disability of a spontaneous fracture. Cases in late middle life, ushered in by backache and progressive kyphosis, form a major group. Deformity of bones other than the vertebrae is usually a late manifestation. In some cases of hyperparathyroidism, particularly those in which renal calculi cause the presenting complaint, skeletal symptoms and bone changes in the roentgenograms may be entirely absent.

Roentgenographic Picture.—The fundamental process of demineralization causes a generalized decrease in roentgenographic density, which may be complicated by the secondary changes of deformity, bone cysts, fractures, and benign giant cell tumors. In addition to the generalized decalcification, roentgenograms of the spine may show cupping, wedging, and crushing of the vertebral bodies, as well as various degrees of kyphosis.

Differential Diagnosis.—The varied clinical picture of hyperparathyroidism leads to simulation of numerous other diseases. Skeletal types of hyperparathyroidism must be differentiated from senile osseous atrophy, osteomalacia, osteitis deformans, solitary cyst and solitary benign giant cell tumor, fragilitas ossium, polyostotic and monostotic fibrous dysplasia, cystic angiomas of bone, myasthenia gravis, multiple myeloma, and metastatic malignancy. The biochemical and roentgenographic examinations are usually of chief differential value.

Treatment.—The treatment of choice is parathyroidectomy. After excision of the proper amount of parathyroid tissue, marked improvement in both symptoms and general nutrition is to be expected, and usually regression of the bone changes also occurs. Irradiation of the parathyroid glands has not usually proved efficacious. Diets rich in calcium and phosphorus may cause clinical improvement but sometimes lead eventually to kidney complications. Benefit from a high vitamin diet is questionable. Orthopaedic treatment consists of appropriate measures, such as braces and splints, for the prevention of deformity. Support is especially indicated when the spine is involved. In some cases after parathyroidectomy has been performed and recalcification has occurred, corrective bone operations, such as osteotomy, may be indicated.

Polyostotic Fibrous Dysplasia (Albright's Syndrome)

Polyostotic fibrous dysplasia is a syndrome characterized by typically unilateral bone lesions. When the bone lesions are accompanied by unilateral pigmentation of the skin (café au lait spots) and, in females, by precocious puberty with or without early skeletal maturation, the disorder is called Albright's syndrome. Polyostotic fibrous dysplasia is more common in girls than in boys. It is seldom seen in infants but develops usually during the later years of the growth period; the lesions progress slowly or not at all after growth has ceased. The unilateral aspect of the disease, which is almost always present, suggests that its cause is an abnormality of embryonic development. For many years polyostotic fibrous dysplasia was not distinguished from hyperparathyroidism and other cystic diseases of bone.

Roentgenographically the lesions, which are static with little or no progression, consist of cystic, rarefied, and deforming changes in the bones, with thin cortices and frequent fractures. The fractures usually heal well with the exception of those of the upper third of the femur, which cause some of the most crippling features of the disease (Fig.

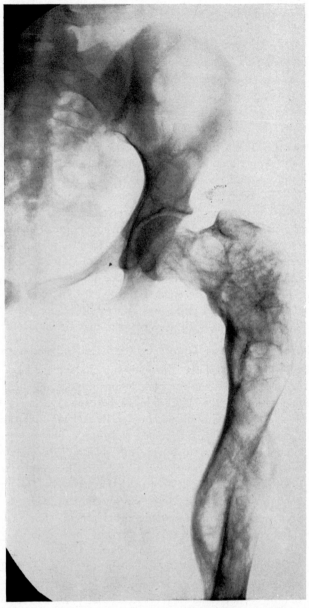

Fig. 47*A*.—Roentgenogram showing polyostotic fibrous dysplasia. Note the extensive cystic changes in pelvis and femur, thickening and distortion of the upper end of the femur, and malunited fracture of the femoral shaft.

47*A*). The unilateral bone lesions tend to be segmental, leaving normal bone adjacent to the involved areas.

Typically, the cystic bone defect (hypo-ostosis) and the new bone formation (hyperostosis) are seen together. Significantly, the growing epiphyses are not involved. An important characteristic is increased density of the bones of the base of the skull, suggested by Thannhauser as a possible etiologic factor because of their relationship to the pituitary gland.

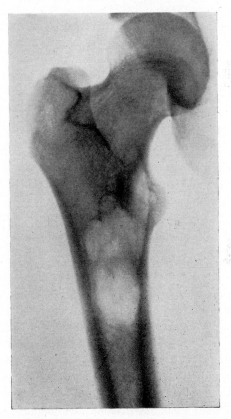

Fig. 47*B*.—Roentgenogram showing monostotic fibrous dysplasia of femur. Note the multiloculated cystic area extending from above the lesser trochanter down into the shaft.

The blood chemistry findings are normal except after a major fracture or in the presence of extensive skeletal involvement, when the alkaline phosphatase may be elevated. This, along with the unilateral and segmental nature of the syndrome, differentiates it from generalized bone diseases such as hyperparathyroidism and osteomalacia.

The unilateral skin pigmentation when present has a typically irregular, jagged contour which is in contrast with the smoothly outlined café au lait spots of neurofibromatosis. The static nature of the disorder distinguishes it from the lipoid granulomas, although some observers have been impressed by the lipoid-containing foam cells sometimes found.

Histologically the bones show proliferation of spindle cells, fibroblasts, osteoblasts, osteoclasts, and lymphocytes, with areas of cartilage, newly formed osteoid, and new bone. Collagen fibers associated with the spindle and stellate cells make up the bulk of the tissue. The spongiosa and marrow of the bone are replaced by fibrous tissue which may be highly vascular. Grossly the tissue of the early lesion is gray-white and soft; when more mature it is yellow and firm.

Treatment.—The fractures and deformities often need orthopaedic treatment, especially the bowing and pseudarthrosis of the upper femur. The latter may require osteotomy and grafting. There is no treatment for the underyling disease.

Monostotic Fibrous Dysplasia

This condition, described as an entity in the past decade, is characterized by a single isolated cystic bone lesion (Fig. 47*B*) and has no known relationship to Albright's syndrome. It is not associated with other anomalies or defects. It apparently represents a local defect in bone formation, the nature of which is unknown. About half of the reported lesions have involved the ribs (possibly because of the frequency of routine chest roentgenograms), although lesions have been reported in many other bones, long and flat, membranous and enchondral. Notably, the bones of the hands and feet seem to escape.

Monostotic fibrous dysplasia may be asymptomatic or may present itself by local swelling, pain, or tenderness. It is neither progressive nor destructive. Grossly the lesion is a symmetrical fusiform cystic enlargement, sometimes similar to that of a benign bone cyst. Histologically there is a typical pattern of vascular connective tissue, arranged in bundles and crossed by fine trabeculae of bone, apparently formed by connective tissue metaplasia. The connective tissue bundles have raised the question of a possible relationship to neurofibromatosis.

Treatment.—Biopsy is indicated when the diagnosis is in doubt, at which time the lesion may be curetted and filled with bone chips, as in the treatment of a bone cyst.

Osteomalacia

Under the term *osteomalacia* there have been described in the past a variety of clinical syndromes with the common characteristic of progressive softening of the skeleton due to decalcification, followed by the development of deformity. It is likely that many of these cases would on further study be found to represent atypical varieties of better known diseases; there is considerable evidence, for instance, that some of these cases should be ascribed to hyperparathyroidism. On the other hand, one group of such cases possesses features which are sufficiently uniform and characteristic to define at the present time a clinical entity, for which the designation of *idiopathic osteomalacia* has been recommended.

Occasionally there are observed in osteomalacic bones transverse bands of rarefaction called *pseudofractures* or *Looser's transformation zones.* Pseudofractures are to be distinguished from fatigue or march fractures (see p. 485). Typical fatigue fractures usually occur in normal bones upon excessive activity, whereas pseudofractures may develop in a patient confined to bed. When multiple pseudofractures, which are often bilaterally symmetrical, are associated with osteomalacia, the condition is sometimes called milkman's syndrome.

Idiopathic Osteomalacia

Incidence.—Idiopathic osteomalacia is seen infrequently in the English-speaking races but is said to be of common occurrence among the inhabitants of Central Europe and of the Far East. Typically it appears in multiparas who have passed through their pregnancies under unfavorable hygienic and nutritive conditions; yet it may occur also in children.

Etiology.—The cause of idiopathic osteomalacia is unknown. There is much evidence for the belief that it is an adult form of rickets caused by a deficiency of vitamin D. An endocrine imbalance has been postulated but is unproved.

Pathology.—The decalcification may become so extreme that the bone is grossly soft and flexible and is cut easily with a knife. The cortex is thinned, the internal structure is greatly altered, and microscopically much of the bone is replaced by osteoid tissue. Characteristic gross deformities of the skeleton are the "heart-shaped pelvis" from pressure at the acetabula, the shortened or "telescoped spine," and marked bowing of the tibias and femurs.

Clinical Picture.—The patient complains of shooting pains referred to the pelvis, back, or hips, and on examination shows tenderness in these regions. Severe progressive muscular weakness may be present. The softened spine, pelvis, and long bones develop deformities from muscular and gravitational stresses, and pathologic fractures are common. The roentgenograms demonstrate a striking loss of calcium.

Diagnosis.—In differential diagnosis hyperparathyroidism and occasionally fragilitas ossium, metastatic carcinoma, multiple myeloma, and senile osteoporosis must be considered.

Treatment.—Exhaustive diagnostic studies should be carried out in an effort to find the causative factor, and associated disorders, such as foci of infection, should be treated. Vitamin D concentrate should be given in large doses. A radical change in environment and diet may prove helpful, and an abundance of nutritious foods, calcium, fresh air, and sunshine should be assured. Protective measures to forestall deformity should be combined with careful exercise or physical therapy adequate to counteract the atrophy of disuse.

Prognosis.—Most cases pass through a chronic progressive course lasting for many years. Some are rapidly fatal. However, a few cures have been described.

Posttraumatic Painful Osteoporosis

(Sudeck's Atrophy, Posttraumatic or Reflex Sympathetic Dystrophy)

Occasionally an injury of an extremity or of a peripheral nerve is followed by prolonged local pain, vasomotor instability, trophic changes in the soft tissues, and bone atrophy. The trauma may be of quite minor nature, and the disturbance of function is always greater than that which would be expected from the injury alone. This condition, termed posttraumatic painful osteoporosis and first described as an

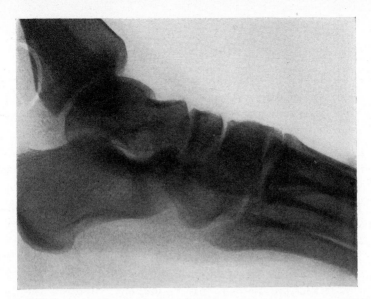

Fig. 48A.—Lateral roentgenogram of normal left foot of girl sixteen years of age with tuberculosis of twelfth dorsal vertebra. There were a rapidly developing compression of the vertebral body, spastic paraplegia, and intense pain in the left foot and leg for several weeks prior to roentgenogram. Roentgenogram shows normal calcification of all body structures.

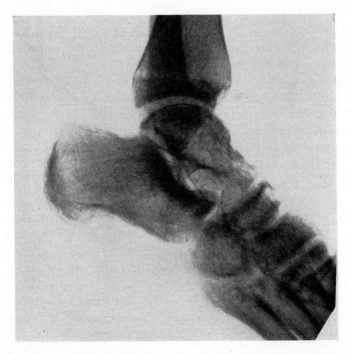

Fig. 48B.—Lateral roentgenogram of left foot of same patient as in Fig. 48A, three months later, during which time pain in foot and leg had persisted. Note spotty irregular decalcification with many small cystic areas in lower tibia, tarsal bones, and proximal end of metatarsals. This is characteristic of Sudeck's atrophy.

entity by Sudeck in 1900, must be distinguished carefully from simple disuse atrophy of bone with or without malingering, and from causalgia due to a lesion of a peripheral nerve. The bone atrophy may have an irregular and spotted appearance (Fig. 48B).

Etiology.—The pathogenesis is not well understood. Much of the evidence suggests that disturbed function of the sympathetic nerve supply is the major factor.

Treatment and Prognosis.—Although the period of disability is always long, most patients recover spontaneously or with simple treatment such as immobilization followed by physical therapy and active use of the extremity. In the more intractable cases, sympatholytic drugs, repeated procaine block of the sympathetic ganglia, ganglionectomy, or periarterial sympathectomy may be indicated. Rarely a permanent deformity and disability result despite treatment.

Secondary Hypertrophic Pulmonary Osteoarthropathy (Bamberger-Marie Disease)

This condition, called also *pulmonary osteoarthropathy of Marie* and evidenced clinically by the common clubbed fingers, is always secondary to a chronic wasting disease. Pulmonary tuberculosis, empyema, lung abscess, bronchiectasis, and cardiac disease are the common causes; intrathoracic tumors and long-standing infections elsewhere in the body are occasionally responsible. The mechanism by which these diseases produce the bone changes is not understood but is probably of either circulatory or toxic nature. The characteristic pathologic process is a thickening of both soft tissues and bone; the bony proliferation is brought about by a very chronic ossifying periostitis.

Clinical Picture.—The first clinical sign is a generalized, symmetrical, and painless enlargement of the distal portion of the fingers, due to thickening of the soft tissues (Fig. 49). The nails become slightly cyanotic. They may show thickening, ridges, and an increased convexity. Analogous changes may appear in the toes and toenails. Later the hands and feet, and in extreme cases even the lower portion of the forearms and legs, may be similarly involved. Wrists and ankles also may become swollen, and the joints may contain increased fluid. Rarely is the spine affected. The roentgenograms show proliferative bony changes, sometimes with spurring, and in severe cases the shafts of the bones of forearm and leg may be obviously thickened from sub-periosteal formation of new bone.

Treatment.—The primary visceral disease must be investigated and treated. If this is cured promptly, the clubbing may regress. In the majority of cases, however, the bone lesions when once established either remain unchanged or show a very gradual progression.

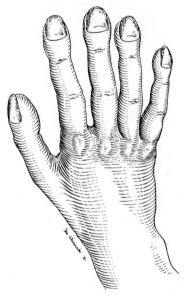

Fig. 49.—Secondary hypertrophic pulmonary osteoarthropathy. Note the club-shaped appearance of the ends of the fingers and thumb with a broadening of the nails.

Acromegaly

The bone changes of acromegaly are believed to represent the reaction of the adult skeleton to hyperactivity of the anterior lobe of the pituitary gland. Acromegaly in the adult thus corresponds in etiology to *gigantism* in the youth.

Clinical Picture.—The characteristic changes of acromegaly usually appear first in early or middle adult life and are slowly progressive. They include a gradual enlargement of the bones of the skull, jaw, spine, hands, and feet, and an associated involvement of the soft tissues.

The lower jaw protrudes. The orbital and zygomatic arches are prominent, and the nose, ears, lower lip, and tongue are large. Kyphosis of the thoracic spine is commonly present, the hands and feet become massive, and the fingers and toes may be strikingly thickened (Fig. 50).

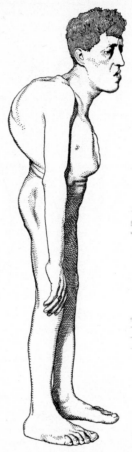

Fig. 50.—Acromegaly. Note prominence of supra-orbital areas, protuberance of jaw, kyphosis, and enlargement of hands and feet. (From clinical material of Dr. Walter E. Dandy.)

The costo-chondral junctions become enlarged, forming the acromegalic rosary, and with advancing ossification the ribs lengthen and the chest thickens. There may be marked rarefaction of the bones due to nitrogen deficiency or insufficient intake of calcium and phosphorus. The thyroid gland may be enlarged. The urinary excretion of calcium may be doubled.

Diagnosis and Treatment.—The typical deformities are often associated with other evidences of endocrine disorder and with progressive symptoms, such as disturbances of vision, which are secondary results of the local intracranial changes. These associated symptoms are of diagnostic value, as are roentgenograms of the sella turcica. Myxedema, osteitis deformans, and leontiasis ossea are to be excluded. Treatment by surgery, irradiation, or a combination of the two is the prerogative of the neurologic surgeon. The administration of thyroid and sex hormones may be followed by improvement.

Leontiasis Ossea

Leontiasis ossea is a rare bone disease which causes a massive thickening of the osseous structures of the face and cranium. It makes its appearance in childhood or adolescence and is slowly progressive. Its cause is obscure. Some observers believe it to be related to osteitis deformans. Current treatment is symptomatic and unsatisfactory.

Pathologically, leontiasis ossea may be divided into two types. The *periostitis* type is the result of a chronic inflammatory process in the periosteum, possibly of infectious origin, starting usually about the nose or paranasal sinuses, spreading slowly to involve other bones of the skull, and causing an enormous overgrowth of subperiosteal bone. No means of arresting the process is known, and as the disease advances, nasal obstruction, lachrymal disorders, exophthalmos, and blindness may develop. The disease is usually fatal in comparatively early life as a result of cerebral complications.

The *osteitis fibrosa* type of leontiasis ossea usually follows an episode of local trauma and pursues a slowly progressive course. An overgrowth of connective tissue in the interior of the affected bone or bones is followed by excessive new bone formation, resulting in extreme osseous thickening and in a marked increase of bone density.

CHAPTER VI

INFECTIONS OF BONE (EXCLUSIVE OF TUBERCULOSIS)

Acute inflammatory reactions in bone involve as a rule the entire structure. Chronic inflammatory reactions may be localized in one part of the bone. Both are commonly designated by the term *osteomyelitis*. Under infections of bone, exclusive of tuberculosis, are grouped those forms of osteomyelitis which are caused (1) by the pyogenic organisms *(Staphylococcus, Streptococcus, colon bacillus, typhoid bacillus, Pneumococcus, Clostridium welchii, and Gonococcus)*, (2) by the fungi *(Actinomyces bovis, Blastomyces, Sporotrichum, and Coccidioides immitis)*, (3) by the parasite *Echinococcus granulosus*, and (4) by the *Spirocheta pallida*.

Pyogenic Osteomyelitis

The term pyogenic osteomyelitis is used to include all infections of bone which are caused by pyogenic organisms.

Incidence.—Pyogenic osteomyelitis is most common in children between one and twelve years of age, the period during which bone growth is most active. It is four times as common in boys as in girls. The lower extremities are much more often affected than the upper extremities. The bones most commonly involved, in their order of frequency, are the tibia, femur, humerus, and radius. The spine, pelvis, and scapula are less frequently affected. Osteomyelitis is more common in rural than in urban areas. The incidence of hematogenous osteomyelitis has declined sharply following the advent of chemotherapy and antibiotics for the control of primary pyogenic infections.

Etiology.—In at least 75 per cent of the cases the infecting organism is the *Staphylococcus aureus. Streptococcus hemolyticus* is the next most common organism. There is no doubt that trauma sometimes determines the site of infection. This is true in from 25 to 33⅓ per cent of the cases. It is known definitely that fevers and debilitating diseases predispose bone toward infection, as do states of chronic fatigue and of malnutrition.

Most of these infections are bloodborne from a distant focus, often located in the skin and very commonly consisting of a furuncle or an infected abrasion. The mouth and nasopharynx may also be portals of entry. The bacteria may be carried by the lymphatic vessels. Infection sometimes enters the bone by direct spread from a nearby infected area or by direct introduction of surface organisms into a compound wound.

Pathology.—Osteomyelitis usually starts in the metaphysis, or cancellous end of the diaphysis. The circulation in this region is relatively sluggish, and here are found end arteries in which the bacteria, especially staphylococci which characteristically form clumps, are thought to lodge, causing a septic infarction. The organisms may be transported to this point through the nutrient arteries or through the perforating periosteal vessels. The site of localization, as has been mentioned, is often influenced by trauma. Injury causes hemorrhage and cell destruction, which furnish an ideal culture medium for the bacteria.

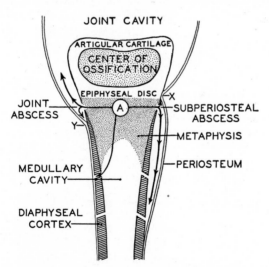

Fig. 51.—Diagram showing direction of possible spread of infection from focus *A* in metaphysis. *X* and *Y* mark the junction of synovial membrane and periosteum in subperiosteal abscess and joint abscess respectively. (After Hart.)

There is uncertainty regarding the method by which the infection spreads through the bone from the point of original involvement (Fig. 51). One hypothesis is that the organisms pass from the cancellous bone into the periosteum, form subperiosteal abscesses, and then by way of minute vascular channels enter the medulla and spread through its cavity. A second hypothesis is that the organisms go directly into the medullary cavity from the metaphysis, then travel outward through the vascular channels to the periosteum, there to form subperiosteal abscesses. In either case the infection spreads with great rapidity.

In children the epiphyseal cartilage plate acts as a barrier to the infection, preventing or delaying extension into the epiphyseal end of the bone and thence into the joint. When the metaphyseal area is intracapsular, however, infection may spread quickly into the joint. Often the joints develop a secondary synovitis before they become actually infected.

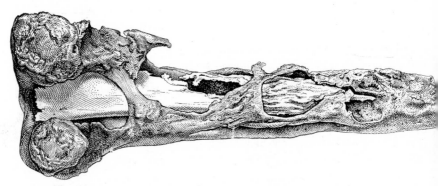

Fig. 52.—Chronic osteomyelitis of femur, showing large sequestrum and surrounding involucrum. Drawing from museum specimen.

With the formation of pus beneath the periosteum, new bone is laid down on the entire inner surface of the periosteum, forming an *involucrum*. In this new bone numerous openings or *cloacae* for the discharge of pus and bone débris appear. Certain areas of bone may become ischemic from the stripping up of periosteum and the thrombosis of cortical capillaries. These areas become necrotic and separate, forming *sequestra* (Fig. 52). Small bits of this necrotic bone are extruded through the involucral cloacae into sinuses draining upon the skin surface. It is impossible, however, for the larger sequestra to be extruded, and they may have to be removed surgically. The sequestra may become surrounded by granulation tissue and may gradually be disintegrated and absorbed by the action of proteolytic ferments liberated in the purulent exudate.

In extensive osteomyelitic involvement of the shaft of a long bone pathologic fracture occasionally occurs. This is particularly likely to happen if strain is placed upon the bone before sufficiently strong involucrum has restored the bony continuity and stability.

All pyogenic osteomyelitis is not accompanied by the formation of sequestra. The resistance of the body, with or without the aid of chemotherapy and antibiotics, may early overcome the infection, which then completely subsides. Osteomyelitis in infancy rarely results in gross sequestration.

Phemister has classified osteomyelitis into acute and chronic forms of diffuse and of localized processes. There is no hard and fast rule for differentiation of the various types, since they may merge gradually one into another. The acute diffuse form is most frequently encountered. It produces extensive pathologic changes not only in the affected bone but also in distant bones and viscera by metastatic infectious foci.

Clinical Picture.—Acute osteomyelitis usually starts with malaise, general weakness, and aching, followed by an elevation of body temperature and pain in the affected region. In the early stages, if the infectious process is within the bone and does not come to the surface, there may be no sharply localized tenderness. Usually, however, pain is later referred constantly to one area. Nearly always a septicemia is associated with acute osteomyelitis, and the patient is extremely ill. He is generally apprehensive. A leucocytosis of from 15,000 to 40,000 cells, depending upon the severity of the infection, may be present. Ordinarily there is protective muscle spasm and flexion of the joint nearest the disease focus. As the infection advances, there may be localization of the process, with swelling, redness, and acute tenderness about the infected area. At times, however, extensive infection of the shaft of a bone may be unaccompanied by evidence of localization. If the resistance of the body is sufficient to overcome the infection, the acute inflammatory symptoms will subside; if not, they will persist until pus is released by a surgical procedure or liberates itself spontaneously. Afterwards the fever gradually decreases, but even in the presence of adequate drainage the body temperature may not become entirely normal for as long as six weeks. The local signs of acute inflammation usually subside slowly after evacuation of the pus.

Often after the liberation of pus and subsidence of the acute symptoms, a chronically draining sinus or sinuses develop. Such a sinus is evidence of chronic osteomyelitis. The drainage will persist as long as dead bone and infected granulation tissue remain. Accumulation of pus from inadequate drainage may cause periodic exacerbations of septic symptoms. Prolonged disuse of the infected parts leads to muscle atrophy, and, if the joints are not properly splinted, contractures often develop. There may be at first no general symptoms, but, when purulent drainage has continued for a period of years, nephritis or amyloid disease may develop.

Roentgenographic Picture.—Evidence of bone changes is seldom visible in the roentgenograms in less than ten days from the time of onset. Roentgenographic changes are seen later in adults than in children, and several weeks may elapse before definite abnormality of the affected bone can be demonstrated. Often the first roentgenographic change is an area of haziness or of mottling in the metaphysis with new bone formation under the periosteum. This may be followed by destructive changes in the shaft and later by evidences of sequestration (Figs. 53A, 53B, and 54).

Differential Diagnosis.—Acute osteomyelitis in its earliest stages is sometimes confused with acute rheumatic fever. In acute rheumatic fever multiple joint involvement is more common than in osteomyelitis. Erysipelas and cellulitis about the joints are sometimes confusing, and rheumatoid arthritis must be considered. Pyogenic arthritis is always to be kept in mind and must be distinguished from acute osteomyelitis. Secondary synovitis of the neighboring joints, especially of the knee or hip, may make differentiation difficult. Pyogenic arthritis can usually be recognized by aspiration of the joint followed by smear and culture of the aspirate. Acute osteomyelitis may also be confused with acute anterior poliomyelitis, especially if it occurs at the time of an epidemic. In the diagnosis of subacute or chronic osteomyelitis, tuberculosis, syphilis and fungus infections must be considered.

Prognosis.—The course varies with the type and virulence of the organism, the resistance of the patient, and the response of the patient to antibiotics. When repeated positive blood cultures are obtained, the prognosis for survival is poor. The younger the individual, the greater the likelihood of fatality. The nearer the infection is to the hip or shoulder, the less favorable is the outlook. Even with thorough treatment of the original focus, exacerbations may occur subsequently, due to pocketing off of the infection. It is possible that in these areas of lowered resistance a second infection takes place years after the original inflammatory reaction has subsided. When there are

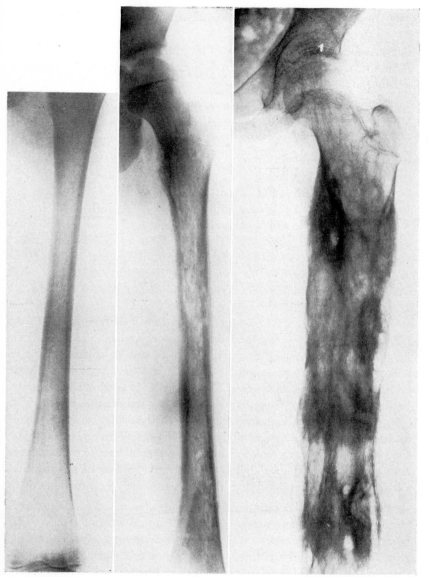

Fig. 53*A*. Fig. 53*B*. Fig. 54.

Fig. 53*A*.—Osteomyelitis of the femur in a boy nine years of age. This anteroposterior roentgenogram, taken three weeks after onset of acute infection of the bone, shows no definite abnormality.

Fig. 53*B*.—Osteomyelitis of the femur. Anteroposterior roentgenogram of patient in Fig. 53*A*, three weeks later. Note the irregular areas of absorption with fuzzy appearance of the bone, elevation of the periosteum, and irregular calcification beneath portions of the periosteum.

Fif. 54.—Osteomyelitis of the femur. Anteroposterior roentgenogram of same patient, three and one-half years later. Note the tremendous thickening of the shaft of the femur due to massive involucrum formation, and the irregular areas of bone absorption and bone proliferation. The light areas of punched-out appearance mark the sites of draining sinuses.

multiple foci the prognosis is not so favorable as when there is a single focus. In chronic cases of long standing the complications of nephritis and amyloid disease are often fatal.

Treatment.—The type of treatment depends upon the type of infecting organism and whether the infectious process is acute or chronic.

1. *In the acute stage,* the patient is suffering not only from a local bone infection but also from a blood stream infection with severe general reaction. He therefore requires constant nursing care and complete rest both of the affected part and of the whole body. Repeated small transfusions are of the greatest benefit. A high fluid intake must be maintained, with intravenous injections of 5 per cent glucose or isotonic saline if necessary. The importance of adequate systemic chemotherapy with antibiotics, preferably penicillin and sulfadiazine, or with both of these agents, cannot be overestimated, as in every series of cases recently reported the mortality rate has been markedly lower than before these drugs were available. The dosage is subject to wide variation in the individual case and must be regulated according to the clinical response and the laboratory findings. If the infecting organism is resistant to penicillin as shown by clinical response and laboratory tests, other antibiotics such as aureomycin, terramycin, and streptomycin should be tried. The patient's general condition must be followed closely by means of frequent determinations of blood levels of the antibiotic, cell counts, Schilling index, hemoglobin, and urinary findings, and repeated blood cultures should be made. In severe staphylococcic infections with toxemia evidenced by a preponderance of immature leucocytes in the blood, which is not responding to antibiotic therapy, the administration of staphylococcus antitoxin may be of great value.

With early intensive treatment of the patient's general condition, and antibiotic therapy, it is possible to delay surgical operation upon the infected bone and in many cases to avoid it altogether. At the onset of pain and tenderness the affected extremity should be put at rest by traction or splinting and hot moist dressings should be applied constantly. In some clinics ice bags are thought to be preferable to hot applications. After the local signs, of which the most useful is fluctuation, indicate that a subperiosteal abscess has formed, it should be aspirated of as much pus as can be obtained. This should be cultured. Into the abscess cavity a solution of penicillin or of one of the sulfonamides may be instilled. If there is a recurrence of the subperiosteal abscess, it is best to effect surgical drainage. Operation upon the bone itself is inadvisable in the early stage of the disease but later may become necessary. It should include drilling, lifting a small window in the cortex, or both. As the acute condition subsides, a cast must usually be applied to protect the weakened bone. The patient must be followed carefully during his convalescence.

2. *In the chronic stage,* the patient is no longer obviously ill, but has a local infection of low grade which may be manifested by persistent drainage from one or more cutaneous sinuses and by recurrent episodes of local pain, increased heat, and swelling. In these cases also a thorough course of treatment with an antibiotic or a sulfonamide or both agents is indicated; some patients may be cured by this measure alone. Transfusions are often helpful. A high caloric diet and supplementary multi-vitamin capsules should be given. Surgical removal of dead bone, or *sequestrectomy,* is indicated when the patient is in good general condition, the necrotic bone is roentgenographically well separated, and an adequate involucrum has been formed. In the absence of persistent diffuse infectious changes in the affected bone, individual sequestra are best removed through sinuses or small incisions. If roentgenograms show most of the bone to be still involved by chronic infection, however, the much more extensive surgical procedure of *saucerization* is necessary. It includes removal of all scar tissue, infected granulation tissue, sequestra, sclerotic bone, and overhanging bone edges and leaves a long flat depression in the bone with a grossly clean and freely bleeding surface. A sulfonamide or penicillin may be put into the wound, although this type of therapy is not advocated in some clinics. In most cases closure of the soft tissues is practicable, while in some it may be necessary to fill the wound with petrolatum gauze (the *Orr* method) ; in either case an ample cast is applied to rest the affected structures and protect the weakened bone. In the Orr method the cast and dressings should be changed only at long intervals when the odor becomes offensive or the cast softened. The wound exudate is believed to stimulate the formation of autogenous bacteriophage which increases the patient's chances of overcoming the infection. In some cases it is advisable to administer staphylococcus toxoid in an effort to increase staphylococcus antitoxin in the blood.

In the chronic stage it is often difficult to obliterate large cavities, especially when they occur at the lower end of the femur. Sometimes it is possible to close these cavities by removing completely the superficial layer of bone lining the cavity, together with all infected soft tissue, and allowing the remaining soft tissues to collapse into the cavity. If this proves unsuccessful, it may be necessary to carry out the "bone-filling" operation of transplanting muscle and fascia or fat into the cavity. Sometimes cancellous bone chips may be packed into the cavity after complete saucerization.

Rarely is amputation of an extremity necessary in osteomyelitis. However, there are a few adult patients in whom chronic infection over a long period of years has responded poorly to the usual treatment and has produced such serious kidney damage that amputation may prove a lifesaving measure.

Brodie's Abscess (Chronic Localized Osteomyelitis)

Brodie's abscess is a localized form of osteomyelitis caused usually by a staphylococcus of low virulence (Fig. 55). The infecting organisms are brought by the blood stream from a primary focus elsewhere and lodge in the bone just as in diffuse osteomyelitis, but remain localized in a single portion of the bone. The lesion may be secondary to a diffuse osteomyelitis and is then the result of attenuation of the organism. A thin wall of fibrous tissue and sclerotic bone forms around the abscess. The most common site is in the lower end of the tibia. These abscesses occur most often in older children and young adults, and affect males more frequently than females. Clinically the onset is gradual. The chief symptom is local pain, often worse at night, and usually there is slight tenderness over the site of the lesion. A slight increase in local heat and in body temperature and a feeling of general malaise may be present.

Diagnosis.—The history and clinical signs and the roentgenographic appearance of an area of decreased density surrounded by sclerotic bone provide the basis for diagnosis. Brodie's abscess is to be differentiated from osteogenic sarcoma, syphilitic periostitis, Garré's osteitis, osteoid-osteoma, eosinophilic granuloma, bone cyst, and monostotic fibrous dysplasia.

Treatment.—The treatment is similar to that of chronic osteomyelitis of more diffuse type and consists of operation and of local and systemic chemotherapy. The abscess should be thoroughly cleaned out or excised. A sulfonamide or penicillin may be placed in the wound, after which it is either closed or packed with petrolatum gauze and a cast is applied.

Chronic Diffuse Sclerosing Osteitis of Garré

Etiology.—The exact cause of chronic diffuse sclerosing osteitis is unknown but is thought to be an infection of low virulence. The disease occurs most often in late childhood, in boys more often than in girls, and usually in the shaft of a long bone, particularly the tibia or femur.

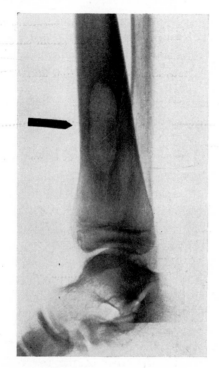

Fig. 55.—Lateral roentgenogram showing Brodie's abscess of the lower end of the tibia in a boy fourteen years of age. Note well-demarcated area of decreased density indicating the site of the abscess.

Pathology.—The cortex is greatly thickened by hyperplasia of both the periosteal and the endosteal surfaces. Roentgenographic examination shows the bone to be of increased density and of spindle-shaped contour. Microscopically an inflammatory reaction can be demonstrated in the medulla. There is no evidence, however, of actual suppuration.

Clinical Picture.—A dull ache is usually present in the region of the affected bone. In other cases the pain may be intense. It is usually worse at night. At times there is an elevation of local temperature with redness over the affected area. When the process is located near the surface, ulceration of the skin may take place.

Differential Diagnosis.—Garré's osteitis is to be differentiated from syphilitic periostitis, osteogenic sarcoma, Ewing's sarcoma, localized osteitis deformans, and osteoid-osteoma.

Treatment.—Conservative treatment alone is never satisfactory. Two operative procedures have proved of value: one is the drilling of holes through the dense cortical area, and the other is extensive excision of the thickened cortex with its periosteal and endosteal surfaces. These measures relieve the pain, presumably by releasing tension within the bone. Occasionally even after the cortex has been removed, however, the pathologic bone reforms and the pain returns.

Typhoid Infections of Bone

Osteomyelitis or periostitis caused by the typhoid bacillus is an occasional complication of typhoid fever. Typhoid infections of bone are now rare in this country.

Clinical Picture.—The bone involvement is a localized process which may occur with acute symptoms during the later stages of typhoid fever or may make its clinical appearance as a chronic low-grade inflammation a number of years after recovery from the systemic infection.

Typhoid osteitis of the vertebrae, called for brevity *typhoid spine,* characteristically affects two adjacent vertebrae at the lower dorsal or upper lumbar level. Its onset is marked by fever, pain, tenderness, and muscle spasm, and kyphosis or scoliosis may develop. The infectious process usually results in narrowing of the intervertebral space and fusion of the affected vertebral bodies. After *undulant fever* a metastatic infection of the vertebrae very similar to that of typhoid spine is occasionally seen.

Typhoid osteomyelitis of the bones of the extremities is usually a low-grade localized process similar in clinical and pathologic characteristics to a Brodie's abscess.

Treatment.—Typhoid spine is treated by immobilization of the back with plaster, followed by a brace. The functional result after spontaneous fusion of the involved vertebrae is usually very satisfactory. Typhoid abscess of a long bone may be treated by excision and closure;

the patient should also receive chloramphenicol. The prognosis of permanent cure is good.

Brucellosis (Undulant Fever, Malta Fever)

In brucellosis, involvement of bones and joints by the bacillus melitensis is not uncommon. Joint involvement appears to occur more often than osseous disease. Migratory arthralgia and transitory synovitis are frequently observed. Acute monarticular arthritis with swelling and reddening of the joint is rare. When the spine or the sacroiliac joint is infected, healing usually takes place with bony ankylosis. Skeletal complications usually occur in the subacute stage of the disease, weeks after the acute onset. Some investigators report most skeletal involvement in the spine, while others believe the ankle, hip, elbow, and sacroiliac joints to be the most frequent sites. Rarely is infection seen in long bones, where it may cause an osteitis, periostitis, or abscess formation similar to a Brodie's abscess. When a long bone is involved, multiple abscesses are also common, with perhaps less bone destruction and a greater tendency to repair than in staphylococcus osteomyelitis; however, some observers state that involvement of bone is most often in the nature of a localized process with abscess formation.

Diagnosis.—Although the correlation of clinical brucellosis with bone and joint changes supports the tentative diagnosis, a positive culture of the organism is necessary for absolute diagnosis. A special culture medium is required; routine media will not grow the organism. The agglutination reaction, when positive in a titer of 1:100 or higher, is an indication of infection or of recent or past exposure. Skin testing with brucellergin furnishes similar information.

Prognosis.—Although reports are few, the skeletal disease seems to be controlled in the great majority of cases by routine measures. Chronic draining sinuses are rarely, if ever, a complication of brucellosis. The outlook for healing is good.

Treatment.—Rest, splinting, and antibiotics are used. Streptomycin, with or without aureomycin or sulfadiazine, appears to be the most effective antibiotic in curing or controlling the disease.

Fungus Infections of Bone

Although osteomyelitis caused by fungi is uncommon, occasional cases of infection by the organism of actinomycosis, blastomycosis, sporotrichosis, or coccidioidomycosis are seen. Of these, actinomycosis is the most common; it is seen most often in the jaw, where it may involve primarily either soft tissue or bone to produce the so called "lumpy jaw." In approximately 2 per cent of all cases of actinomycosis the spine is involved. In blastomycosis of bone the mortality rate may be as high as 89 per cent.

Pathology.—Suppuration occurs through sinus tracts, and through these, in actinomycosis, the sulphur granules are extruded. Involvement of the vertebrae by actinomycosis is frequently secondary to actinomycosis of the gastrointestinal tract. When these fungus infections involve the spine, the anterior part of the vertebra is most often affected, just as in tuberculosis of the spine. Destruction is more characteristic than new bone formation and is usually very extensive. Large areas of soft tissue are involved, with resultant formation of numerous draining sinuses. In blastomycosis of bone the most frequent bone lesions occur in the vertebrae and skull, and it is very common to find associated abscesses in the skin and lungs; a positive intradermal test with blastomyces vaccine is helpful in diagnosis. Bone involvement due to sporotrichosis resembles in roentgenographic appearance that of multiple myeloma.

Treatment.—Surgical treatment consists of incision and, when practicable, extensive removal of the infected areas. Medical treatment includes the administration of large doses of potassium iodide. Iodides are specific for sporotrichosis. Penicillin and sulfadiazine are of great value in actinomycosis. In blastomycosis, desensitization with vaccine is indicated if an intradermal test shows the patient to be sensitive to the organism.

Coccidioidomycosis

Involvement of bone or joint by *Coccidioides immitis,* a moldlike organism which produces cutaneous, pulmonary, and generalized lesions, is occasionally seen. In this country it occurs most commonly in California. The primary benign infection may be followed by a malignant or systemic phase which has a mortality rate of 80 per cent. The bone and joint lesions, which occur in the systemic phase, are usually multiple. The joints become swollen, red, and painful. When the bones are affected, the lesions very closely resemble those of tuberculosis; the infectious process is similar to that of blastomycosis but involves the spine less often. Intradermal testing with coccidioidin and biopsy are of value in establishing the diagnosis.

Treatment.—Early resection or amputation may be followed by permanent cure.

Echinococcus Cyst

Occasionally cysts caused by the parasite *Echinococcus granulosus* are formed within bone. The process usually starts within the marrow cavity and extends outward to the cortex. Little pain is associated with the invasion until secondary infection takes place. When a joint is involved, it becomes swollen and painful. Pathologic fracture may be the first indication of the disease. Eosinophilia is present in 25 per cent of the cases. Hydatid fluid may be used for complement fixation, precipitation, and intradermal tests to aid in establishing the diagnosis. Statistics have shown that from 1 to 9 per cent of echinococcus infections involve bone and that the pelvic bones are affected most commonly.

Treatment.—Complete excision of the cyst is the treatment of choice.

Syphilis of Bone

Bone lesions may occur in both the congenital and the acquired forms of syphilis. Fifty per cent of all children with congenital syphilis show osseous lesions at some stage of the disease. The most common varieties of bone involvement are osteochondritis, periostitis, and osteoperiostitis.

1. Osteochondritis

Pathology.—In early infancy syphilitic infections may cause characteristic changes in the epiphyses. An irregular deposit of lime salts appears along the epiphyseal line. The cartilage cells are of abnormal appearance and multiply in a disorderly manner with the production of many immature forms. Areas of necrosis are present. If the disease is unchecked, it may cause suppuration and the development of frank syphilitic osteomyelitis. Occasionally the epiphysis separates from the shaft and extreme distortion results. The neighboring joint may exhibit a synovitis or even a destructive arthritis. The joints are practically always involved to some extent.

Clinical Picture.—The lesions of syphilitic osteochondritis are most often of symmetrical distribution and involve, in order of frequency, the lower end of the femur, the lower ends of the tibia and fibula, and the lower ends of the radius and ulna.

The joints become swollen, and muscle spasm may be present. There is always nonfluctuant swelling at the lower end of the diaphysis, with which pain and tenderness are associated, but no local or general febrile reaction is present. Often the infant appears to be partially paralyzed; this condition has been called *pseudoparalysis.*

Diagnosis.—Syphilitic osteochondritis is to be differentiated from rickets, tuberculosis, scurvy, infantile paralysis, and cerebral palsy.

Prognosis and Treatment.—If proper antisyphilitic therapy is instituted, the prognosis for recovery is good. If adequate treatment is not given, however, the epiphyses may sequestrate, and marked bony deformities may develop.

2. Localized Periostitis

There is a form of syphilitic periostitis, called *periostitis ossificans,* in which thickening of the periosteum causes the formation of a hard, dense, circumscribed swelling. This swelling is always found on the convex side of the bone. When the tibia is involved, the condition is sometimes spoken of as *saber shin.*

3. Diffuse Periostitis and Osteoperiostitis

In the late stage of syphilis a gummatous periostitis and osteitis causing necrosis of bone are sometimes observed. Involvement of the skull is common, with the development of craniotabes. The process may lead to suppuration and may simulate pyogenic osteomyelitis. There may be diffuse thickening of the bony cortex with the formation of small hyperostoses which present a characteristic appearance. Pathologic fractures are encountered not infrequently in syphilitic osteomyelitis. In the acquired form the tibia is most often affected; in the congenital form the upper ends of the ulna and radius and the nasal bones are frequently involved. When the nasal bones are affected, the characteristic *saddle nose* of congenital syphilis is produced.

Clinical features typical of syphilis of bone are the multiplicity of the lesions and the absence of pain. Most characteristic in the roentgenogram of this type of bone syphilis is the abundance of newly formed bone.

CHAPTER VII

INFECTIONS OF JOINTS (EXCLUSIVE OF TUBERCULOSIS)

The acute infectious reactions of joints are caused by pus-forming organisms, of which the staphylococcus and streptococcus are the most common examples. The gonococcus, before the advent of antibiotics, caused one of the three most common types of acute infection of joints. The chronic infectious reactions include those caused by the same organisms in attenuated form and those caused by the tubercle bacillus and the *Spirocheta pallida*.

Pyogenic Arthritis (Pyarthrosis; Purulent, Septic, or Suppurative Arthritis)

Incidence.—Pyogenic arthritis is more common in children than in adults, but is seen frequently in both. Males are affected from two to three times as commonly as females. The hip and knee are the most common sites of infection. Since the advent of antibiotics, the incidence of pyogenic arthritis, like that of pyogenic osteomyelitis, has sharply decreased.

Etiology.—Trauma unquestionably influences the localization of the infection. As in osteomyelitis, the *Staphylococcus aureus* and the *Streptococcus hemolyticus* are the most common infecting organisms. Next in order are the pneumococcus, the gonococcus, and the meningococcus; as these organisms produce characteristic joint reactions, each of them will be discussed separately. Rarely are joint infections caused by the organisms of diphtheria, undulant fever, influenza, and typhoid fever, and by the colon bacillus.

Routes of Infection.—Organisms reach the joint by one of three routes: (1) by vascular transfer from a distant focus, such as an infected abrasion, furuncle, or upper respiratory tract infection; (2) by direct inoculation of infected material through a compound wound into the joint; or (3) by direct or lymphatic extension from a neighboring infected area, such as an epiphysitis or osteomyelitis.

Pathology.—Depending upon the virulence of the organism, the resistance of the patient, and the duration of the infection, three distinct types of joint effusion are to be noted.

1. *Serous Effusion.*—If the infection is mild there may be only moderate increase of synovial fluid. The fluid may, however, become cloudy and show an increased cell count.

2. *Serofibrinous Effusion.*—The second stage of inflammation is more serious. A layer of fibrin forms over the synovial membrane. The fibrinous exudate is usually followed by the formation of intra-articular adhesions.

3. *Purulent Effusion.*—This is the most severe stage of inflammatory reaction. All articular structures rapidly become involved. The cartilage becomes eroded, especially at points of pressure, leading to inflammatory changes in the underlying bone and later to frank osteomyelitis. The amount of destruction depends upon the virulence of the organism and the length of time during which the infection has been present. Septic joints of this type often progress to a fibrous or bony ankylosis (Fig. 57).

In addition to the local inflammatory process, the widespread pathologic changes associated with septicemia may be present.

Clinical Picture.—The symptoms vary with the degree of the joint reaction. In the serous type of reaction there may be only moderate swelling and slight pain. There is an increase of local heat, and the joint becomes flexed because of protective muscle spasm. Palpation of the distended joint capsule yields the sensation of fluctuation, and often the outline of the distended capsule can be defined. Attempts to move the joint are accompanied by pain. Fever and leucocytosis are present but not of great degree.

In the serofibrinous type of arthritis the joint is much more painful and all of the signs of inflammation are more intense.

In the suppurative type of inflammation the symptoms are still more severe. There is usually an extreme systemic reaction with a marked elevation of temperature (104° to 105° F., 40° to 41° C.) and leucocytosis. The patient is usually apprehensive. The joint is extremely painful on examination. The infection may spread to the neighboring structures, giving rise to brawny induration and thickening of the periarticular tissues.

Differential Diagnosis.—Osteomyelitis, periarticular cellulitis, and purulent bursitis are often confused with pyogenic arthritis. Gonococcal arthritis may require careful differentiation. Whenever the diagnosis of pyogenic arthritis is in doubt, it is advisable to aspirate the joint fluid, examine a smear microscopically, and culture the fluid. Frequently pyogenic arthritis must be differentiated also from acute rheumatic fever. Normal cardiac findings and failure of the patient to respond to large doses of salicylates are important differential points. Rheumatoid arthritis, tuberculosis, scurvy, hemophilia, and infantile paralysis must also be excluded.

Acute appendicitis may cause psoas spasm, resulting in flexion of the right hip which may suggest pyogenic arthritis of the hip. Acute pelvic inflammatory disease may cause symptoms referable to either hip joint.

Treatment.—Therapy is determined by the degree and duration of the joint involvement. Every case should have immediate diagnostic aspiration and bacteriologic study of the aspirate. Systemic chemotherapy with penicillin or a sulfonamide or both agents should be started at once and modified later according to the bacteriologic findings and the clinical course. In severe infections blood transfusions may be indicated. Roentgenograms should be made early to rule out old infectious bone lesions and for comparison with later films.

In the milder, serous types it may be necessary only to aspirate the excessive fluid, to instill penicillin or a sulfonamide and to apply heat. In some clinics ice bags are considered preferable to hot applications. If a serofibrinous exudate is present, however, the joint will probably require daily aspiration, thorough lavage with saline solution, and instillation of a chemotherapeutic agent. Injection of a small quantity of air or oxygen into the joint also seems to be helpful in many cases. Traction, which provides rest and yet allows some motion, is another most important part of the treatment.

If the exudate is purulent, multiple aspirations and instillations may not suffice to overcome the infection; prompt surgical drainage and thorough irrigation are then indicated. This is particularly true of infections of the hip joint, which is difficult to aspirate completely and may be permanently damaged if the infection is not promptly controlled. Insertion of drainage tubes into the joint is considered injurious. In the case of a septic knee, incisions should be made on either side of the patella and soft rubber drains should be inserted down to the synovium; later the drains are allowed gradually to extrude themselves. Active motion should be started as soon as the acute symptoms will permit.

In the Willems treatment of joint infections one or more openings are made into the joint, and when possible the synovial membrane is brought out and sutured to the skin. In the knee joint this is a comparatively simple procedure. Immediately after operation the patient is encouraged to move the joint voluntarily. Everidge has added a most practical improvement to the Willems method; he employs an overhead splint counterpoised with weights and pulleys, which lessens the effort and pain of active motion. Many patients, however, find the pain too great to permit of the desired amount of active exercise.

In pyogenic arthritis which has progressed to destruction of adjacent bone, it is useless to attempt the Willems method. After drainage has been carried out, the application of traction and subsequent splinting of the joint to prevent deformity is the best method of treatment. In any infection of the hip joint which involves danger of spontaneous dislocation, traction should be applied to the leg in an abducted and extended position, and subsequently a cast is often necessary.

Following the subsidence of an acute pyogenic arthritis, it is essential that physical therapy be instituted as soon as the patient can tolerate it. This should consist of local heat, massage of the muscles, and active and passive motion with emphasis upon restoring muscle tone and strength. Physical therapy should be continued as long as there is clinical improvement; this period may last for several months. If ankylosis becomes inevitable following pyogenic arthritis, care should be taken that it take place in the position of maximum usefulness.

Prognosis.—Serous effusions are rapidly absorbed and recovery takes place quickly and completely. If a serofibrinous or purulent exudate is present, however, some limitation of motion is almost certain to result and in many cases the final outcome is bony ankylosis. In the case of the hip joint there is always the danger of pathologic dislocation. When the pyarthrosis is associated with a septicemia, which happens more frequently in children than in adults, there is grave danger of a fatal outcome.

Acute Pyogenic Epiphysitis

In acute pyogenic epiphysitis the infecting organisms lodge at the epiphyseal line or in the bony portion of the epiphysis. This type of infection is most often found in young children and frequently is the precursor of pyogenic arthritis. The affected joint, which is very frequently the hip, is extremely painful and tender, and there is a tremendous amount of muscle spasm and flexion deformity. A great many cases diagnosed as epiphysitis, however, probably start in the metaphysis and involve the epiphysis and joint by extension.

Treatment.—In acute pyogenic epiphysitis, antibiotic therapy should be started at once, and incision and drainage of the purulent focus are usually indicated in an effort to prevent the infection from extending into the adjacent joint. If the hip is involved, traction should be applied until all signs of infection have disappeared and weight-bearing should be begun slowly. The hip may require protection for from six to twelve months to prevent the development of a flexion-adduction deformity or a pathologic dislocation. If the knee is involved, care must be taken to splint the joint in extension to prevent the muscle spasm of the acute stage from causing a flexion deformity.

Pneumococcal Arthritis

Incidence.—Pneumococcal arthritis is relatively rare and, with the advent of more effective chemotherapy for the primary infection, is probably becoming still less common. In 75 per cent of the cases of pneumococcal arthritis the involvement is monarticular, the hip joint being most commonly infected. Pneumococcal arthritis is usually secondary to pneumonia, the arthritis often beginning about two weeks after the onset of pneumonia. The joint complication is particularly common among infants and alcoholics.

Pathology.—The least serious form of pneumococcal arthritis is a serous inflammation which may subside quickly. The commonest type, however, is a severe suppurative infection. In this type the pus is greenish yellow and usually contains flakes of fibrin. Pneumococcal arthritis may cause severe destruction of the joint structures and may be followed by bony ankylosis.

Clinical Picture.—The symptoms are those of a fulminating joint infection; they are usually superimposed upon the symptoms of pneumonia. The diagnosis is confirmed by bacteriologic study of fluid aspirated from the affected joint.

Treatment.—The treatment is the same as that outlined for other types of acute pyogenic arthritis. In addition, an antipneumococcal serum has sometimes proved beneficial.

Prognosis.—Before the advent of the sulfonamides and antibiotics the mortality was at least 50 per cent and in the severer types there was little hope of preserving joint motion, even with early drainage. The prognosis is now much more favorable as regards both survival and preservation of function.

Meningococcal Arthritis

Meningococcal arthritis occurs as a complication of the epidemic form of cerebrospinal meningitis. Sometimes joint involvement has followed the administration of antimeningococcal serum. Meningococcal arthritis is usually monarticular, the knee being most often affected. Most of the pathologic changes may be extra-articular. The infection usually runs its course in from one to four weeks, with relatively good recovery of joint function. Occasionally the infection is of polyarticular nature; this type usually subsides very quickly. The local treatment is the same as that described for other types of pyogenic arthritis. Antibiotics and the sulfonamides have proved to be of great value in treating meningococcal infections.

Sites for Incision of Infected Joints

The most useful surgical approaches for drainage of infected joints are the following:

Hip.—A posterior approach is by far the most useful as dependent drainage can be established, facilitating rapid subsidence of the infection (Fig. 56,*A*).

Knee.—Small incisions on either side of the patella, which do not involve the joint ligaments, are to be preferred (Fig. 56,*B*). These can be incorporated later into the "U"-shaped incision for radical drainage if an unfavorable clinical course makes it necessary to sacrifice the joint.

Ankle.—Incision is made just below the fibular or tibial malleolus. It is necessary usually to divide a portion of the external or internal lateral ligament in order to secure proper drainage.

Shoulder.—An anterior approach is most frequently used.

Elbow.—Incision is made on the lateral aspect of the elbow over the radiohumeral portion of the capsule. If through-and-through drainage is desired, another incision may be made anterior to the medial condyle of the humerus.

Wrist.—The wrist is best drained through a longitudinal incision made on the dorsum of the joint after careful separation of the tendons.

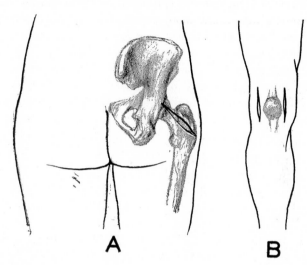

Fig. 56.—*A,* Posterior incision for drainage of hip joint; *B,* parapatellar incisions for drainage of knee joint.

Gonococcal Arthritis

Incidence.—Before the advent of the sulfonamides and antibiotics, metastatic joint involvement complicated from 2 to 5 per cent of all gonococcal infections. Now, however, gonococcal arthritis is uncommon. In 75 per cent of the cases of gonorrheal arthritis the joint involvement appears within two or three weeks after the onset of the primary gonorrheal infection. Gonococcal arthritis is seen usually in individuals whose resistance is low and who have had repeated gonorrheal infections. Males between twenty and thirty years of age are most often affected.

In about 40 per cent of the adult cases the arthritis is monarticular. In infants it is more often polyarticular. The knee is by far the most frequently affected joint. Next in order of frequency are the ankle, the hip, and the wrist.

Clinical Picture.—The symptoms depend largely upon the degree of joint involvement. There are usually fleeting pains in multiple joints before the infection becomes localized in a single joint. This is most characteristic of the dry form, which is sometimes called *gonorrheal rheumatism*. In mild cases there may be slight swelling and discomfort in the joint with weakness and stiffness throughout the extremity. In more severe cases there are extreme pain, redness, marked increase in local heat, swelling, a glossy appearance of the skin, and marked muscle spasm. These joints may be exquisitely tender, and the slightest movement may cause excruciating pain. The more severe and advanced types are usually followed by partial or complete ankylosis. Often the periarticular infection involves the periosteum, the tendon sheaths, and the bursae.

Diagnosis.—Diagnosis is made from the clinical picture and from identification of the organisms in the urethral or vaginal discharge. It is important to exclude staphylococcus and streptococcus infection and acute rheumatic fever. Early diagnostic aspiration of the affected joint and bacteriologic study of the aspirate should be carried out. Within the first ten days of the infection gonococci will often be found in the joint fluid. In chronic or subacute cases there may be some difficulty in finding the organisms and in differentiating the condition from tuberculosis and from rheumatoid arthritis. The gonococcal complement fixation test is positive in a large percentage of the cases.

Treatment.—Therapy should be directed toward cure of the primary focus as well as the inflamed joint. Penicillin in large doses should be given systemically at once. In the milder cases this may result in very rapid relief of the symptoms. If the organism is resistant to penicillin, other antibiotics should be tried. Sulfonamides also may be used.

In more severe cases, the joint should be elevated and supported in good functional position by traction or splinting; hot wet dressings should be applied constantly. Joints suitable for therapeutic aspiration, such as the knee or ankle, should have prompt removal of the excess fluid and gentle lavage. It is usually advisable to instill a strong solution of penicillin into the joint, and air or oxygen may be injected also to aid in relieving painful friction and preventing the formation of adhesions. In the more severe cases repeated aspirations and instillations may be needed. Gonorrheal joints should not be incised.

Following the acute stage the affected joint should receive thorough physical therapy consisting of heat and active exercise. Although the response is sometimes slow, the functional result will usually be good unless the articular cartilages have been destroyed. In cases of long standing it is sometimes advisable to manipulate the joint gently under anesthesia in order to break adhesions. Manipulations should always be preceded and followed by physical therapy.

Infectious Myositis

Infectious myositis, or infection of muscle tissue, is conveniently described here because it is usually secondary to the more common pyogenic infections of joints or of bone.

Etiology.—Primary infection of a muscle is extremely uncommon except as a result of penetrating wounds; involvement of muscle by gas gangrene in *Clostridium welchii* infections is an important example. Metastatic involvement of muscle and fascia occasionally occurs in pyemia. Infection by extension from a neighboring focus, as in pyogenic arthritis or osteomyelitis, is more common, but usually the muscular involvement is of less importance than the primary infectious process. Acute infectious myositis may occur in typhoid fever, scarlet fever, and hemolytic streptococcal infections, while chronic infectious myositis occurs in syphilis and tuberculosis.

Pathology.—Inflammatory changes are not demonstrable in muscle fibers themselves. Changes take place, however, in the connective tissue sheaths which cover bundles of muscle fibers and in the fasciae which enclose the muscles. The term *infectious fibrositis*, which is descriptive of the pathologic changes, has been suggested as preferable to that of *infectious myositis*.

Clinical Picture.—Myositis is evidenced by acute pain throughout the muscles, which are tender and in a state of spasm. There may be an associated general reaction of malaise, chills, and fever. Abscesses within muscle are seen most often in the pectorals, the triceps, and the adductors of the thigh.

Differential Diagnosis.—Lumbago and stiff neck, which have a rather vague etiology, are to be differentiated. They are most often the result of fatigue and exposure to cold and are thought to be due to an obscure chemical reaction within the muscles. Occasionally intramuscular calcification or true myositis ossificans is to be differentiated.

Treatment.—In acute suppurative myositis, prompt and intensive chemotherapy directed at the invading organism is essential. Since the suppurative process spreads extensively through the muscle sheaths and fascial planes, wide incision may be necessary in order to insure adequate drainage. In subacute conditions heat, rest, and splinting are indicated for relief of the intense pain. In extensive and long-standing infections, scar tissue may cause contractures of muscles and deformities of joints. The development of contractures should be prevented by appropriate traction or splinting.

Syphilis of Joints

Syphilitic infection of joints is not so common as that of bones. When joint infections do occur, they may be mistaken for rheumatoid arthritis or proliferative synovitis. They are found most often in the early stages of acquired syphilis.

Syphilitic joint involvement may be of several types:

1. *Symmetrical Serous Synovitis (Clutton's Joints).*—This condition, a manifestation of congenital syphilis, was first described by Clutton in 1886. It is a painless hydrarthrosis without bone changes, more often bilateral than unilateral, coming on usually between the ages of eight and fifteen years, and terminating by spontaneous regression at about the twentieth year. It is to be distinguished principally from gummatous synovitis, early tuberculosis, and rheumatoid arthritis. Accurate diagnosis is important since useless exploratory operation may be prevented and effective medical treatment instituted.

2. *Arthralgia.*—Mild pains in the joints, not accompanied by objective signs of inflammation, may accompany the other phenomena of secondary syphilis.

3. *Gummatous Arthritis.*—This affection is occasionally observed in the late stage of syphilis and usually involves the perisynovial tissues. Seldom is there pain in the joint, but a feeling of weakness is common.

4. *Chronic Synovitis (Hereditary Synovitis).*—This affection is seen in children and usually involves both knees. It causes a moderate amount of pain, slight tenderness, and only moderate disability.

Prognosis.—With adequate antisyphilitic treatment the prognosis for recovery in all types of syphilitic synovitis and arthritis is excellent.

Ankylosis

Ankylosis is a restriction of the normal range of motion by tissue changes within or without the joint cavity. Ankylosis may occur with the joint in a position favorable for function or in an attitude of deformity.

Etiology.—Ankylosis is usually secondary to an infectious process within the joint. It is a fibrous, partial, or false ankylosis when the fibrous adhesions between the articular surfaces are not accompanied by actual bony union. These adhesions are formed across the joint as the end-result of the presence of hemorrhage or exudate. Fibrous ankylosis is common in young patients. The most common extra-articular causes of ankylosis are contractures of ligaments or of nearby soft tissues following infection, trauma, or prolonged immobilization. Bony, complete, or true ankylosis exists when solid new bone has been formed between the articular surfaces. This is usually the result of a more advanced infectious process within the joint, which has destroyed the cartilaginous surfaces and allowed the apposition of denuded bone. Ankylosis may at times follow severe intra-articular trauma, as when fracture fragments enter the joint cavity. A severe burn about a joint sometimes results in bony ankylosis.

Clinical Picture.—In fibrous ankylosis a small amount of motion may be present and pain may be experienced when the joint is manipulated. In bony ankylosis no joint motion is possible. Often it is difficult to determine whether the ankylosis is true or false. Roentgenograms of the joint should always be examined but at times are deceptive. The films may suggest solid bony fusion when definite joint motion can be elicited clinically or can be demonstrated later at operation. The most reliable roentgenographic criterion of bony ankylosis is the presence of fine bony trabeculae which can sometimes be seen to extend directly across the region of the former joint space (Fig. 57,*B*).

Treatment.—In the early stages of joint involvement the best assurance against the development of ankylosis is proper treatment of the original disease. There is no doubt that in pyogenic arthritis which does not respond quickly to antibiotic therapy, the Willems treatment is best for preserving joint function. In some instances, contrary to the usual practice, it is advisable to place the joint absolutely at rest in order to avoid injury of the delicate joint surfaces. When the knee or the hip is involved, traction applied below the joint and designed to lessen the pressure of the adjacent articular surfaces is often an effective aid in preventing joint destruction and ankylosis. In treatment of fractures, casts should immobilize no joint without good reason, should be discarded as soon as early union will permit, and should be followed by physical therapy with emphasis on active exercise of all affected joints.

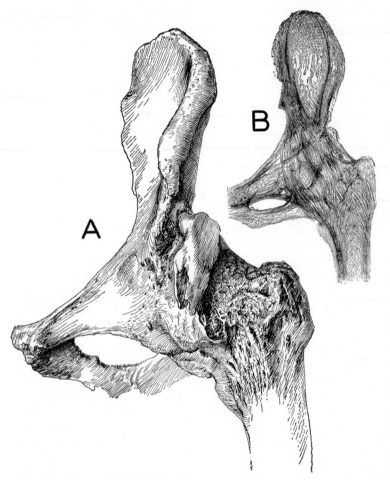

Fig. 57.—Bony ankylosis of hip, the end result of a severe pyogenic arthritis (Museum specimen). *A,* Specimen showing complete obliteration of the joint by new bone; *B,* drawing from roentgenogram showing bony trabeculae traversing the former joint space.

If fibrous ankylosis has taken place, it may be possible by means of physical therapy to preserve a useful range of motion in the joint. Heat, massage, and strenuous active motion are essential. Passive motion should not be forced if the movement is accompanied by severe pain, since additional damage and stiffening may result and since the discomfort may serve to discourage further endeavors. Electrical stimulation of muscles about the joint and insistence on active contraction of these muscles will often help. A joint which by gentle physical therapy can be restored even partially to motion will usually preserve its regained function. On the other hand, a joint which has undergone forcible correction, with the breaking of adhesions and subsequent intra-articular hemorrhage, will often become less mobile than before manipulation.

When it becomes necessary to break up adhesions, the manipulation should be done gently under anesthesia. In some cases it is necessary to perform repeated manipulations. If the adhesions can be broken with a minimum of effort, the prognosis for improved joint function is good, provided that muscle tone and strength are adequate, but if considerable force is used the outcome is at best doubtful. About these partially ankylosed and little used joints there is a tremendous amount of bone atrophy and consequent weakening of the bony structures. Care should therefore be taken not to exert too much force, as the bones fracture easily. The danger of fat embolism following manipulation must also be considered. Of great importance is the patient's cooperation in a program of vigorous active exercise after the manipulation.

If the ankylosis has occurred with the joint in good position, arthroplasty, or other operations for mobilization, may be considered. When the ankylosis has occurred in a faulty position, however, operations for improvement of the deformity, as well as those for restoration of joint motion, must be kept under consideration. In a partial extension ankylosis of the knee such as sometimes occurs following a fracture of the lower half of the femur, with contracture of the quadriceps muscle, a lengthening of the quadriceps tendon (Bennett operation) or a resection of the scar tissue about the quadriceps tendon and muscle fibers (Thompson operation) will sometimes result in a very useful increase of the range of flexion.

Optimum Positions of Joint Fixation

In many patients with joint disease it becomes impossible to prevent ankylosis. Should ankylosis become inevitable, the position most suitable for future function of the extremity must be determined early, and efforts must be made to prevent ankylosis from occurring in any less favorable position. This is a vital factor in the preservation of function.

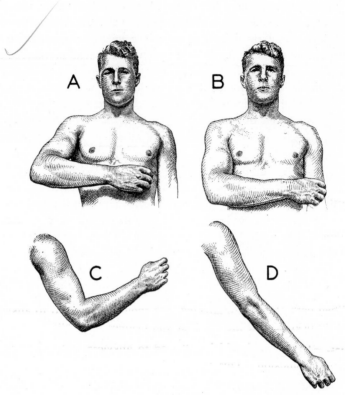

Fig. 58.—Correct and incorrect positions for ankylosis. Shoulder: *A*, Correct; *B*, incorrect. Elbow: *C*, Correct; *D*, incorrect.

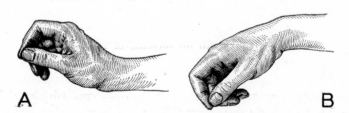

Fig. 59.—Correct and incorrect positions for ankylosis of wrist. *A*, Correct; *B*, incorrect.

A great number of orthopaedic operations are made necessary only because ankylosis in poor functional position has been allowed to take place. The therapeutic procedure of producing a bony ankylosis by surgery is called *arthrodesis*. It is frequently indicated in tuberculosis of joints and whenever intractable pain or permanent instability render the joint useless. In arthrodesis, also, care must be taken that the ankylosis occurs with the joint in the position most favorable for function.

The most favorable positions for ankylosis are as follows:

Spine.—The vertebral column should be so supported that the curves remain relatively normal. Ankylosis should never be allowed to take place with the spine in a flexed or laterally deviated position.

Shoulder.—In children the shoulder should be allowed to ankylose in from 50 to 75 degrees of abduction; in adults abduction of 50 degrees is preferable. The arm should also be brought forward 45 degrees from its resting position at the side of the body (Fig. 58).

Elbow.—The elbow should be allowed to ankylose at a right angle with the forearm in a position midway between supination and pronation. When both elbows are affected, one should be allowed to ankylose at about 80 degrees and the other at 100 degrees (Fig. 58).

Wrist.—The wrist should be allowed to ankylose in from 15 to 35 degrees of dorsiflexion. This is most important, as ankylosis in volar flexion causes marked limitation of the usefulness of the hand (Fig. 59).

Hip.—The hip is ankylosed preferably in about 5 degrees of abduction, 5 degrees of external rotation, and 10 to 25 degrees of flexion. The most suitable degree of flexion depends largely upon the habits of the individual. If the patient's occupation is of sedentary nature, ankylosis of the hip in full extension would obviously be undesirable (Fig. 60).

Knee.—The knee may be ankylosed in full extension, but in women and in men of sedentary occupation flexion of from 20 to 30 degrees forms a less awkward position. In children full extension is essential, however, because with growth an increase of flexion is likely to occur (Fig. 61).

Ankle.—The ankle should be allowed to ankylose with the foot at a right angle to the leg or in very slight equinus (Fig. 62). If the affected leg is shortened, however, slight equinus provides a more serviceable extremity. Care should be taken to avoid rotation deformity by aligning the foot with the ankle. When the ankle or knee undergoes ankylosis, the position should be such that a line drawn from the anterior superior iliac spine to the middle of the patella and projected to the foot passes either through or close to the second toe.

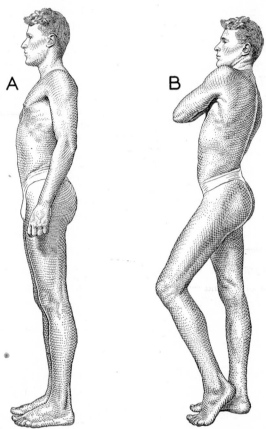

Fig. 60.—Correct and incorrect positions for ankylosis of the hip. *A*, Correct; *B*, incorrect.

Arthroplasty

Arthroplasty is a surgical procedure for restoring to a stiffened joint the ability to move. At the same time the necessary stability of the joint and its freedom from pain must be preserved. In properly selected cases the results of arthroplasty are sometimes satisfactory. The best results

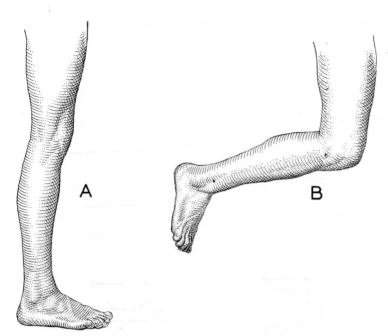

Fig. 61.—Correct and incorrect positions for ankylosis of the knee in a child. *A*, Correct; *B*, incorrect. In adults, slight flexion is often desirable.

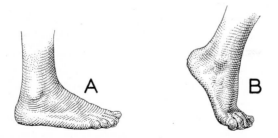

Fig. 62.—Correct and incorrect positions for ankylosis of the ankle. *A*, Correct; *B*, incorrect.

are obtained in the hip and jaw. Many different types of procedure have been described, but seldom is the detailed anatomy of the normal joint restored.

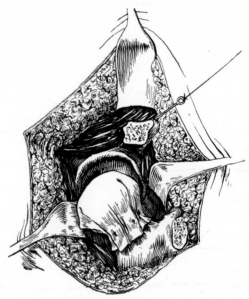

Fig. 63.—Arthroplasty of the hip. Head of the femur has been reshaped and covered with an interposing material and is ready to be replaced into the remodeled acetabulum. (After Baer.)

The cases most favorable for arthroplasty are those in which the ankylosis has been the result of trauma or an acute pyogenic infection. However, before this operation is to be considered, the infection must have remained quiescent for at least six months and preferably for a year or more. The most favorable case is that of the young adult with ankylosis of only a single joint and with good musculature above and below the joint. Ankylosis following tuberculous arthritis is ordinarily unfavorable for arthroplasty. In selected late tuberculous cases, however, the operation very rarely may be advisable. In joints ankylosed from rheumatoid arthritis the results of arthroplasty are not so good as in joints ankylosed as a result of pyogenic infection.

Arthroplasty is most likely to be successful in cases in which the joint has become ankylosed in a relatively normal position. When there is a large amount of bony overgrowth about the joint, the outlook for a successful functional result is not good. Arthroplasty is contraindicated in children before the epiphyses have united. It is usually inadvisable to perform arthroplasty on any weight-bearing joint of an individual whose occupation requires heavy manual labor.

In arthroplasty sufficient bone must be removed from between the bone ends to permit free movement in the desired directions. This separation of the bone ends should measure ½ inch or more. The bone ends should be shaped, smoothed, and covered with some type of interposing material (Fig. 63). In most clinics, fascia lata is the tissue of choice. In arthroplasty of the hip, Smith-Petersen's technic of inserting a Vitallium cup over the head of the femur has given good results. Vitallium, which was developed and has been extensively studied by Venable and Stuck, is an alloy of cobalt, chromium, and molybdenum which causes no electrolytic reaction in the tissues and can be left in place permanently. After closure of the arthroplasty wound, sufficient traction should be applied to hold the bone ends apart. Early mobilization is essential and should be encouraged by an extended program of physical therapy with emphasis upon active exercise. If these basic principles of the indications and technic of arthroplasty are observed, the prognosis for a useful degree of joint function may be good.

In recent years, for hip ankylosis and for degeneration following infection, arthritis, or fracture, replacement of the head of the femur with a plastic or metal prosthesis has become popular, especially in European clinics. The most commonly used prosthesis is the Judet acrylic head. These prostheses are usually attached to the neck and shaft of the femur by a projection from the prosthetic head which is inserted into a tunnel running through the neck to the shaft below the greater trochanter. Some prostheses are placed in the neck and down into the medullary canal of the upper end of the shaft. It is too early to evaluate the long-term results of these procedures, but it can be stated that the results to date are encouraging.

CHAPTER VIII

TUBERCULOSIS OF BONES AND JOINTS:
THE SPINE AND PELVIS

Tuberculosis of bones and joints is a localized, progressively destructive disease resulting from the activity of tubercle bacilli in bone or articular structures.

Incidence.—Tuberculosis is the most frequently observed of the chronic bone and joint infections, and before the campaigns against tuberculosis were waged it was one of the most common of all orthopaedic conditions. Tuberculosis of bones and joints constitutes approximately 3 per cent of all tuberculous conditions. It is commonest in childhood, occurring most frequently during the years when growth of the bones is most active. In one series of 5,000 cases, 87 per cent were in children under fourteen years of age. Bone tuberculosis is most common in the poorer classes. Males are affected slightly more often than females.

Tuberculosis of the spine is more common than that of the extremities. Statistics show that from 40 to 50 per cent of all bone and joint tuberculosis occurs in the spine and approximately 30 per cent in the hip. The lower extremities are affected 18 to 35 times as often as the upper extremities. This fact possibly indicates that trauma and strain are definite factors in the localization of the tuberculous infection. The upper extremities are affected relatively more frequently in adults than in children. Approximately 30 per cent of the cases show multiple joint involvement.

Predisposing Factors.—It is known that individuals with low resistance to infection show a tendency to develop bone tuberculosis. Susceptibility to the disease may be hereditary. Tuberculosis of bone cannot arise unless there is a focus of tuberculous infection elsewhere in the body. Trauma undoubtedly plays a part in the etiology. It has been shown experimentally that there is a tendency for tuberculous infection to localize in joints which have been injured. In actively growing children who suffer frequent falls and blows, small hemorrhages may appear about the epiphyseal lines where normally there is a rich blood supply. Such injuries prepare fertile soil for the localization of the tubercle bacilli.

Types of Infection.—Three types of tubercle bacilli may cause bone and joint tuberculosis; viz., the human, the bovine, and the avian; however, each provokes the same pathologic reaction in the tissues. In certain countries where raw milk is extensively used, the bovine type is the most common. This is not true, however, in the United States, where the human type is most frequent. The avian type is very rare.

Modes of Infection.—Infection with the human type of tubercle bacillus is usually transmitted by the sputum. The organism may enter the respiratory passages, be carried to the lungs, and later lodge in the peribronchial lymph nodes. Either the human or the bovine type of bacillus may be ingested with infected milk or other food. The organism then penetrates the wall of the gastrointestinal tract and ultimately finds its way into the retroperitoneal lymph nodes. It appears certain that bovine tuberculosis could be completely abolished as a disease of humans by adequate control of the milk supply. Great protection is given at the present time by routine inspection and periodic tuberculin testing of the herds of dairy cows and by the pasteurization of milk.

Pathology.—The outstanding characteristic of tuberculous infection of bone is destruction with little tendency toward the formation of new bone. The process may involve the bone alone without entering the joint, but more often it starts in the articular end of the bone and then by gradual extension along the line of least resistance enters the joint. In some instances it starts in the synovial membrane and involves secondarily the bone beneath the joint surface. Primary synovial tuberculosis is observed more commonly in adults than in children.

Tubercle bacilli are usually blood-borne from a primary focus such as infected peribronchial or abdominal lymph nodes. Localization of the bacilli in the cancellous end of the bone is followed by the formation of typical tubercles. Granulation tissue appears, tuberculous pus forms, ischemic necrosis takes place, and neighboring bone is destroyed. When the infection enters the joint, a fibrinous exudate forms over the cartilage and becomes organized into granulation tissue. The cartilage may be invaded directly by the granulation tissue on its articular surface or undermined at its synovial margins, gradually separated from the underlying bone and destroyed. These changes are accompanied by the formation of a purulent, cheesy exudate containing remnants of necrotic tissue. The bone becomes disintegrated and destroyed on its exposed joint surfaces as the result of the formation and coalescence of tubercles. The purulent exudate dissects the surrounding joint structures along the planes of least resistance and enters the soft tissues. If the infection is overcome, the exudate is slowly absorbed and replaced by fibrous tissue. The bone about the edges of the infected area is stimulated to proliferate, and gradually the evidences of an active infectious process subside.

Tuberculous abscesses are called "cold abscesses" because an acute inflammatory reaction manifested by marked increase in local heat, redness, and pain is not present. Deep tuberculous abscesses sometimes heal completely by calcification. Sometimes they become secondarily infected, especially when they rupture or are incised, and may then show all the signs of an acute inflammatory reaction.

Tuberculosis of the metaphyseal bone without involvement of the joints is rare. The incidence of bone tuberculosis without extension to the joints is about the same in adults as it is in children. The femur and the tibia are the bones most often affected. Fraser of Edinburgh has described four types of metaphyseal tuberculosis:

1. *Encysted.*—The infection is well localized and surrounded by sclerotic bone. When multiple cystic foci are present the affection is called *osteitis tuberculosa multiplex cystica (Jungling's disease)*. However, it is thought by some observers that this is not a true tuberculous process but an osteal sarcoid.

2. *Infiltrating.*—This type develops in early youth and progresses with great rapidity. Before rarefaction becomes extreme, there may be extensive caseation, necrosis, and sequestration.

3. *Atrophic.*—Gradual wasting of the bony lamellae characterizes this type.

4. *Hypertrophic.*—This type, marked by extensive formation of new bone, is extremely rare.

An arborescent synovial tuberculosis, in which synovial villi formed of adipose and fibrous tissue proliferate, is occasionally seen, most frequently in the knee. This condition must be differentiated from syphilis and villous arthritis. Occasionally "rice bodies," consisting of the hypertrophic and detached synovial villi, are found in the tuberculous joint fluid.

Tuberculous bone infections have been thought by some observers to be accompanied by the formation of tuberculous toxins sometimes capable of exciting multiple joint reactions which resemble those of acute rheumatoid arthritis. This type of affection has been called *tuberculous rheumatism.*

Clinical Picture.—The symptoms depend upon the region involved. In general, however, tuberculous bone and joint infections are preceded by a state of malaise, poor general health, loss of weight, and repeated respiratory infections. All of the symptoms are variable and may not be present in the individual case. Spontaneous pain, pain on motion, and restriction of motion of the affected joint are often the first evidences of tuberculosis. The pain is accompanied by muscle spasm and pronounced muscle atrophy. Occasionally, however, these symptoms are entirely absent. In joints of the extremities, swelling is common. Later, because of bone destruction or epiphyseal changes, the extremity may become shortened. There may be gross deformity of the joint and contracture due to muscle spasm. Rarely the joint is acutely sensitive on palpation. In children night cries and night sweats are characteristic symptoms, and there is usually a slight afternoon elevation of temperature. A mild leucocytosis may be present.

Diagnosis.—A positive diagnosis cannot be made unless (1) the presence of tubercle bacilli is demonstrated, (2) microscopic examination of excised tissue reveals the presence of tubercles, or (3) inoculation of tissue or pus into guinea pigs produces tuberculosis. In many cases the tubercle bacilli can be demonstrated in regional lymph nodes.

The intracutaneous tuberculin test is of great value. Intramuscular injections of old tuberculin have been recommended by some authors but are not considered safe by those specializing in tuberculosis, because of the danger of activating a latent acid-fast infection. A positive tuberculin skin test is suggestive but not conclusive evidence that tuberculosis is present. A negative tuberculin skin test is of more significance. Rarely is tuberculosis present if the results remain negative even when the tests are repeated with increased concentrations of tuberculin.

Roentgenographic Picture.—The bones show atrophy, faint joint outlines, and irregular notching with occasional displacement of the joint surfaces. There is sometimes a circumscribed area of decreased density which has the appearance of a Brodie's abscess. In tuberculosis of the spine, erosion of the vertebral bodies is seen. The most characteristic feature of the roentgenograms, however, is the almost complete lack of bone regeneration in the early cases. In later stages of the infection, however, new bone may be seen, and the joint outlines again become sharply defined. Sequestra are occasionally visualized.

Treatment.—The object of all treatment is to secure *rest* for the affected part or parts and to build up the resistance of the body. In addition, streptomycin is of proved value.

General Measures.—Good food, fresh air, and hygienic surroundings are essential. The patients with bone and joint tuberculosis do better when living out of doors. It is surprising how much tolerance to cold weather can be developed by the body, especially in the case of a child. The diet should be well balanced and should include foods of high vitamin content. Cod liver oil is a valuable adjunct.

Wherever possible, heliotherapy should be given. The body should be exposed to the sun for increasing periods each day until several hours of exposure can be tolerated. This should be continued until the disease is arrested. Remarkable improvement and cures of bone and joint tuberculosis have been effected with heliotherapy and general supportive measures alone. Heliotherapy is the most important form of treatment in certain special hospitals. The most famous of these has been that of Rollier, located high in the Alps at Leysin, Switzerland. Artificial heliotherapy or ultraviolet light therapy also has definite value in the treatment of patients with bone tuberculosis. Ultraviolet irradiation may be obtained from any of several types of lamp, of which the mercury vapor arc and the carbon arc are most used.

Numerous reports have been made on the use of streptomycin in the treatment of tuberculosis of bones and joints. It is of greatest value in cases with draining sinuses. This drug may be given by deep subcutaneous or intramuscular injection every four to six hours for several months. Recent investigators have advised adult doses of 1 Gm. daily or twice weekly. Few toxic reactions have been reported. To prevent the bacilli from developing resistance to streptomycin, para-aminosalicylic acid should be given in large doses by mouth. For adults, 12 Gm. daily in divided doses have been recommended.

Local Measures.—The affected part should first be put at rest with traction or in a splint or brace. Fixation allows the tuberculous granulation tissue to be replaced by fibrous tissue. In the case of the hip or knee, fixation can be obtained satisfactorily with traction, which also relieves the muscle spasm and pain. When the convalescent patient is allowed to be up, special protection should be given the lower extremities to prevent the strain of too early weight-bearing from aggravating and prolonging the disease.

Concerning the wisdom of operative treatment, there is some variance of opinion. It has been established, however, that a stabilizing operation will often result in complete rest of the joint, thereby tending to hasten recovery and to prevent recurrence. These operations are done particularly upon the spine and hip. Removal of the tuberculous soft tissue, cartilage and bone from the knee joint very often leads to quick recovery, but after such a procedure there is no possibility of preserving motion. In children radical surgical treatment should not be performed so early in the course of the infection as in adults. Surgical methods are justified in adults only when the convalescent period can thereby be materially lessened. The presence of active pulmonary tuberculosis is a definite contraindication to operation. Amputation of an extremity for tuberculosis, except in the case of the ankle or foot, should be done only in extremely late cases or as a life-saving measure.

Cold abscesses should not be aspirated or incised unless they are about to rupture or are causing marked pain, because 50 per cent of them disappear with complete rest of the tuberculous bone or joint. Rarely they become completely separated from the joint and lie free in the soft tissues. When this happens, excision of the abscess can sometimes be effected. If, however, the tension in the abscess becomes great and is accompanied by pain, the pus may be aspirated. In order not to cause the formation of a chronic sinus, aspiration should be done through a long needle which is inserted through healthy tissues. If repeated aspirations do not relieve the symptoms, the abscess should be evacuated through a small incision. A drain should be left in for a day or two, and in dressing the wound great care should be taken to prevent secondary infection. In spite of all care secondary infection often occurs. Curettage of tuberculous sinuses in the soft tissue and bone to secure healing of the lesion is nearly always futile and is usually to be condemned as ill-advised surgery. Streptomycin is very helpful in the treatment of tuberculous sinuses.

Prognosis.—The prognosis in bone and joint tuberculosis depends much upon the resistance of the individual. In negroes the resistance is notably poor. The more acute the symptoms, the poorer is the prognosis. In the presence of active pulmonary tuberculosis the outlook is unfavorable. Involvement of multiple joints makes the prognosis worse. Adults are less favorable risks than children. The mortality rate is higher in involvement of the spine and hip. If prolonged suppuration occurs, there may be amyloid changes throughout the liver, spleen, kidneys, and other organs, and in cases of this type the prognosis is poor. Statistics show that in the presence of abscess formation the mortality rate is doubled. Abscesses may rupture and extend to adjacent organs or even into the spinal canal, in which case a fatal meningitis is likely to result. Tuberculosis of the ankle is especially serious because the infection tends to spread to other areas. The prognosis for recovery of joint function is extremely poor in adults and only fair in children.

Tuberculosis of the Spine

The most common site of bone and joint tuberculosis is the spine, which is involved in 40 to 50 per cent of the cases. It is spoken of as *Pott's disease* because in 1779 Sir Percival Pott first described a painful deformity of the spine, accompanied by paralysis of the legs, which is considered to have been due to tuberculosis. Paralysis develops, however, in only about 10 per cent of the cases of tuberculosis of the spine.

Predisposing Factors.—More than 50 per cent of the tuberculous lesions of the spine occur in the segment of greatest mobility of the back; viz., from the tenth dorsal to the first lumbar vertebra. Greater mobility leads to greater trauma, a factor very important in determining the localization of the lesion. In 50 per cent of the patients the onset is between the third and fifth years of age. Boys are affected more often than girls.

Pathology.—The anterior part of the vertebral column is most often involved by the disease (Figs. 64 and 65), but the laminae or transverse processes may also be the sites of pathologic changes. Pathologic studies have shown that the disease usually begins in the vertebral body, despite the fact that narrowing of an intervertebral disk is one of the earliest roentgenographic signs. When the vertebral body is attacked the focus of infection may be in the central portion of the spongy bone at a point close to the epiphysis or in an extreme anterior position beneath the periosteum whence it spreads into the body. The strength of the vertebral body is so undermined that finally it collapses when continued stress is exerted upon it. Following collapse there may be a dorsal protrusion of the spine, or *kyphosis*. As in tuberculosis elsewhere, the local blood supply is impaired by the inflammatory changes, resulting in degeneration of the marrow, absorption of the bone lamellae, and ultimately caseation. Other parts of the vertebra may undergo a sclerotic type of necrosis due to ischemia rather than infection; lesions of this type may not be apparent in the roentgenogram. During the early stages of the disease there may be no evidence of subperiosteal deposition of new bone. The changes are destructive, and the process may extend beneath the anterior spinal ligaments to invade the vertebrae above

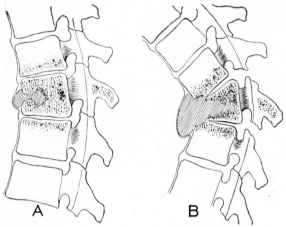

Fig. 64.—Tuberculosis of the spine. Stages in the process of bone destruction and abscess formation: *A*, early; *B*, late. (After Calot.)

and below. Usually from three to six vertebrae are involved, but the most extensive destructive changes are confined to the vertebra first affected. More than one level of the spine may be involved. In the dorsal spine, which has normally a moderate posterior convexity, a sharp gibbus or angular deformity is often seen as a result of the disease. In the cervical and lumbar portions of the spine, where the convexity is normally anterior, kyphosis following collapse of the vertebral bodies may not be noticeable until the disease is far advanced. Healing takes place by gradual fibrosis and by new bone formation with a resulting bony ankylosis of the collapsed vertebrae.

As the destructive process advances and the vertebral bodies collapse, abscess formation becomes pronounced. An abscess can be demonstrated in 20 per cent of the cases by roentgenographic or physical examination, while at autopsy abscess has been found in 80 per cent of the cases. Abscesses are most frequently seen in involvement of lower levels of the spine. There is little doubt, however, that abscess formation occurs at one time or another in every case of tuberculosis of the spine. In cases of long standing, complete calcification of the abscess may take place.

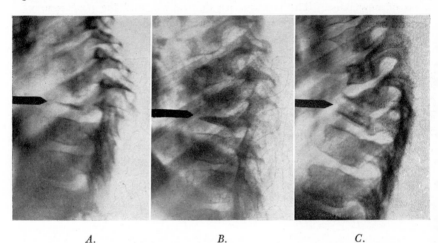

A.   B.   C.

Fig. 65.—Lateral roentgenograms showing tuberculosis of spine. *A*, In boy three years of age. Note destruction of the bodies of the seventh and eighth dorsal vertebrae and kyphosis.

B, In same patient as shown in *A*, two years later. Treatment had consisted of rest on a Bradford frame and immobilization in a plaster body cast. Note the sharp, well-demarcated areas of the diseased vertebral bodies. There has not been an advancement of the destructive lesion.

C, In same patient as shown in *A*, three and one-half years later. Note fusion of vertebral bodies and well-demarcated outlines in the affected areas. Also note the anterior cupping of the two vertebral bodies above the tuberculous lesion, which is frequently observed. This can also be noted in *A* and *B*.

As the destruction and kyphosis increase, compression of the spinal cord may occur from the presence of an abscess, a mass of granulation tissue, or the formation of tuberculomas, resulting in partial or complete paralysis of the lower extremities. If an abscess ruptures through the dura mater, pachymeningitis or myelitis may develop and lead to a fatal outcome.

Clinical Picture.—The premonitory symptoms of loss of weight, weakness, and fatigue are usually present before the lesion becomes demonstrable.

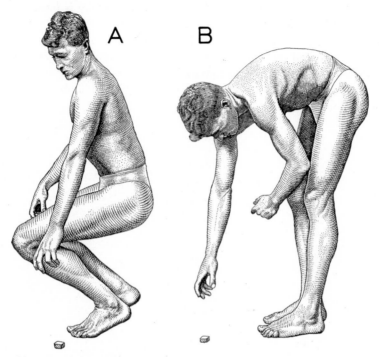

Fig. 66.—Tuberculosis of the lumbar spine. Note the contrast between the rigidity of the tuberculous spine *(A)* and the flexibility of the normal spine *(B),* as shown in the manner of picking up an object from the floor.

The symptoms vary according to the portion of the spine involved. Weakness or pain is often the first indication of a beginning tuberculous process. Next the patient may develop stiffness and muscle spasm. In children night cries may be present at this time. Painless kyphosis may be the first evidence. There are usually weakness of the legs and awkwardness of gait. The patient walks with extreme caution and is careful not to bend over or take sudden steps which may jar the spine. If he is asked to bend over to pick up an object from the floor he will usually assume a squatting position, being very careful to keep his spine straight (Fig. 66). Occasionally when there is acute pain in tuberculosis of the cervical spine, the patient may walk supporting his head with his hands, while with tuberculosis of the dorsal or lumbar spine he may walk with the vertebral column hyperextended.

Upon careful examination it may be noted that there are changes in the anteroposterior curvatures of the spine. Deformity is most marked when the lesion is located in the dorsal portion of the spine (Fig. 67). In advanced tuberculosis of the dorsal spine, the respiration may be embarrassed and of grunting type. Muscle atrophy can be demonstrated, but swelling is not obvious early unless there is an abscess pointing posteriorly. Such an abscess occurs occasionally in the lumbar region and rarely in the dorsal or cervical spine.

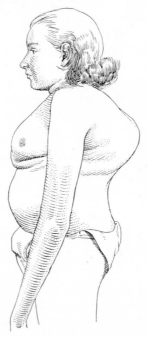

Fig. 67.—Extreme kyphosis resulting from tuberculosis of the dorsal spine. (From clinical material of Dr. G. E. Bennett.)

Abscess Formation.—An abscess presenting in a retropharyngeal position is often evidence of a tuberculous infection of the cervical spine or of a similar process between the occiput and the first cervical vertebra. Such an abscess may, by pressure upon the pharynx, produce severe respiratory embarrassment. Torticollis associated with spasm of the cervical muscles may be a sign of irritation caused by an abscess in the lower portion of the cervical spine. The abscess may point in the deep muscles on either side of the neck.

Tuberculous abscesses of the upper dorsal spine point into the posterior mediastinum. As the abscess increases in size it may occasionally rupture into the pleura or lung, or it may traverse the intercostal muscles to point on the posterolateral aspect of the chest. Thoracic abscesses have been known to follow along the course of the aorta to the diaphragm and to localize in the pelvis as iliac abscesses, but as a rule they are stopped by the diaphragm. In the lower dorsal and upper lumbar spine the abscess may enter the sheath of the psoas muscle and follow its course to (1) point in the area of the lumbar muscles, (2) point on the inner side of the thigh, (3) point on the outer portion of the groin about the attachment of Poupart's ligament, (4) extend back to point in Petit's triangle (formed by the quadratus lumborum, midline, and crest of the ilium), or (5) point in the gluteal region below the sacrosciatic notch (Fig. 68). When the abscess enters the psoas muscle sheath it often causes an irritation of the muscle which results in flexion contracture of the hip. In such flexion contracture, any attempt at extension is painful. The spasm and pain often cause an obvious limp.

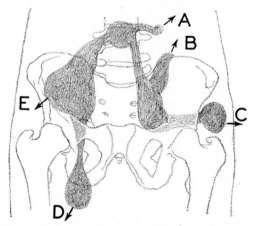

Fig. 68.—The most common sites of localization of abscesses in tuberculosis of the lumbar spine. *A,* Lumbar; *B,* in Petit's triangle; *C,* gluteal; *D,* femoral; *E,* inguinal. (After Calot.)

Neurologic Changes.—Compression of the spinal cord occurs in from 6 to 24 per cent of the cases of tuberculosis of the spine. It is most likely to complicate lesions of the upper and middorsal portions of the spine, where the spinal canal is narrow and kyphosis is normally present.

The symptoms of cord compression may appear as early as six months after the onset of the tuberculosis. The first symptom may be awkwardness in gait, followed by stumbling and inability to control the legs. Usually spastic paralysis of the legs then develops. The extensor muscles are particularly affected, and the deep reflexes are markedly hyperactive. Occasionally when compression of the cord is more complete the paralysis may be temporarily of the flaccid type. Incontinence of bladder and bowels is sometimes present. There are usually no sensory disturbances.

Diagnosis.—The diagnosis of tuberculosis of the spine is based upon the history and the findings on clinical and roentgenographic examination. A positive tuberculin test is corroborative evidence. In advanced cases, the abscess formation and paraplegia provide further confirmation.

Differential Diagnosis.—In all portions of the spine, chronic arthritis, osteomyelitis, fungus infections, benign and malignant tumors, and fracture are to be differentiated from tuberculosis. Of other affections which should be considered, the following are the most common; (1) in the cervical spine, torticollis and tuberculosis of the glands of the neck; (2) in the dorsal spine, osteochondritis, rickets, and scoliosis; (3) in the lumbar spine, tuberculosis of the hips and sacroiliac joints, lumbosacral sprain, rupture of an intervertebral disk, congenital anomaly, spondylolisthesis, retroperitoneal infection, and injury of the soft tissues.

Treatment.—The object of treatment is to arrest the disease while the spine is in the best possible position for function.

Conservative Treatment.—The general treatment must receive first consideration. It consists of ensuring proper rest, food, fresh air, sunshine, hygienic surroundings, and appropriate medication to build up the resistance of the body.

The local treatment falls into three chronological phases: (1) recumbency, (2) ambulation, and (3) convalescence.

Recumbency eliminates the strain upon the diseased vertebrae. In the active stages of the disease recumbency is imperative to prevent increase of the deformity. The affected part of the spine should be fixed in a position of slight hyperextension to allow healing to take place with as nearly normal a restoration of the general alignment of the spine as possible. The back may be supported on a Bradford or Whitman frame

(Fig. 69), or it may be splinted in a position of hyperextension by means of plaster shells (Fig. 70). For lesions of the cervical spine in children, nine months of recumbency are often sufficient. It these cases it may be advisable to apply traction to the head with the neck in hyperextension. When the upper dorsal spine is involved, it is difficult at times to obtain adequate immobilization without the use of a posterior plaster shell which covers the trunk and shoulders and extends up over the neck and

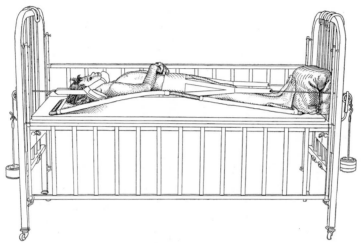

Fig. 69.—Whitman frame with head and pelvic traction for treatment of tuberculosis of the lumbar spine. Note fracture board in place of mattress.

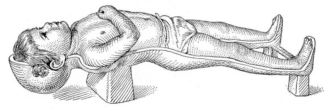

Fig. 70.—Full length posterior plaster shell for treatment of tuberculosis of the upper lumbar or dorsal spine.

head. The period of recumbency in tuberculosis of the upper dorsal vertebrae is longer than in lesions at any other level of the spine. Eighteen to twenty-four months is the average period for children. In disease of the lumbar spine, plaster shells or a Bradford or Whitman frame will provide adequate immobilization. The period of recumbency should be from sixteen to eighteen months. In all instances recumbency should be continued until: (1) all pain has disappeared; (2) the general condition of the patient is good; (3) no increase of the kyphosis is taking place; (4) the temperature is normal; and (5) most important of all, roentgenographic evidence of new bone formation is unquestionably present. Occasionally the period of recumbency must be continued for as long as five years or more.

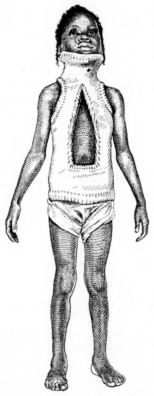

Fig. 71.—Modified Calot plaster jacket for treatment of tuberculosis of upper dorsal or lower cervical spine.

The period of ambulation should extend over at least two years, during which time the patient wears either a plaster cast or a brace. For the cervical spine either a Calot jacket (Fig. 71) or a brace which immobilizes the head, neck and back is used. For the upper dorsal spine, the body and neck must be included in a carefully moulded plaster support or reinforced leather brace. For the lower dorsal and lumbar spine the cast (Fig. 72) or brace (Fig. 73) should be sufficiently large and strong to immobilize the entire trunk.

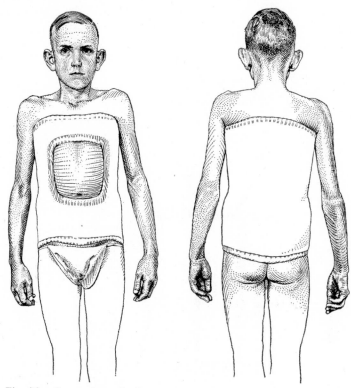

Fig. 72.—Sayre plaster body jacket for ambulatory treatment of tuberculosis of lumbar spine.

The period of convalescence begins when sufficient progress has been made to allow gradual removal of the brace. The patient should now be observed periodically for at least ten years. If at any time during this period there is unusual fatigue, loss of weight, or complaint of pain in the back, the patient must again be made recumbent and kept so until the symptoms have completely subsided. This is most important, as the recurrence of an old tuberculous process may be more severe than the original infection. Periodic roentgenographic examination of the affected portion of the spine should be made.

In early cases correction of the kyphosis may sometimes be obtained by gradually increasing the hyperextension during recumbency. In older cases, in which the tissue changes are fixed, little can be done to reduce the deformity.

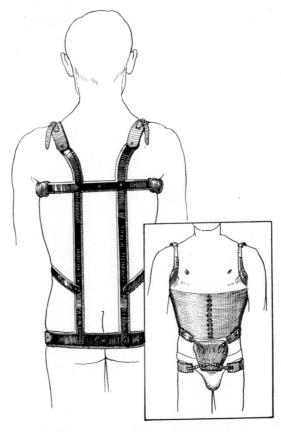

Fig. 73.—Large spinal brace for treatment of tuberculosis of lower dorsal or upper lumbar spine (modification of Bennett brace).

Operative Treatment.—In tuberculosis of the spine an operative stabilization may be indicated to lessen the period of convalescence. It is performed more often in adults than in children, although enthusiastic supporters of arthrodesis have advocated its use in patients of all ages.

Some orthopaedic surgeons believe, on the other hand, that an operative stabilization is indicated only when the patient is over twelve years of age.

The functional result after conservative treatment with a long period of recumbency is thought by some to be better than that following operative stabilization followed by early ambulation. In 62 per cent of the cases the kyphosis undergoes gradual increase regardless of whether arthrodesis has been performed. If it has been decided that an operative stabilization should be performed, a preliminary period of recumbency, during which the general condition of the patient may be studied and improved, is always advisable.

Hibbs and Albee in 1912 were the first to describe effective methods of of arthrodesis of the spine. They reported that about 90 per cent of the tuberculous processes treated with their respective stabilization operations were arrested.

The Hibbs method consists of splitting the spinous processes into small fragments, chipping up the outer surfaces of the laminal arches, removing the cartilage from the articular facets, and placing the bone chips as bridges across the denuded bone of the posterior surfaces of the vertebral arches (Fig. 74). It is often advisable, especially in adults, to reenforce this bridge of bone chips with additional autogenous bone from the iliac crest or the tibia or bone from a bone bank. The Albee method, which is now seldom used, comprises longitudinal splitting of the spinous processes and inserting a long cortical bone graft from the tibia between their two halves. There is a difference of opinion as to the necessary after-care. Some surgeons allow walking in five or six weeks with or without a brace. The absence of a back support is believed by some surgeons to stimulate bone formation. In most clinics, however, the patients are kept at rest in bed for at least twelve weeks after operation, following which an ambulatory brace is worn for a period of a year from the time of operation.

It has been demonstrated that with any form of treatment ossification of the tuberculous lesion may not take place for three years from the time of onset of the disease. Some clinics report that the average period of treatment for tuberculosis of the spine is seven and one-half years.

Treatment of Tuberculous Abscess.—As a rule tuberculous abscesses should not be opened unless there is severe pain or embarrassment from pressure. The principles of treatment of such abscesses have been described. Abscesses at times become walled off from the original tuberculous focus and may become calcified or completely absorbed. During the stage of recumbency 70 per cent of the psoas abscesses regress and do not require aspiration or incision. After an abscess has been opened, it may drain for an indefinite period and secondary infection is unavoidable; hence it is advisable to postpone intervention as long as possible.

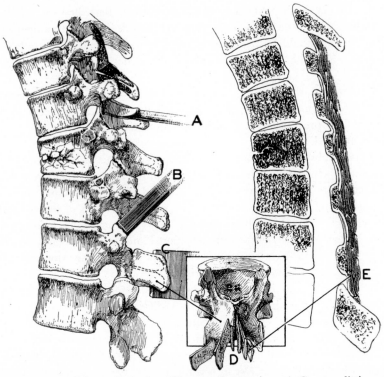

Fig. 74.—Hibbs method of stabilization of the spine. *A*, Gouge splitting off and turning down chips from spinous processes and laminae; *B*, chisel removing cartilage from articular facets; *C*, splitting spinous processes; *D*, posterior view showing splitting of spinous processes; *E*, sagittal section of spine showing continuous layer of small grafts posterior to the denuded laminae.

The treatment of tuberculous abscess varies somewhat according to the portion of the spine involved. A retropharyngeal abscess may have to be opened because of its exerting pressure on the throat. For a mediastinal abscess which is causing pressure on the heart or lungs, costotransversectomy is occasionally indicated to allow for drainage. Psoas abscesses which point in the iliac and inguinal regions are frequently mistaken for hernias or appendiceal abscesses and may be opened under a mistaken diagnosis. Streptomycin is most effective in the absence of undrained pus; it should therefore always be used when an abscess is evacuated or drained.

Treatment of Paralysis.—The treatment of paralysis of the lower extremities secondary to vertebral tuberculosis is absolute recumbency with the spine in slight hyperextension. It may take from six months to five years for complete function of the legs to return. Ninety per cent of these patients, however, recover with no residual muscular weakness. Occasionally, aspirating an abscess may relieve the pressure upon the spinal cord. A laminotomy or laminectomy may be done if there is no return of muscle power. Some surgeons advocate performing this operation early, others after waiting at least eighteen months, and others only when sensory symptoms are present. It may be necessary to follow laminectomy with a bone graft. Patients who do not recover after the pressure has been relieved by operation may have developed a tuberculous infection of the meninges or spinal cord. A paralysis may recur many years after apparent cure; this sometimes results from a latent abscess which has never completely healed.

Prognosis.—Tuberculosis of the spine is unquestionably the most serious form of bone and joint tuberculosis. Statistics indicate that it is fatal in from 15 to 50 per cent of the cases. The mortality statistics may prove to be somewhat lower since the advent of streptomycin. The prognosis is most serious in lesions of the dorsal spine, from which the rupture of an abscess into the lung or pleural cavity is always a possibility. Spinal tuberculosis is always attended by the danger of tuberculous meningitis, which is often fatal. In tuberculosis of the spine which persists over a period of years with secondarily infected draining sinuses, amyloid disease of the liver, spleen, kidneys, and other organs may form a fatal complication. Severe thoracic deformity distorts vital organs and lowers the patient's resistance to intercurrent disease.

Tuberculosis of the Sacroiliac Joint

The sacroiliac joint is seldom involved by tuberculosis. When the infection does occur, however, it is sometimes bilateral. It is rare in children, occurring usually in young adults.

Pathology.—The disease usually starts in the sacrum and spreads to the ilium or into the lumbar spine. Abscess formation is extremely frequent; the abscess points forward more often than backward. Following the line of least resistance the pus may form a sinus tract and point (1) in the groin, (2) on the medial side of the anterosuperior spine of the ilium, (3) in the buttocks after coming through the sacrosciatic notch, or (4) in the ischiorectal fossa. Occasionally the abscess ruptures into the rectum.

Clinical Picture.—The onset is extremely insidious. Abscess formation may be the first evidence of disease. Slight pain may be present in the back. It may be referred to the hip and cause limitation of hip motion. There may be increased pain upon sitting, climbing, or walking. Coughing, laughing, and sneezing may cause pain in the sacroiliac joint. Radiating pain occasionally occurs in the back of the thigh. In other cases the pain radiates down the lateral aspect of the thigh or the front of the leg. The characteristic signs and symptoms of a low back sprain may be present, including deviation of the lumbar spine from the affected sacroiliac joint, lumbar muscle spasm, and marked limitation of all motion in the lumbar spine, with pain referred to the sacroiliac joint on attempts to flex the spine. There may also be a positive straight leg-raising test on the affected side, pain in the affected side on straight leg-raising on the opposite side, and complete inability to bend forward with the knees in full extension. Pressing the iliac crests firmly together will cause pain in the affected sacroiliac joint. The patient tires easily and loses weight. In late stages the gait is characteristic, as the patient walks with extremely short steps, keeping his knees close together and shuffling his feet.

Diagnosis.—Roentgenographic changes may be late in appearing. The earliest finding is haziness or loss of definition of the joint line. The articular surfaces then become irregular with areas of erosion. The disease is to be differentiated from a low back sprain or arthritis, rheumatoid arthritis of the hip, early Strümpell-Marie arthritis of the sacroiliac joints and lumbar spine, sciatic neuritis, rupture of an intervertebral disk, and myositis.

Treatment.—General therapy, including proper diet, fresh air, and hygienic surroundings, is essential. Streptomycin and para-aminosalicylic acid are helpful.

Conservative treatment is indicated first. Rest can be obtained by fixation in plaster. This should be accomplished by the use of a double spica cast, carried to the knees and incorporating at least two-thirds of the trunk. Occasionally simple recumbency upon a Bradford frame provides sufficient immobilization of the pelvis and sacroiliac joints. Plaster, however, permits much more efficient fixation.

A stabilization operation is indicated if conservative therapy has not proved successful. It is advisable to curette away the infected tissue within the joint at the time of the stabilization operation. The following methods are satisfactory for fusing the sacroiliac joint:

1. Removing the posterosuperior spine and adjacent crest of the ilium, exposing the joint, curetting away the infected tissue, and then placing the resected bone between the upper portions of the joint surfaces (Picqué).

2. Removing a rectangular section of bone from the ilium over the lower margin of the sacroiliac joint, curetting away the infected tissue, and replacing this rectangular section to act as a bone graft after its inner surface has been denuded of cartilage (Smith-Petersen).

3. Placing an extra-articular graft across the sacroiliac joint at its upper margin (Campbell).

Prognosis.—In adults with abscess formation the mortality rate is high. Cases treated early have a much more favorable prognosis.

CHAPTER IX

TUBERCULOSIS OF BONES AND JOINTS: THE EXTREMITIES

Tuberculosis of the Hip

Incidence.—Involvement of the hip constitutes about 30 per cent of all bone and joint tuberculosis. It is more common in early childhood, 88 per cent of the cases occurring in children under ten years of age and 45 per cent between the ages of three and five years. It is slightly more common in the male than the female and is seen more frequently in the right than the left hip.

Pathology.—The lesion may first appear near the epiphyseal cartilage of the head of the femur where the blood supply is poorest and where newly formed bone has least resistance. However, the original focus of tuberculosis may be in the acetabulum. Occasionally the tubercle bacilli first lodge in the synovial membrane. Usually the bacilli are borne by the blood stream to the small terminal vessels of the bone, where tubercle formation takes place and is followed by the appearance of tuberculous granulation tissue. The disease process usually extends into the joint, where tuberculous granulations either undermine the cartilage or spread from the joint margins over the cartilaginous surfaces and destroy them. At first there is an increase of joint fluid, but, as the infection progresses, a purulent exudate is formed and rapidly fills the joint. The periarticular tissues become edematous and thickened, appear grayish, and show necrotic changes. Because of muscle spasm the head of the femur exerts an increased upward pressure upon the upper acetabular margin; this may result in erosion of the femoral head and of the acetabulum (Fig. 76). The acetabulum becomes enlarged about its superior border as it erodes and has been termed the "wandering acetabulum." As the disease progresses the purulent exudate increases in volume and often breaks through the capsule and spreads in the lines of least resistance. It may go (1) forward to point in the groin, (2) toward the greater trochanter to point either in front of or behind it, (3) back into the buttock, or (4) through the acetabulum to form a pelvic abscess. Abscesses are demonstrable in 50 per cent of the cases of tuberculosis of the hip. If there is sufficient tension in the abscess, it will dissect to the skin and rupture.

Healing of the hip lesion takes place by absorption of the exudate, replacement with fibrous tissue, and laying down of new bone. The new bone is first seen in the roentgenogram as a line of increased calcification about the margins of the joint.

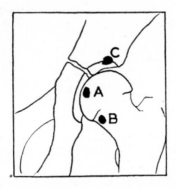

Fig. 75.—Common points of origin of tuberculosis of the hip. *A,* Head of femur; *B,* medial portion of femoral neck adjacent to the epiphyseal line; *C,* upper margin of acetabulum.

Clinical Picture.—As in tuberculosis of other joints, the premonitory symptoms of malaise, loss of appetite, and loss of weight are usually present.

One of the first characteristic symptoms is slight stiffness of the hip, accompanied by a limp in the morning. The limp may rapidly pass off during the day to return later. The patient has a tendency to protect the affected extremity. The stiffness may be followed by pain referred down the courses of the obturator and the femoral nerves to the knee. In children pain may be evidenced by night cries, which are caused by sudden discomfort due to rubbing together of the inflamed bony surfaces following relaxation of the muscles in sleep. These symptoms are followed by a noticeable loss of weight and afternoon fever, both of which are greater in the presence of abscess formation. Deformity may quickly follow the development of pain but is more often a late sign.

Limitation of motion of the hip is one of the first signs to appear and one of the last to disappear. It often precedes any abnormality of gait.

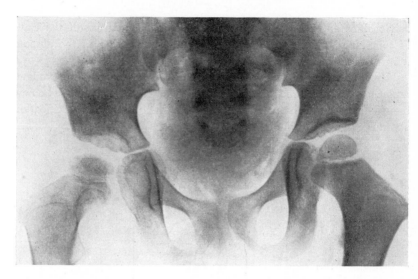

Fig. 76A.—Anteroposterior roentgenogram showing tuberculosis of right hip in boy three and one-half years of age. Note the osteoporosis or decalcification of upper end of femur and acetabulum, a flattening of the capital epiphysis, and a circumscribed oval area of increased calcification in the inferior portion of the neck. There is lateral displacement of the head of the femur from the acetabulum.

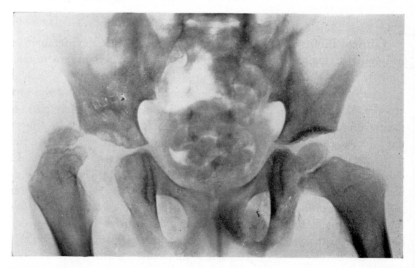

Fig. 76B.—Anteroposterior roentgenogram showing tuberculosis of hip in patient in Fig. 76A, one month later. Note the upward dislocation of the right hip. This followed the removal of skin traction and is a true pathologic dislocation.

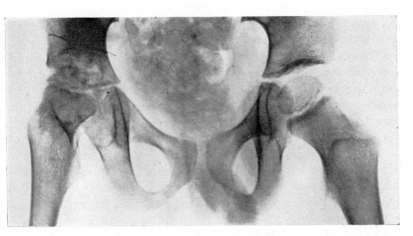

Fig. 76C.—Anteroposterior roentgenogram showing tuberculosis of hip in patient in Fig. 76A, two years later. Patient had been immobilized continuously in plaster. Note the erosion in the superior portion of the acetabulum, the upward displacement of the femoral head and the irregular calcification of the epiphysis.

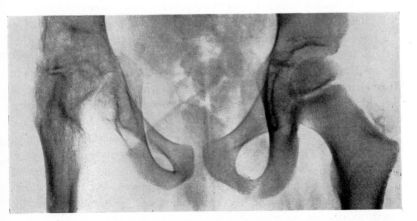

Fig. 76D.—Anteroposterior roentgenogram showing tuberculosis of hip in patient in Fig. 76A, four and one-half years later. An extra-articular arthrodesis had been done two and one-half years previously. Note the continuous bony structure from the upper end of the femur to the acetabulum, upward displacement of the head, and marked atrophy of the shaft.

In the early stages the limitation of motion is usually due to reflex muscle spasm. Later it may be caused by actual pain on motion of the joint and finally by destruction of the joint surfaces. Another of the early signs is a palpable thickening of the tissues about the hip.

The type of hip deformity is characteristic of the stage of the disease. Following the initial increase of joint fluid, which distends the capsule and results in pain, the extremity is flexed at the hip, abducted, and outwardly rotated. In this position the joint capsule is relaxed, and the pain is relieved. There is an apparent lengthening of the extremity in this stage due to the abduction, and the patient walks carefully on the toes so that most of the weight falls upon the anterior part of the foot. Seldom is the heel brought down, since any jarring causes pain. As the disease progresses, the hip becomes adducted and internally rotated as well as flexed, which results in an apparent shortening. Several factors produce this change. Spasm of the strong adductor muscles is one cause; in adduction the leg is less likely to be suddenly jarred or injured; and because of destruction of the acetabulum and head of the femur there is an upward displacement of the femur. This displacement may progress to result in a posterior dislocation. In the position characteristic of the second stage, the pelvis is elevated on the affected side while the lumbar spine develops a convexity toward the unaffected side. Above the lumbar region compensatory curves are usually observed.

Examination is best carried out with the patient upon a hard table. The normal hip should be placed in a position symmetrical with that of the affected one. The range of passive motion is gently tested; any abnormal restriction is suggestive of inflammation within the joint. Measurements are then taken from the anterior superior iliac spine of each side to the corresponding medial malleolus. The difference between these measurements is the real or actual shortening of the leg. In late cases in children the shortening may be due to retardation of growth at all the epiphyses of the long bones of the extremity as well as to the destructive process in the hip. It is known also that disuse of an extremity causes retardation of its development. Rarely, however, lengthening of the affected leg occurs because of stimulation of the growth at one or more epiphyses.

Atrophy of the muscles of the affected limb is a constant finding in tuberculosis of the hip. The degree of atrophy varies with the duration of the disease. There is often hypertrophy of the sound limb because of its increased use. Nearly always there are changes in the contours about the joint; the gluteal fold is shallow and often obliterated. Swelling due to periarticular inflammation or an abscess may occur in any area about the hip.

Occasional cases of tuberculosis limited to the greater trochanter or its bursae are seen. They do not present the extensive clinical signs of tuberculosis of the hip joint and are usually best treated by excision of the diseased tissue.

Roentgenographic Picture.—Early tuberculosis of the hip shows in the roentgenogram osteoporosis and a haziness of the joint margins; in the later stages there may be evidence of destruction of the joint surfaces, narrowing of the joint space, and bone atrophy. Destructive changes are usually seen first in the lower side of the neck of the femur adjacent to its head. An erosion of the upper portion of the head and of the upper portion of the acetabulum may be observed later (Fig. 76,*C*). In the early stages there is little evidence of new bone formation. When this is present the healing process is definitely taking place. Occasionally sufficient new bone is produced to effect spontaneous fusion of the joint.

Diagnosis.—A tentative diagnosis is made from the history, physical signs, and roentgenogram. A final diagnosis cannot be made, however, until (1) tubercle bacilli have been found in the joint fluid, (2) tubercle formation has been demonstrated at biopsy, or (3) a guinea pig inoculated with fluid or with a tissue emulsion obtained from the hip has developed tuberculosis. In many instances the clinical diagnosis of tuberculosis of the hip is later proved erroneous.

Differential Diagnosis.—There are many affections which may be confused with tuberculosis of the hip. The most common of these is coxa plana or Legg-Perthes' disease. Before this affection was found to be of nontuberculous origin, it was repeatedly diagnosed as a low-grade tuberculous coxitis. Subacute pyogenic epiphysitis, low-grade osteomyelitis of the upper end of the femur or of the pelvis, or pyogenic arthritis may give all the symptoms and signs of an early tuberculosis of the hip. Rheumatoid arthritis may start in the hip joint with the same symptoms. Traumatic synovitis of the hip is often confusing. Tuberculosis of the spine, with abscess formation causing psoas irritation and contracture of the hip, must be excluded. The same is true of inflammation of the retroperitoneal lymph nodes, perinephritis, and appendicitis, all of which may cause irritation of the psoas muscle.

Less common conditions sometimes confused with tuberculosis of the hip are inflammation of the iliopsoas muscle or the deep trochanteric bursa, extra-articular infection, slipping of the upper femoral epiphysis, congenital coxa vara, congenital dislocation of the hip, scurvy, rickets, and hemophilia.

Infantile paralysis, hysterical joints, and certain upper motor neurone lesions may on rare occasions give rise to symptoms similar to those of tuberculosis of the hip. In adults osteoarthritis of the hip sometimes simulates an old tuberculous arthritis.

Treatment.—The treatment may be divided into general and local measures. General treatment should include rest, a well-balanced and nourishing diet, hygienic surroundings, fresh air, sunshine, and the administration of streptomycin and para-aminosalicylic acid.

As in all bone and joint tuberculosis, rest is the essential principle of local treatment. Rest for the hip may be obtained through conservative or operative means. The objectives of treatment are (1) to relieve acute pain and muscle spasm, (2) to prevent the development of deformity or to correct any deformity which is already present, and (3) to promote healing of the destructive infectious process.

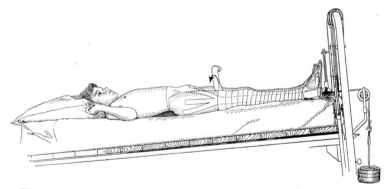

Fig. 77.—Adhesive traction used in the treatment of tuberculosis of the hip.

During the acute stage traction applied to the leg is the best means of relieving the pain and muscle spasm (Fig. 77). The necessary tension may be obtained by the use of weights with the patient in bed or by use of a hip spica cast incorporating a traction windlass. Traction relieves the pressure on inflamed contiguous surfaces within the joint and so tends to prevent destructive changes and allow healing to take place.

It should be continued until (1) there is no pain in the joint, (2) there is no evidence of abscess formation, (3) the night cries have ceased, (4) the deformity has been reduced, (5) there is no afternoon fever, (6) the general condition is definitely improving, and (7) there is roentgenographic evidence of recalcification in the diseased area.

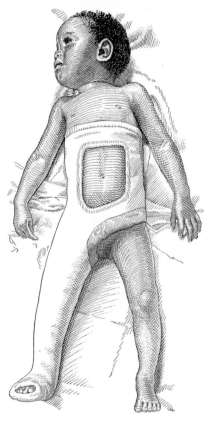

Fig. 78.—Single hip spica cast for immobilization in tuberculosis of the hip in a young child. It is often preferable to use a bilateral spica cast extending to the toes on the affected side and only to the knee on the unaffected side, as shown in Fig. 27.

When no indication of active infection within the joint remains, the second stage of treatment is started. A single or bilateral plaster spica cast is by far the best means of securing immobilization (Figs. 27 and 78). Occasionally it is desirable to incorporate adhesive traction straps in the plaster. During this stage use may be made of hip traction splints, such as the Jones abduction splint, which is widely used in England. When the patient is allowed up on crutches in this splint or cast, he should wear a high-sole shoe on the sound leg, which prevents weight from being borne on the affected hip. When the patient can be allowed greater freedom, an accurately fitting Thomas ischial-bearing walking caliper splint may be applied. This takes the weight off the hip and puts it upon the tuberosity of the ischium. Ambulation without weight-bearing should be continued for at least a year if there is any indication whatever that the infection is still active. A gradual return to weight-bearing is then permitted; this period should extend over at least another year. The hip should be observed every three months for three years after the patient starts unrestricted walking. If there is a tendency toward recurrence, the patient should at once be put back to bed and the strain of weight-bearing taken off the hip. Especial care should be taken to forestall the development of a deformity of the hip. When a tuberculous hip has not undergone bony ankylosis, the danger of its developing a deformity is always present.

Operative Treatment.—Arthrodesis of the hip is often indicated in an effort to secure strong bony ankylosis in good position with as little loss of time as possible after the process of healing has begun. While some surgeons advocate operative treatment for adults only, others employ it for children as well. Before surgery is performed, it is advisable that the patient be in the best possible physical condition and gaining weight. It is often helpful to perform the operation through a large window in the cast; this insures good position and minimizes shock. Operation must be followed by an ample and closely fitting bilateral spica cast for at least six to nine months, or until roentgenograms show strong bony union, after which a gradual return to weight-bearing under supervision is allowed.

Hibbs in 1926 first reported a fusion operation for the treatment of tuberculosis of the hip; his method consisted of transplanting a portion of the upper end of the femur across to the upper margin of the aceta-bulum. Modifications of the Hibbs procedure are now more popular than the original technic. From 60 to 70 per cent of the primary opera-tions of this type result in bony fusion. These operations are done without destroying the structures within the diseased joint. In performing the operation, it is often impossible, however, to avoid exposing the tuberculous tissue. Exposure of the operative field to the infection does not necessarily result in unsuccessful fusion.

An alternative method of iliofemoral fusion, perfected by John C. Wilson, is the turning down of a large flap of bone from the outer table of the iliac wing and fixing this securely into the split greater trochanter. This technic is particularly suitable for the relatively plastic bone of children.

A method of fusing the upper portion of the femoral shaft to the ischium by osteotomy and bone graft has been described by Trumble and modified by Brittain. Direct ischio-femoral transplantation has been described by Bosworth. These operations have the advantage of permanently relieving the diseased hip joint of the pressure of weight-bearing. They are particularly useful when there has been extensive destruction of the ilium or the upper end of the femur.

Prognosis.—In tuberculosis of the hip, the prognosis both as to survival and as to joint function is better in children than in adults, and especially when there is complete ankylosis. Tuberculous meningitis is a frequent complication.

Tuberculosis of the Knee

Incidence.—In frequency, tuberculosis of the knee ranks next to that of the spine and hip. Eighty-seven per cent of the cases occur in childhood; 51 per cent occur in children under five years of age.

Pathology.—The infectious process may begin either in bone or in the synovial membrane. When bone is the site of origin, the infection starts either in the epiphysis of the femur or in that of the tibia. Apparently it occurs as frequently in one as the other. From the primary site the process may spread into the joint. Before the infection reaches the joint cavity, there is a secondary synovitis; after it enters the cavity, the synovium becomes thickened, adhesions form, and tuberculous granulations cover and destroy the articular cartilages. Often there is a tuberculous infiltration of the periarticular tissues which gives them a boggy consistency.

Abscesses occur in about one-third of the treated cases and in a larger percentage of untreated cases. In patients with abscesses the mortality rate is doubled. Occasionally the abscess may rupture into the surrounding tissues, infiltrating the muscles, tendons, and fascial planes, and causing extensive and serious soft tissue infection. Occasionally the abscess ruptures through the skin to form a chronically draining sinus.

Clinical Picture.—The first symptoms are usually a slight limp and limitation of motion caused by protective muscle spasm. This is followed by swelling of the knee, increase in local heat, and slight pain and tenderness. Muscle atrophy is severe in the later stages, and a flexion deformity may develop. The tendency toward flexion may be a result of pain when the articular surfaces are in contact, the area of contact being least when the knee is flexed. Secondary changes, such as outward rotation of the tibia on the femur or posterior subluxation of the tibia, are not uncommon. If erosion of one condyle takes place without a symmetrical erosion of the other, genu valgum or genu varum may develop.

Shortening of the affected extremity is a frequent finding. In children the shortening may be caused by the presence of infection at the epiphyseal lines, since most of the growth of the extremity normally takes place at the epiphyses about the knee. An additional cause of shortening is actual destruction of the joint surfaces. Occasionally the infection causes a stimulation of epiphyseal growth and results in lengthening of the extremity. In children, however, the influence of weight-bearing tends to result in gradual equalization of the length of the legs.

Diagnosis.—As in the case of other tuberculous infections the diagnosis should be made from the history, physical signs, roentgenograms, and demonstration of tubercles or tubercle bacilli by culture or biopsy. Occasionally it is difficult to differentiate between tuberculosis of the knee and rheumatoid arthritis.

Other affections which may cause symptoms simulating those of tuberculosis and must be excluded when the diagnosis is being made are traumatic or pyogenic synovitis; traumatic hemarthrosis; gonococcal arthritis; acute rheumatic fever; bursitis; rickets; scurvy; syphilis; and hemophilic, neuropathic, and hysterical joint syndromes.

Treatment.—The treatment may be divided into general and local measures. A nutritious diet, fresh air, rest, and heliotherapy are essential. Streptomycin and para-aminosalicylic acid are indicated.

The local treatment depends much upon the age of the individual. In children conservative treatment is indicated, and recumbency upon a Bradford frame with the leg in adhesive traction is a very satisfactory form of immobilization. This treatment should be continued for twelve months. Some clinics make use of the Thomas knee splint with a knee flexion attachment permitting of a moderate amount of motion. If the tuberculous process is advanced and there is a marked amount of joint destruction, immobilization in plaster is indicated in the hope of obtaining spontaneous fusion. The plaster may be applied as a leg cast or a hip spica cast. After the subsidence of pain, tenderness, increased local heat, muscle spasm, and other evidence of active infection, and after the roentgenograms have begun to show recalcification, the patient may be allowed to walk without bearing weight upon the affected leg. The combination of a Thomas knee splint applied to the affected leg, a high-sole shoe on the normal leg, and crutches should be employed for about eighteen months. After this period a gradual return to weight-bearing is allowed. The patient should then be observed at intervals for at least three years.

Flexion deformity may usually be corrected by simple adhesive traction and recumbency. It is necessary at times, however, to apply forcible correction or gradual extension by means of wedged plaster casts. The use of great force is to be condemned.

Operative Treatment.—Arthrodesis of the knee is the procedure of choice for the adult in all clinics and for the child in most clinics. It must be borne in mind that in children an arthrodesis may be followed by marked shortening of the extremity, and also that disturbances of epiphyseal growth may produce a varus, valgus, or recurvatum deformity. If such a deformity develops, an osteotomy may be indicated for its correction.

The arthrodesis is of intra-articular type. The synovial membrane, as well as the tuberculous portion of the bone, is removed; the ends of the femur and tibia are shaped to fit together accurately after their cartilaginous articular surfaces have been removed; and the denuded patella is fitted into an especially prepared bed on the anterior surface of the tibia and the femur. After operation the joint should be fixed in plaster at an angle of 170 degrees in adults or of 180 degrees in children. If in four months the union is solid, a walking caliper brace may be applied. This should be worn for from six to nine months. It has been reported that in 88 per cent of the cases this method of arthrodesis has been followed by firm bony ankylosis.

In adults excision of the knee is at times the best procedure. It always results in slight loss of length. The rapidity with which excision can be performed, however, makes it the operation of choice in patients whose condition is relatively unfavorable for operation.

Amputation should be done only as a lifesaving measure when the patient's condition is becoming progressively worse even under diligent treatment. Occasionally it is impossible to correct a flexion deformity by traction or wedged casts; in such cases supracondylar osteotomy may be indicated. Its results are usually very satisfactory.

Prognosis.—Death seldom comes as a direct consequence of tuberculosis of the knee but rather as a result of the development of tuberculosis elsewhere in the body. In children under favorable conditions of early treatment a movable joint may sometimes be obtained. In adults firm ankylosis is preferable.

Tuberculosis of the Ankle and Foot

Incidence.—From 10 to 15 per cent of the tuberculosis of the lower extremity involves the ankle and foot. It is uncommon in children under ten years of age. Males are affected more frequently than females.

Pathology.—Tuberculosis of the ankle and foot usually begins in the bone in children and in the synovium in adults. When it starts about the ankle, it arises more often in the astragalus than in the tibia or fibula. Abscesses are present in 85 per cent of the cases.

Infection of the tarsal bones without involvement of the ankle joint is commonest in the astragalus, os calcis, and cuboid bone. When a single tarsal bone is involved, a walled-off cavity similar to that of a Brodie's abscess may form. There may be a definite condensation of bone about its margins. Occasionally tuberculosis of the foot or ankle starts as a tenosynovitis. Because of the close association of the various structures of the tarsus, there is a distinct tendency for tuberculosis of a single bone to spread progressively and finally involve the whole tarsus.

Clinical Picture.—A history of minor injury preceding the onset usually can be obtained. At first there may be a slight limp, spontaneous pain at night, and pain on weight-bearing. Tenderness, muscle spasm, and restriction of motion become more marked as the disease progresses. Swelling most often appears behind the malleoli and in front of the Achilles tendon, particularly in the synovial type of infection. If the process starts in bone, swelling may be present anteriorly at the ankle. This is followed by an increase of local heat and often by redness. The patient has a tendency to walk on the heel with the foot everted and the thigh rotated outward. The deformity is first one of dorsiflexion but later changes to plantar flexion with the foot in a valgus position. If the infection starts in bone, the pain is more severe and the limp is noticeable at an earlier period. The infection may spread to cause a tuberculous synovitis and abscess formation. The abscesses often rupture and produce sinuses on the skin surface.

Often the subastragalar joint may be affected primarily; symptoms are similar to those of involvement of the ankle joint. If the astragalo-scaphoid joint is affected, the foot assumes a position of marked abduction.

When the infection is primary in a tarsal bone, limitation of motion and pain on weight-bearing are marked. They are followed by muscle spasm and atrophy. The resultant deformity is again one of plantar flexion. Infection of tarsal bones usually causes a slightly tender swelling over the bone first involved. A roentgenogram is helpful in determining in which bone the focus of infection is located.

Differential Diagnosis.—Chronic ankle or foot sprain, traumatic arthritis or synovitis, rheumatoid arthritis, chronic osteomyelitis, fracture of a tarsal bone, and Köhler's disease of the scaphoid are conditions to be differentiated from tuberculous infection of the ankle region. The signs and symptoms of any one of these conditions may simulate those of an early tuberculosis of the ankle or foot.

Treatment.—General therapy, as outlined, is most important. Streptomycin is given if sinuses are present. In the child, local therapy should be conservative. It should consist of immobilization of the foot for a period of at least twelve months by means of a plaster cast extending from the toes to above the knee. If sinuses are present, a celluloid or special metal splint sufficiently large to allow for dressings should be applied for the same length of time. This should be followed for a period of about six months by a walking caliper knee splint to relieve the foot from the strain of weight-bearing.

In the presence of deformity, such as talipes equinovalgus, attempts should be made to correct the malposition gradually by wedged plaster casts or by casts applied following gentle manipulation. Painful subcutaneous abscesses which sometimes develop during this stage may require incision.

When the infection is limited to a single tarsal bone, excision of the affected bone may result in cure. When the ankle joint alone is involved, arthrodesis is often satisfactory. In certain cases amputation in the lower third of the leg is necessary to save life. Amputation is more often necessary in the adult than in the child and especially in fulminating tuberculosis of the tarsal bones because of a tendency for the infection to metastasize to other parts of the body. In such a case delay may jeopardize the life of the patient.

Prognosis.—When the infectious process remains limited to the ankle, the prognosis is good for both life and function, especially in the younger child. The prognosis is poor, however, when multiple sinus formation occurs, since it is then often impossible to arrest the infection. Frequently the growth of the foot is much retarded. The prognosis is always better when the disease is treated early. In a considerable percentage of the cases, tuberculosis of the ankle is complicated ultimately by the development of generalized tuberculosis.

Tuberculosis of the Shoulder

Tuberculosis of the joints of the upper extremity is uncommon as compared with that of the lower extremity and constitutes only from 1 to 2 per cent of the tuberculous infections of the extremities. Involvement of the shoulder is especially uncommon in children.

Pathology.—The infection is much more frequently of bony than synovial origin. It starts most often in the head of the humerus near the bicipital groove. The infectious process may assume a dry form, *caries sicca,* in which there is no enlargement, swelling, or abscess formation. Instead there is a gradual destruction of the head of the humerus followed by a replacement of the bone by tuberculous granulation tissue. Such a process is sometimes spoken of as the "quiet type" of tuberculosis. The destruction of the bone is caused by a gradual wearing away of its joint surface rather than a caseative disintegration. The dry form is seen more frequently than the wet form, which is accompanied by abscess formation.

Clinical Picture.—The symptoms are much less severe than in involvement of the lower extremity. The onset is usually insidious. The pain is often of dull, aching character and frequently is referred to the front of the arm as far down as the elbow. It is difficult sometimes to recognize abnormal limitation of motion because of the mobility of the scapula. Abduction and external rotation are the first movements to be limited. As the restriction of motion grows more pronounced the scapula becomes fixed with the arm in adduction. With the resulting severe muscle atrophy there may be flattening and angulation of the shoulder and occasionally a subluxation of the joint. If an abscess forms it usually points anteriorly.

Differential Diagnosis.—Rheumatoid arthritis, subacromial bursitis, syphilis, osteogenic sarcoma, bone cyst, and traumatic arthritis are to be considered in the differential diagnosis.

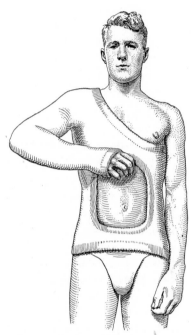

Fig. 79.—Plaster spica cast for immobilization in tuberculosis of the shoulder.

Treatment.—General therapy should be carried out as previously described. Conservative local therapy consists of immobilization of the joint, preferably in a shoulder spica cast with the arm in 45 degrees forward flexion and in a position of at least 50 degrees of abduction (Fig. 79). When the joint becomes fixed, this is the position of optimum function. Some authors advise abduction of 75 degrees in adults, and of 90 degrees in children. The cast should be worn for several months after the subsidence of all signs of active infection and may be followed by an abduction brace for several additional months.

Operative Treatment.—In adults the most satisfactory surgical procedure is arthrodesis of the shoulder. At operation the tuberculous tissue is first thoroughly excised. Several satisfactory methods of securing fusion between the upper end of the humerus and the scapula have been described (see page 256).

Prognosis.—Treatment may extend over a period of from two to five years before recovery takes place. Healing usually results in stiffening of the joint. If recovery occurs in childhood, the arm may be shortened. Tuberculosis of the lungs is a common complication.

Tuberculosis of the Elbow

Incidence.—Tuberculosis of the elbow is more frequently observed than tuberculosis of the shoulder. It is much more common in adults than in children, and in England than in America.

Pathology.—It has been reported that 93 per cent of the lesions start in bone. The focus of infection is most often in the olecranon process of the ulna, and the next most frequent site is the external condyle of the humerus. The head of the radius is very infrequently involved. The infection often spreads to the remaining parts of the joint.

Clinical Picture.—The first symptoms may be very slight discomfort, stiffness, and swelling of the joint. When swelling appears, it is usually first noticeable behind the joint, and as it becomes more marked the elbow acquires a fusiform or spindle shape. Extensive periarticular involvement is usually present and leads to a doughy, elastic consistency on palpation of the elbow. Motion is painful. At first only the extremes of motion are limited; as the condition progresses, muscle spasm becomes marked, abscess formation is very common, and sinuses are likely to develop. The abscess usually points near the external condyle. There is practically always an elevation of the local temperature. Above and below the swollen joint, muscle atrophy may be conspicuous (Fig. 80).

Treatment.—General therapy as outlined previously is important. The early case should be treated by absolute rest in plaster with the forearm in a position of 90 degrees flexion and midway between pronation and supination. If the elbow has become extended more than 90 degrees, the forearm should be brought up gradually to a right angle. The "collar and cuff" method of treatment is popular in England: a bandage is applied around the wrist and the neck with the elbow flexed. This method may also be used to secure an improved functional position of the elbow.

Operative Treatment.—In adults the tuberculous focus should be removed surgically when possible. Occasionally an excision of the joint is indicated. Some authors suggest an arthrodesis by removal of the articular surfaces, while others recommend an extra-articular arthrodesis by placing an osteoperiosteal graft posteriorly from humerus to ulna.

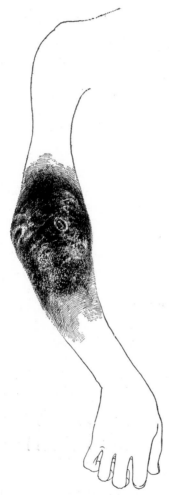

Fig. 80.—Untreated tuberculosis of the elbow in the late stage. Note the swelling, sinus formation, and muscle atrophy.

Prognosis.—If treatment is begun early in the course of the disease the prognosis for a useful elbow is good. Life is seldom endangered. In childhood 50 per cent of the treated cases retain fair mobility.

Ankylosis in the optimal position of 90 degrees flexion and midway between pronation and supination is compatible with good function of the extremity.

Tuberculosis of the Wrist

Tuberculosis of the wrist is uncommon in children and is the least frequent form of joint tuberculosis in the upper extremity.

Pathology.—The infection usually starts in the lower end of the radius, in the os magnum, or in the synovium. It becomes rapidly disseminated through the synovial membrane and tendon sheaths. Abscess formation soon occurs and is followed by the development of many draining sinuses.

Clinical Picture.—Swelling appears early because of the superficial position of the bony structures. It is usually the first indication of disease and is followed by pain and tenderness. Muscle spasm develops, motion becomes restricted, and the deformity of volar flexion often results. The joint sometimes becomes subluxated. A picture typical of tuberculosis of the wrist is that of a large spindle-shaped swelling with draining sinuses situated between an atrophied forearm and hand; the fingers are likely to be held in full extension.

Diagnosis.—With the characteristic symptoms and roentgenograms the diagnosis is not difficult. Tuberculosis of the wrist may occasionally be confused, however, with the disintegrated wrist joint of rheumatoid or severe gonococcal arthritis, with subacute osteomyelitis of the carpal bones, or with a neurotrophic arthropathy.

Treatment.—General therapy should be carried out. The forearm should be put in a plaster cast or upon a splint with the wrist in a position of 35 degrees of dorsiflexion. The splint should extend to the metacarpophalangeal joints but should not go beyond this point because of the danger of ankylosis of the phalangeal joints. Early movement of the fingers is imperative. The support should fit closely and must be worn for at least eighteen months. In children the cast should extend above the elbow in order to provide more thorough immobilization. Flexion deformity should be corrected by gradual stretching with wedged casts. After eighteen months of immobilization a leather brace should be worn on the wrist for six months. If sinuses are present, a metal cock-up splint is useful and will allow for drainage and dressings.

Operative treatment may consist of excision of all of the carpal bones. If indicated this procedure is best done early; however, it should seldom if ever be done in children. Arthrodesis is often advisable. If treatment is started before an abscess or sinuses form, extra-articular grafts from the lower end of the radius to the third metacarpal bone may result in firm bony ankylosis of the wrist and aid in arrest of the tuberculous process. Amputation should be performed only as a last resort.

Prognosis.—Tuberculous arthritis of the wrist is extremely resistant to treatment, and the prognosis for recovery of function is not so good as in other joints. The infection is often found in debilitated people of low resistance and is frequently complicated by pulmonary disease. In children who are treated early, however, the prognosis for function is good.

Tuberculous Dactylitis (Spina Ventosa)

Tuberculous dactylitis is a form of bone tuberculosis involving the metacarpals, metatarsals, or phalanges. It occurs usually in children under the age of five years. It is often associated with other tuberculous lesions, is often multiple, and may involve corresponding bones on both sides of the body.

Pathology.—The tuberculous focus is within the shaft of the bone. The medullary cavity is gradually replaced by tuberculous granulation tissue. Within the shaft, bone destruction takes place while new bone is produced beneath the periosteum. Draining sinuses frequently develop.

Clinical Picture.—The lack of acute pain is characteristic. There may be a dull ache through the swollen part, which usually becomes fusiform or spindle-shaped. There is little increase of local temperature. Occasionally an involved finger or toe may enlarge to such great size that mechanical discomfort is more troublesome than pain.

Diagnosis.—The diagnosis is usually made from the roentgenogram. Within the shaft of the bone is a cystlike area similar to that of an enchondroma or of a syphilitic dactylitis. A biopsy is sometimes indicated.

Treatment.—Prolonged fixation is often followed by arrest of the tuberculous process. When sinuses have formed, amputation may be advisable. Even when sinuses are not present it is sometimes desirable to remove the diseased member; this applies particularly in adults.

CHAPTER X

CHRONIC ARTHRITIS

The problem of chronic arthritis belongs to almost every branch of medicine. The general practitioner, the diagnostician, and the specialist all have a part in the examination of the patient. If the disease fails to respond to general and specific medical treatment, the patient often looks to the orthopaedic surgeon for advice and assistance. However, in many university and private clinics and in larger communities there are now physicians who limit their work to the diagnosis and treatment of chronic arthritis and other rheumatic diseases. These physicians are known as rheumatologists. Because of the large numbers of arthritic patients seen in orthopaedic clinics and private practice, a discussion of both the medical and surgical aspects of chronic arthritis is appropriate in an orthopaedic text.

Introduction.—Because of its frequency, chronic arthritis forms a vital problem economically as well as medically. In Massachusetts, where a careful survey of the situation has been made, there are more cases of chronic arthritis than of heart disease, tuberculosis, and cancer combined. There can be no doubt that chronic arthritis does not receive the attention which its prevalence demands. The treatment unfortunately is not simple, and every patient suffering from chronic arthritis looks in vain for the magic drug which will suddenly cure his disability. On the part of most doctors there is a distinct lack of appreciation of the true pathologic and physiologic changes of arthritis. In their enthusiasm for a favorite method of treatment they have often neglected the broader principles of therapy. There is no specific treatment for chronic arthritis. Although this has long been recognized, it is being appreciated more and more by those responsible for the care of chronic arthritic patients.

Great confusion has existed in the classification of chronic nonspecific joint affections. There can be no satisfactory etiologic classification of the arthritides so long as our knowledge of their many causes is so meager. The two most common and distinct types of chronic arthritis may, how-

Note.—This chapter is adapted from the *Primer on Rheumatism* prepared by the American Rheumatism Association and published by the American Medical Association.

ever, be differentiated by clinical examination, the type depending upon whether a proliferative or a degenerative pathologic process has taken place within the joint. These two types are called (1) *rheumatoid (atrophic* or *proliferative) arthritis* and (2) *osteoarthritis (hypertrophic* or *degenerative arthritis* or *degenerative joint disease).*

Incidence.—Both types are very prevalent in the temperate zones. There is no doubt that in chilly, damp climates the incidence of the rheumatoid type is greater than in regions which are warm and dry.

Each type of chronic arthritis is found among both rich and poor. The worries of life favor the onset of the rheumatoid type; occupational strains and injuries lead toward osteoarthritis.

The rheumatoid type is found from infancy to middle life and is three times as common in women as in men. Osteoarthritis is most often found in obese individuals over forty years of age and is perhaps more common in men.

Rheumatoid arthritis is more common in slender individuals; osteoarthritis more often affects persons of stocky build.

Classification.—The terms "rheumatoid arthritis" and "osteoarthritis" are used (1) because of the need for a simple classification which will be applicable despite conflicting opinions concerning the more specific etiologic factors, (2) because by physical examination and roentgenograms the essential differences between these two types can easily be recognized, and (3) because at the present time this terminology is more generally used in the United States and Great Britain than any other. The following are the more common synonyms for the two chief types of chronic arthritis: *rheumatoid arthritis—atrophic, infectious, proliferative, ankylosing,* or *Type I arthritis; osteoarthritis—hypertrophic, degenerative, nonankylosing,* or *Type II arthritis.* The term *arthritis deformans* may refer to either rheumatoid arthritis or osteoarthritis.

Rheumatoid Arthritis

Rheumatoid arthritis is a generalized disease characterized by chronic inflammatory changes in the synovial membranes and periarticular structures, by migratory swelling and stiffness of the joints in the early stage, and in the later stage by more or less deformity and ankylosis. Eighty per cent of the cases occur between twenty-five and fifty years of age.

Etiology.—It is said that 50 per cent of the persons affected by arthritis have a familial history of the disorder. Physical make-up may have something to do with this, since the slender individual is more commonly affected by rheumatoid arthritis than the stocky. The individual of thin type usually has ptosis of the abdominal viscera, which leads to abnormalities of the gastrointestinal tract. It is known that persons of this type suffer early from fatigue, from infection, from the wear and tear of life, and from intestinal disorders, all of which may favor the development of arthritis. Variations in temperature and moisture undoubtedly increase the susceptibility to arthritis; fatigue exerts a similar predisposing influence. It has been shown that severe nervous depressions or worries have preceded the onset of exacerbations of rheumatoid arthritis in over 50 per cent of the cases.

There can be no doubt that there are a great many contributory causes, such as poor general physical condition and subnormal weight. Injuries play a part in lowering the resistance of the individual joints and so promoting localization of the affection. Infections, such as tonsillitis, sinusitis, abscessed teeth, head colds, and influenza, are definite predisposing factors. The development of infection in the presence of lowered resistance sets the stage for the onset of rheumatoid arthritis.

Rheumatoid arthritis is considered by most authorities to be a disease of unknown etiology. Their opinion is based on the fact that rheumatoid arthritis is variously claimed to be (1) an infectious process, (2) a metabolic disease, (3) an endocrine disease, (4) a disease of the peripheral circulatory apparatus, (5) a disease of the nervous system, (6) a psychogenic disease, and (7) an allergic phenomenon.

Despite extensive knowledge of the clinical manifestations of the disease, its mode of onset, and the various etiologic factors aiding its development, little is known with certainty regarding its fundamental cause. Almost every investigator believes that there is an unknown or "x" factor present in the body of the individual who develops arthritis. Whether this factor is of the nature of a chemical or biological constituent of the blood is problematical. It is thought, however, that with continued research this "x" factor will become known and will be the key to both prevention and treatment of the disease. When Kendall of the Mayo Clinic isolated from the adrenal cortex the 17-ketosteroid first called compound E and later cortisone, and when in 1949 Hench of the same clinic obtained dramatic results in rheumatoid arthritis by the use of this hormone, many observers thought that the "x" factor had been found. Although the clinical and experimental effects of cortisone and of ACTH (adrenocorticotropic hormone, from the lobe of the pituitary gland) are very encouraging, it cannot be said that either of these hormones has done more than partly unlock the door to the prevention and treatment of this baffling disease.

Pathology.—The periarticular tissues of rheumatoid arthritic joints undergo a variable amount of swelling, and occasionally there is considerable thickening of the joint capsule. The synovial membrane itself shows constantly a proliferation and thickening, with infiltrating round cells and growth of granulation tissue over the articular cartilage. This proliferation of the synovial membrane represents the initial joint tissue change. Adhesions may later develop and with an increase of fibrous tissue may limit joint motion. The synovial fluid may be clear or cloudy and practically always shows a marked increase in leucocyte count. Investigations have shown that positive cultures can be obtained most frequently from joints with the greatest increase in the leucocyte count of the synovial fluid. Later in the disease the articular cartilage becomes eroded and the soft cancellous bone is exposed. Eventually there may be complete destruction of the articular cartilage. Atrophy of the bone trabeculae and replacement by connective tissue occur early. After erosion of the articular cartilage, fibrous union may occur between the bone ends and progress to bony ankylosis.

Symptoms.—In the acute forms of rheumatoid arthritis there may be involvement of many joints at the onset, but more often only one or two joints are affected in the initial stage. Usually the onset is gradual and slow; in 75 per cent of the cases it is very insidious. The onset of joint symptoms may be preceded by periods of fatigue, lassitude, and muscular stiffness associated with loss of weight. At first there may be fleeting joint pains. These are followed by joint symptoms of more persistent type, consisting first of constant pain, swelling, and stiffness. Later severe muscle atrophy develops. The joints may become deformed and ankylosed. The proximal interphalangeal and metacarpophalangeal joints of the hands are often affected first, and next the knees. All of the symptoms are definitely worse in bad weather and are increased also by overactivity and fatigue. The pain is usually not limited to the joint proper but may be felt in the adjacent muscles, tendons, and ligaments.

Severe weakness and associated fatigue are often present. Occasionally there is an elevation of 1° or 2° F. in body temperature. Often these systemic symptoms may precede the occurrence of actual pain by weeks. There may be marked disturbance of the nervous system and frequent emotional upsets, sleepless nights, and loss of appetite. There is no doubt that a great many of these patients have complete loss of adaptability to changes in temperature and a particular intolerance of cold.

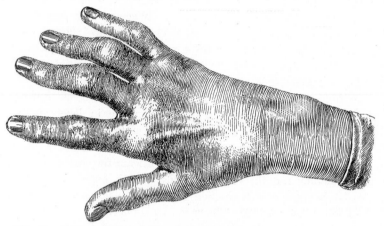

Fig. 81.—Rheumatoid arthritis of the hand, early stage. Note enlargement of the proximal interphalangeal joints. (After Duncan.)

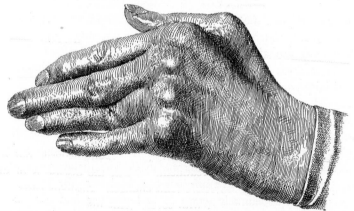

Fig 82.—Rheumatoid arthritis of the hand, late stage. Note enlargement of the metacarpophalangeal joints, ulnar deviation of the fingers, and subluxation of the proximal interphalangeal joint of the ring finger. (After Duncan.)

Physical Signs.—Periarticular swelling is usually the earliest local sign. It is most characteristically found in the smaller joints of the hands and feet, especially in the proximal interphalangeal joints of the fingers, where it produces a spindle-shaped appearance (Fig. 81). In the early stages the joints may be acutely tender, but later they become less sensitive. The tenderness may extend into the adjoining muscles and tendon sheaths. In 15 to 20 per cent of the cases fibrous nodules are found, especially about the elbows and about the phalangeal joints. There is slight increase of surface temperature over these joints, but redness is unusual. Muscular weakness and atrophy are quite characteristic. Flexion deformity may result from spasm of the flexor muscles.

Significant foci of infection may be present in the teeth, tonsils, nasal sinuses, gastrointestinal tract, and genitourinary tract. Occasionally intestinal stasis and associated disorders of digestion are outstanding factors in the clinical picture. The skin and mucous membranes may be extremely pale. At times in the more chronic form of the disease the skin becomes thin and glossy. In the extremities the skin is often cold, and in the acute stage it may be moist. Psoriasis occurs in about 3 per cent of the cases. There is almost always an enlargement of one or more groups of regional lymph nodes, and in children the spleen also may be enlarged (*Still's disease,* Fig. 83).

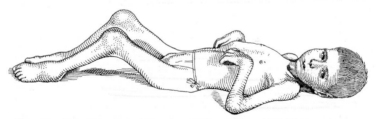

Fig. 83.—Rheumatoid arthritis in childhood (Still's disease). Note enlargement of the joints, muscle atrophy, and contractures. (After Green and Ober.)

Clinical Course.—Many patients improve spontaneously, but their recovery may be hastened by treatment. When the disease is of short duration, there may be no objective joint changes. In many cases, however, the disease is progressive, with severe joint involvement and permanent changes in the joint tissues. Deformity may develop because muscle spasm holds the joint in the position of greatest comfort; thus the knee, for example, is likely to develop a flexion deformity. Maintenance of the flexed position may be followed by capsular contractions and destructive changes within the joint; later the development of adhesions and of partial or complete ankylosis causes a permanent deformity.

However, at this stage the disease may become quiescent, in which event gradual improvement of the general health follows.

Roentgenographic Picture.—Swelling of the tissues about the affected joint is usually visible in the roentgenogram. In the early stages the joint cavity may be distended by the increased amount of synovial fluid. Bone atrophy, evidenced by rarefaction and most marked in the epiphyseal areas, gradually becomes conspicuous. The contour of the articular surfaces is not necessarily altered and remains well defined. The joint space later becomes narrowed, however, and evidences of irregularity can be seen along the joint margins with areas of atrophic bone destruction, referred to as punched-out areas; the edges still remain distinct. In the advanced stages the articular margins may show the presence of bony spurs, ridges, and prominences. These hypertrophic features of the late case resemble the changes of osteoarthritis and tend to obscure the true atrophic character of the bone lesions. In the late stages the articular surfaces may become fused through bony or fibrous ankyloses. There also may be subluxations or dislocations of joints with or without articular bone destruction.

Laboratory Observations.—A slight anemia is usually present, the hemoglobin and red cell content being between 60 and 70 per cent of normal. There may be an increase of the leucocytes, especially when fever is present. Agglutination tests do not yield uniform results. Agglutinins for Group A hemolytic streptococci are usually present in typical cases of six or more months' duration, though the exact significance of their presence is not clear. In cases of osteoarthritis such agglutinins are usually not present. The corrected sedimentation rate of the red blood cells is considerably increased. Cultures of the blood, the joint fluid, and the regional lymph nodes are occasionally positive. Cultures taken from foci of infection elsewhere in the body may show a high percentage of streptococci. The basal metabolic rate is often low. The hydrochloric acid content of the stomach is diminished. Examinations of the urine and stool yield negative results.

The nitrogenous metabolism of the patient is usually found to be within normal limits. The uric acid is within normal limits. There is no change in the calcium content of the blood. This is an indication that the change in the calcium of the bones shown in roentgenograms and by histologic studies is entirely a local process. There is decreased peripheral blood flow as demonstrated by capillary studies. It has been shown that the blood flow in the capillaries is considerably increased following heat, massage, and exercise, and after sympathectomy. Certain metabolites absorbed from the gastrointestinal tract appear in the synovial fluid with great rapidity.

Diagnosis.—At the onset it is sometimes difficult to distinguish acute rheumatoid arthritis from acute rheumatic fever. Tonsillitis may precede the onset of either. However, the temperature is higher in rheumatic fever, with more sweating and frequent cardiac complications. In rheumatic fever the electrocardiogram shows an abnormality in 25 to 50 per cent of the cases. Salicylates afford more effective and lasting relief in acute rheumatic fever than in rheumatoid arthritis.

Osteoarthritis or degenerative joint disease is often confused with rheumatoid arthritis, especially in the aged. The following are the most significant points in differentiation: (1) rheumatoid arthritis is a systemic disease and the patients are sick—in osteoarthritis they are not sick, (2) cutaneous changes are commonly associated with rheumatoid arthritis, (3) weight-bearing joints are more often involved in osteoarthritis, (4) the proximal interphalangeal joints are more often involved in rheumatoid arthritis, the distal interphalangeal joints in osteoarthritis (Heberden's nodes), (5) subcutaneous nodules are not seen in osteoarthritis, and (6) osteoporosis and bony ankylosis are uncommon in osteoarthritis.

Gonococcal arthritis is sometimes confused with rheumatoid arthritis. Careful questioning and thorough examination of the patient are important. Frequently in gonorrheal arthritis the gonococcus can be demonstrated in the joint fluid.

Joint tuberculosis in its early stages may be confused with rheumatoid arthritis; however, tuberculosis is more often monarticular, is more insidious in its onset, and is likely to show more bone destruction roentgenographically. Culture of the joint exudate, inoculation of a guinea pig with it, or biopsy of the synovial membrane may be necessary to establish the diagnosis.

Syphilitic arthritis is sometimes difficult to distinguish, as it may cause multiple joint involvement similar to that of rheumatoid arthritis. A positive complement fixation reaction in the blood and often also in the synovial fluid, as well as the demonstration of spirochetes in the fluid, is helpful in the differentiation.

Gout is occasionally confusing, but its high blood uric acid is characteristic, especially in the absence of an increase of the nonprotein nitrogen. In gout the joints quickly lose their tenderness between attacks, and the great toe is often the first part of the body to be affected. Chronic gout is more often confused with rheumatoid arthritis than is acute gout. Roentgenographically the punched-out areas in bone characteristic of gout are found also in rheumatoid arthritis.

Treatment.—The treatment of rheumatoid arthritis must be suited to the individual patient after a careful survey of the various factors in his particular case. The most important elements in the treatment are the following:

1. *The Individual as a Whole.*—Rheumatoid arthritis is a systemic disease, and local treatment of the affected joints will not result in permanent cure unless the body as a whole is also treated. Rest is as essential to the individual as it is to the joint; placing the patient at complete rest is often productive of marked benefit. It is unwise, however, to put the patient to bed for an indefinite period of time. During the period of rest a carefully supervised regime of general and specific exercise, with particular emphasis upon deep breathing, is important. It is always wise during this period of rest to carry out general massage of the muscles and particularly of those which are the most atrophic. Massage is of especial benefit in improving the local circulation. It should never be given over the affected joints, however, and never to the point of inducing pain or fatigue.

2. *Removal of Predisposing Causes.*—Anxiety and worry, which definitely hinder recovery, should be mitigated insofar as possible. Infections, both general and local, should be treated. Great care should be taken to prevent the patient from becoming fatigued. Care should be taken to prevent exposure to cold and dampness. Anemia and undernutrition should be corrected with the proper diet and medication. Transfusions are sometimes indicated.

3. *Removal of Exciting Causes.*—Foci of infection should be eradicated promptly if the patient's condition will allow the operative procedure. Early removal of foci is undoubtedly desirable and at times arrests the progress of the disease. Often it is advisable, however, to build up the patient's general health and bodily resistance before the abscessed teeth or tonsils are removed. Infected paranasal sinuses should be given a trial of conservative treatment before any radical procedure is undertaken. Infection of the prostate gland and seminal vesicles requires a long series of massage and irrigation treatments. Vaginal discharge should be controlled by douches, and infectious lesions of the cervix

should be cauterized or excised. Systemic administration of penicillin or a sulfonamide may be helpful in the treatment of foci of infection.

Since disordered digestion and constipation often lead to joint pain, the correction of constipation by means of diet and, if necessary, catharsis is indicated.

4. *Diet.*—The diet should be well balanced. The quantity of food should be adequate to maintain the body weight, but not great enough to overload the atonic bowel. Green vegetables and fruits in liberal quantities are usually advised. The carbohydrate and concentrated protein foods should be taken in moderation. Most of the calories required are preferably obtained from fats. The diet is especially important when dysfunction of the gastrointestinal tract seems to be the chief etiologic factor.

A high-vitamin diet planned to suit the needs of the individual patient is desirable. Cod liver oil and haliver oil, as well as wheat germ and yeast preparations, are useful in supplying the necessary vitamin intake.

5. *Drugs and Foreign Protein Therapy.*—No specific drug which will cure rheumatoid arthritis is known. The salicylates are most useful for the alleviation of pain. From ½ to 1 Gm. of sodium salicylate three times a day often gives considerable relief but may upset the stomach if taken over an extended period of time. Aspirin seems to cause digestive symptoms less frequently. Neocinchophen in ½ Gm. doses is sometimes helpful but should be administered with caution because of the possibility of causing acute gastrointestinal symptoms from liver damage. Iron preparations are often useful in treatment of the anemia. Sometimes arsenic, which increases the permeability of the capillary endothelium, seems to be of benefit. It is prescribed in the form of neoarsphenamine or potassium arsenite solution.

A widely used form of treatment is the intramuscular or intravenous injection of gold salts, or chrysotherapy. Their mode of action is not well understood. In many cases of acute rheumatoid arthritis, particularly those treated early in the course of the disease, good results in reducing the pain and swelling of the joints have been obtained when the drug has been given in small doses over a long period of time. The usefulness of gold therapy is distinctly limited at the present time, however, by its occasionally dangerous toxic effects on kidneys, intestines, and skin. Some observers believe, however, that chrysotherapy is the best form of treatment for all early rheumatoid arthritis.

All forms of iodine preparations, including particularly the saturated solution of potassium iodide, are of value in promoting the regression and absorption of pathologic tissues. In patients with a low basal metabolic rate, thyroid extract, given in doses of 30 mg. twice a day, may improve the general nutrition by accelerating the metabolism.

Injections of foreign proteins, such as sterile milk, typhoid vaccine, and various bacterial proteins, when given intravenously, intramuscularly, or subcutaneously, are usually followed by a severe constitutional reaction with chills, fever, and sweating. This type of reaction often seems to increase temporarily the peripheral circulation, and particularly the circulation about the joints, with resultant relief of the pain and swelling, but seldom produces lasting improvement. In the use of intravenous injections, and particularly in the case of typhoid vaccine, care must be taken not to evoke too severe a constitutional reaction, especially in debilitated individuals.

ACTH and cortisone have a definite place in the treatment of the early stage of the disease and in the relief of pain in the later stages. Most patients who have been subjectively improved with ACTH and cortisone find that their symptoms recur when administration of the drugs is discontinued. The use of these hormones is still in the experimental stage, but there can be little doubt that they or their derivatives will eventually have a permanent place in the therapy of rheumatoid arthritis.

After the menopause, especially when it has been artificially produced, arthralgias resembling rheumatoid arthritis are not uncommon. In their treatment, some of the ovarian hormones have proved useful.

6. *Vaccine Therapy.*—Vaccine therapy, which has been so popular in the past, is now seldom used. It has been classified by some authorities as of doubtful value or useless. Vaccines may be stock or autogenous in type and usually contain one strain of streptococcus. There is no doubt that certain cases which have been at a standstill show definite improvement when vaccine treatment is started. Whether the vaccine alone is responsible for the improvement has not been definitely shown. Vaccines are given, in varying dosage, either subcutaneously or intravenously. It is important that the vaccine should not be administered in amounts large enough to cause too severe a general reaction. The unintelligent use of vaccines may do harm.

7. *Local Treatment of Joints.*—Local applications of heat by means of hot moist towels, an electric baker, an infrared lamp, a whirlpool

bath, or diathermy have a beneficial effect in stimulating the circulation and result often in relief of the acute pain. Paraffin baths are often most helpful for arthritic hands and feet. Heat should be followed by gentle massage of the muscles above and below the affected joints. Liniments rubbed lightly on the joints will occasionally stimulate the circulation and ease the discomfort. Voluntary movement of the affected joints, without weight-bearing, should be carried out several times a day. In these exercises the joints should be put through their full range of voluntary motion. The amount of exercise may be increased gradually if there is no unfavorable reaction in the joint. After the acute stage of the disease has passed, some patients can be helped by occupational therapy associated with physical therapy.

Occasionally in acute arthritis the pain is so severe that it is necessary to immobilize the joint with light splints or a plaster cast. Immobilization should be continued no longer than is necessary to relieve the pain, and if possible the joint should be taken out of the splint at least once a day and be put actively through its full range of motion or through as much motion as possible. Occasionally a tremendous amount of relief is obtained from a moderate degree of immobilization by means of large dressings of glazed cotton bound on firmly with elastic bandages.

If intra-articular effusion has occurred, causing the joint capsule to become tense and painful, aspiration is indicated.

8. *Prevention of Deformity.*—The prevention of deformity in rheumatoid arthritis is of the utmost importance because of the frequency of fibrous and bony ankylosis. If an ankylosis cannot be averted, care should be taken that the joint become stiff in the best position for function (see page 153-155). This can be accomplished by fixing the joint in the optimal position by means of traction, a plaster splint or cast, or a brace.

9. *Correction of Deformity.*—When a joint has become partially or completely ankylosed in a faulty position, surgery may be indicated in order to improve the position. Very often the deformity, especially when it is in the knees, can be corrected by skin traction or by the use of wedged or turnbuckle casts. If this is not successful, it may be advisable to manipulate the joint firmly and gently under anesthesia. This should be done with extreme care because although the arthritis may have become inactive, the atrophic bones fracture very easily; in the case of the knee it is necessary also to guard against posterior

subluxation of the upper end of the tibia. If contractures cannot be overcome by closed methods, open operations are justified for their release and for lengthening the tendons. *Capsuloplasty,* or operative release of a portion of the joint ligaments at their attachment to the bone, is a satisfactory procedure for facilitating the correction of flexion deformity of the knee. For a joint enlarged by thickening of the synovial membrane, a synovectomy may be indicated. Operative attempts to restore motion to ankylosed joints by means of arthroplasties are not uniformly successful, largely because of the limitations imposed by muscle atrophy. Excellent results occasionally follow arthroplasty, especially when the joint operated upon is the hip or elbow. Successful arthroplasties of the knee with the use of a thin but tough sheet of nylon between the bone ends have recently been reported. Mobility can be restored to an ankylosed jaw by resection of the condyle of the mandible. For the hip joint a reconstruction operation or a subtrochanteric osteotomy to improve alignment may be indicated. A spine ankylosed in a position of kyphosis can sometimes be improved by mobilization with exercises and recumbency in hyperextension; a strong back brace is then applied to maintain the improved position. For the wrists and fingers, intermittent support in functional position and elastic or spring tension splinting to overcome contractures are of the greatest value. A patient who has been severely disabled by arthritis is usually most grateful for any improvement of joint position or motion, even though it be only the ability to put one hand behind the head to comb the hair.

Prognosis.—Rheumatoid arthritis now has a better prognosis than it has had in the past. It is not altogether an incurable disease, as tremendous strides have been made toward checking its progress and many encouraging results and cures have been reported. It has been said that 70 per cent or more of the patients can receive substantial benefit from treatment. This more favorable prognosis is thought to be due to the fact that rheumatoid arthritis is now being looked upon a great deal more as a general systemic disease and is being treated accordingly. If rheumatoid arthritis is promptly recognized, vigorous and long-continued treatment will usually yield gratifying results.

Osteoarthritis (Degenerative Joint Disease)

Osteoarthritis is a form of chronic arthritis found usually in middle-aged and elderly people, and characterized by degenerative and hypertrophic joint changes coming on at the same time in cartilage and in bone.

Etiology.—An hereditary influence is undoubtedly an important factor. In people over forty-five years of age whose parents have suffered from rheumatism late in life there is a greater susceptibility than in those who have no family history of rheumatism. Occasionally osteoarthritis is seen in younger people, under the age of forty years, whose joints have been subjected to continuous strain or to sudden trauma. As has been stated, the stocky type of individual with a sluggish gastrointestinal tract is most susceptible to osteoarthritis. Climate usually seems to have little effect on the disease. Osteoarthritis has been found in tropical climates as well as in cold climates. However, exposure to cold and moisture, sometimes associated with occupational trauma, undoubtedly predisposes toward the affection.

There is no doubt that injury plays a major part in the onset. Repeated minor traumata cause slight pathologic changes in joints, and it is in traumatized joints that the degenerative process progresses most rapidly. Infection plays a part in osteoarthritis, but not as a primary etiologic agent. Infection lowers bodily resistance, thus accelerating degenerative diseases such as osteoarthritis. Products of intestinal putrefaction, which are unfavorable to normal metabolism, may be exciting causes. It can be shown that a disturbance of the glands of internal secretion sometimes plays a part; examples are the hypertrophic joint changes found in myxedema and those developing in women at the menopause. The latter type of joint disease is sometimes spoken of as *climacteric* or *menopausal arthritis*.

Pathology.—The most significant changes appear in the articular cartilage and the bone. The cartilage undergoes splitting, fibrillation, gradual thinning, and widespread degeneration. About the cartilaginous edges chondro-osseous spicules form quite early. These appear in the roentgenograms as spurs and lipping. Occasionally the chondro-osseous deposits become detached and form loose bodies within the joint. As degeneration of the cartilage progresses, the underlying bone usually becomes eburnated and deformed. In osteoarthritis the atrophy of the bone trabeculae occurs quite late and is thought to be partly the result of a decrease in physical activity. There are often marked changes of shape in the end of the bone, increased bony deposits in and about the areas of cartilaginous degeneration, and erosion of bone beneath the destroyed cartilage. In osteoarthritis the periarticular tissues and synovial membrane show much less important and less characteristic changes than in rheumatoid arthritis. The amount of synovial fluid is essentially normal.

Symptoms.—In the early stages of osteoarthritis there is usually stiffness of one or more joints associated with an aching pain in or about the affected joint. The involvement is more often monarticular than polyarticular. This stiffness tends to become less noticeable after moderate use of the joint. Continued use is always followed, however, by marked discomfort, which may be relieved by rest, support and heat. The patient tires easily on exertion. In this stage there is slight enlargement of the affected joints which may be slightly tender about their margins; this is usually most noticeable in the fingers and knees. The bony enlargement of the distal interphalangeal joints *(Heberden's nodes)* is one of the commonest signs (Fig. 84).

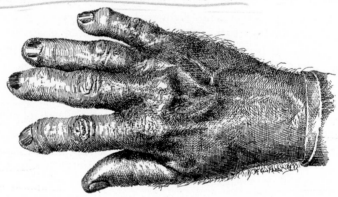

Fig. 84.—Osteoarthritis of the hand. Note enlargement of the distal interphalangeal joints of index, middle, and little fingers. (After Duncan.)

Later in the course of the disease there are marked limitation of joint motion and considerable disability, especially in the larger joints. There may be referred pain from pressure upon nerve roots. Pain may now be present while the joint is resting, as well as when it is in motion. Malalignment of the joint is a frequent result of the irregular degeneration and loss of articular cartilage. Examination at this stage reveals moderate swelling and puffiness and a loss of the normal joint contour.

A tendency to early fatigue is very characteristic of osteoarthritis. Many of the patients are obese. There may be a disturbance of body mechanics with a sagging, protuberant abdomen, a flat chest, and abnormal weight-bearing lines in the feet, knees, and hips, resulting in chronic strain of these joints. Generalized arteriosclerosis is quite often associated, although there is no constant change in blood pressure or kidney function.

Clinical Course.—Remissions and exacerbations are frequent. At times the disease becomes entirely quiescent, and then years later it may become active again. More disability follows involvement of the spine and lower extremities than that of the upper extremities. As the condition progresses in the spine, there may be a limitation of the normal range of motion, localized pain due to impingement of the sensitive bony overgrowths, and radiating pain due to impingement of the bony overgrowths on nerve trunks. The condition may progress to the point of an extreme disability of one or more joints, but, unlike arthritis of the rheumatoid type, seldom results in bony ankylosis except in the spine.

Roentgenographic Picture.—The presence of angular joint margins, lipping, and spur formation progressing to excessive new bone production may be seen in individuals who consider themselves perfectly normal and who have never had pain or disability. When pain makes its appearance, attention is at once called to these growths, and they often are considered to be the cause of the disability. What cannot be visualized in the roentgenograms is undoubtedly an irritation of the soft tissues adjacent to the bony overgrowths, with the probable formation of small bursal sacs which are quite sensitive. As the disease progresses, there will be seen a narrowing of the joint space due to degeneration of the articular cartilage, and occasionally small cystic areas appear in the subjacent cancellous bone. In the case of the head of the femur there is a loss of the normal contour of the articular surface (Fig. 88). In the spine the bony projections may fuse and form osseous bridges between adjacent vertebrae (Figs. 87A and 87B). Calcified loose bodies, broken off from projecting bony edges, may be found within the joint. True bony ankylosis is seldom seen except in the spine, though the roentgenograms may show very close approximation of the joint surfaces. A terminal picture of generalized bone atrophy usually appears. Sclerotic changes in the aorta and large arteries of the extremities are often visible in the roentgenograms.

A barium meal is often retained in whole or in part for more than seventy-two hours; this indicates the presence of intestinal stasis. The cecum is often low; there may be sagging of the transverse loop of the colon; and the haustral markings are partially obliterated. In the descending colon there may be multiple diverticula.

Laboratory Observations.—The blood picture and sedimentation rate are usually normal. Very seldom, if ever, can agglutinins for the hemolytic streptococcus be demonstrated. The uric acid content of the blood may be slightly elevated. Dextrose tolerance curves are frequently of the diabetic type. Certain dietary experiments suggest that calcium is retained, but this has not been proved. The basal metabolic rate is often low.

Diagnosis.—It is important that an accurate diagnosis be made in the early stages of the disease when the findings are most characteristic. Specific diagnosis can usually be made after careful analysis of the history, joint changes as shown by examination, and most important of all, the roentgenographic evidence of hypertrophic bone changes. At times it may be difficult to distinguish osteoarthritis from gout. Syphilis and tuberculosis occasionally may be confusing. Certain trophic joint changes associated with syringomyelia and with tabes dorsalis produce appearances similar to the degenerative changes of osteoarthritis. Osteitis deformans must be excluded. Occasionally neoplasms must be considered in the diagnosis.

Treatment.—1. *The Individual as a Whole.*—Faulty body mechanics should unquestionably be corrected as one of the first steps in the treatment of the individual. The pronated foot should be relieved with appropriate supports and shoes. The painful spine should be supported by means of the proper brace or corset. Postural exercises undoubtedly will benefit the circulatory, respiratory, and digestive systems. As far as possible, worry, mental fatigue, and emotional disturbances should be removed.

2. *Removal of Predisposing Causes.*—Intestinal stasis should be treated by diet, catharsis, colonic irrigation, and similar measures to bring about normal and regular evacuation. Yeast or wheat germ concentrates may be used to increase the tone and motility of the intestines. Weight should be maintained at a normal level, which usually means a decrease from that at the beginning of treatment.

3. *Removal of Exciting Causes.*—Any obvious focus of infection which is suspected of being a contributory factor should be removed.

On the other hand, unnecessary extraction of teeth and major operations for the removal of foci of doubtful significance should be avoided. If the patient's metabolic rate is low, thyroid extract should be administered in small quantities, such as ¼ or ½ grain two or three times a day. Ovarian extracts have sometimes helped cases associated with menopausal changes.

4. *Diet.*—The diet should be well balanced. It should include a great many green vegetables and fruit. The proteins and fats should be consistent with the patient's activity and weight. As a rule, starches and sugars should be decreased or avoided. The reduction of weight should be accomplished slowly and under supervision.

5. *Drugs and Vaccines.*—There are no drugs or vaccines specific for osteoarthritis. Salicylates, as in other joint diseases, relieve pain. Arsenic preparations may be prescribed as a general supportive measure. A saturated solution of potassium iodide often relieves pain about the joints when given in gradually increasing doses. Noneffervescing sodium phosphate is useful when given in small doses about half an hour before meals. Multi-vitamin preparations are always indicated. Cortisone and ACTH have so far proved to be of no permanent value but may at times relieve acute symptoms.

6. *Local Treatment of Joints.*—Usually physical therapy definitely benefits these joints. Heat in the form of baking, hot moist towels, whirlpool or paraffin baths, or diathermy will stimulate the local circulation. Massage of the muscles above and below the affected joints may make the patient more comfortable. Voluntary exercises are indicated but are not to be continued to the point of fatigue or of irritation of the projecting bony overgrowths. Excessive exercise may lead to a tremendous amount of stiffening on the following day. Simple rest usually relieves the pain. The rest may be facilitated by means of a posterior plaster shell, a brace, or other type of support. The sensitiveness associated with the bony spurs often decreases with rest. The joints should not be completely fixed for too long a period since continued immobilization will result in disuse atrophy. Rest in bed, with removable splints and local measures to stimulate circulation, is one of the most satisfactory methods of treatment.

7. *Prevention of Deformity.*—There is much less danger of the development of fixed deformity in osteoarthritis than in rheumatoid arthritis. Most of the deformity is due to changes in the shape of the

articular ends of the bones. At times, however, the hips may become flexed and adducted, the knees flexed, or the feet pronated; selected exercises and splinting will do much to prevent these deformities.

8. *Correction of Deformity by Apparatus and Surgery.*—There is no doubt that foot supports, properly applied to maintain the arches in normal position, make walking more comfortable by protecting the sensitive tarsal joints and preventing lateral strain at the subastragalar joints. Elastic bandages, knee caps, and even light knee braces will relieve a tremendous amount of pain in osteoarthritis of the knee. Back pain may be treated by special belts, corsets, and light braces.

Loose bodies occasionally appear in the knee or hip. They may produce frequent transient pain and may even cause the patient to fall. Their removal often affords distinct relief. Complete cure of the discomfort is scarcely to be expected, however, and, if the arthritis continues to progress, it may be necessary later to remove additional loose bodies. Synovectomy may be indicated if the joint has excessive thickening of the synovial membrane. Forcible manipulation is never advisable because often it provokes a greater overgrowth of bone followed by a greater disability. However, a hip or a knee which has undergone restriction of its range of motion may sometimes be gently manipulated with benefit.

Prognosis.—The prognosis for relief of the joint symptoms and the control of osteoarthritis is unquestionably better than that of rheumatoid arthritis. The damaged joints can be made less disabling and less painful by well-advised treatment. Despite roentgenographic evidence of advanced changes, the patient will experience remarkably little pain when a suitable therapeutic regime is prescribed and diligently followed.

Gout

Gout is characterized by an abnormality of purine metabolism in attacks of monarticular pain. Between attacks the patient is characteristically symptom-free unless permanent joint damage is present. Ninety per cent of the patients are males and they are usually past the age of 30. The attacks are precipitated by excessive intake of meats and other foods high in protein, overindulgence in alcohol, fatigue, and occasionally by trauma or surgery of the involved joint.

Gout is characterized by an abnormality of purine metabolism in which uric acid, the normal end product, is involved. Its cause is unknown.

The joint lesions consist of chalky deposits of sodium urate in the synovium, capsule, articular cartilage, and periarticular bone. The joints most often involved are those of the foot (classically the first metatarsophalangeal joint), hand, wrist, knee, and elbow. For some reason the hip, shoulder, and spine are seldom involved. The involved joint is usually red, tender, and swollen. The veins in the surrounding skin are prominent.

Roentgenographically, there are typical punched-out areas near the ends of the bones at the affected joint. Clinically, tender tophi consisting of deposits of urate are sometimes found in the ears, subcutaneous tissue, and fascia, and occasionally in the heart and other viscera.

The blood uric acid is elevated (5 to 25 mg. per 100 c.c.) during the acute episode only. However, the acute attack is not caused by the high blood level per se, either experimentally or clinically. Thus gout does not develop in uremia.

Treatment.—Although no curative treatment is available for the disease itself, certain drugs give dramatic relief from pain and swelling. Colchicine, ½ mg., may be given hourly, until the pain disappears, although it may cause gastrointestinal upsets. Cinchophen, ½ Gm., may also be used three to four times daily, although it is not so dependable for the relief of pain as colchicine. ACTH in doses of 20 to 25 mg. every six hours for three to five doses may quickly arrest the acute attack. Aspirin is frequently helpful. It is most important for the patient to follow a low purine diet and to obtain sufficient rest. In late cases, large tophi may require surgical extirpation.

CHAPTER XI

CHRONIC ARTHRITIS: SPECIAL JOINTS

Chronic arthritis of the spine, hip, and knee present special problems which can best be considered separately. The classification into rheumatoid arthritis and osteoarthritis has again been followed.

Chronic Arthritis of the Spine (Spondylitis Deformans)

1. RHEUMATOID ARTHRITIS

Incidence.—Rheumatoid arthritis of the spine is more common in men than in women and is most frequent in the early decades of adult life, between the ages of twenty and forty years. Occasionally it is seen in children in association with multiple joint involvement, splenomegaly, and generalized lymphadenopathy (*Still's disease,* Fig. 83).

Etiology.—Rheumatoid arthritis of the spine may be a part of a generalized process. It is believed by some that infection plays an important rôle in its etiology. Statistics have indicated that the focus of infection is most often in the gastrointestinal tract or the pelvis. Faulty body mechanics play a part in adding the element of chronic strain, especially in the highly mobile lumbo-dorsal portion of the spine. Visceroptosis, with resulting intestinal stasis, is an important factor.

Pathology.—The pathologic changes are essentially the same as those described for rheumatoid arthritis elsewhere in the body. There is always an atrophy of the bones, a secondary atrophy of the cartilages, and periarticular swelling. If the condition progresses to ankylosis, the ligaments become ossified, and the intervertebral articulations may become bridged with bone. Ossification or calcification of the intervertebral cartilages and disks may occur, but very seldom, if ever, is there any spur formation or lipping. The changes are most regular and uniform as contrasted with the irregular calcification which appears in certain other forms of arthritis of the spine.

Clinical Picture.—The onset is insidious and slow and is characterized usually by stiffness followed by pain. The discomfort is especially marked on bending over and lifting and is relieved but does not subside completely with recumbency. The pain is located most often in the lower dorsal and upper lumbar levels of the spine. At times it may radiate to the front of the chest and abdomen or down the legs. Coughing and sneezing usually cause sharp pain in the back. It is not uncommon for the symptoms to appear in recurrent attacks which may follow minor infections, excessive exercise, or slight trauma. If involve-

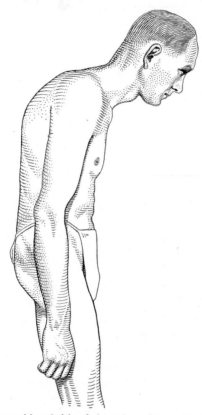

Fig. 85.—Rheumatoid arthritis of the spine with complete ankylosis in faulty position. (After Campbell.)

ment of the costovertebral articulations takes place, there is embarrassment of the respiration. As the condition progresses, lumbar muscle spasm becomes severe. There may be a flattening of the normal lumbar lordosis, with round shoulders and an upper dorsal kyphosis. If involvement of the cervical spine is present, moving the head causes pain. The stiffness becomes gradually more marked as ankylosis takes place (Fig. 85). When the spine finally becomes fused the element of pain disappears.

Diagnosis.—The diagnosis is based upon the character of the onset, the findings on clinical examination, the roentgenographic changes, and the frequent association with characteristic involvement of other joints.

Differential Diagnosis.—Rheumatoid arthritis of the spine must be differentiated at times from other types of arthritis and from tuberculosis, syphilis, malignancy, fracture, ruptured intervertebral disk, back sprain, and diseases of the female pelvic organs.

Treatment.—The treatment is discussed at the end of the section.

Strümpell-Marie Arthritis (Spondylose Rhizomélique)

Strümpell-Marie arthritis, although commonly described under rheumatoid arthritis, is considered by some rheumatologists to constitute a separate type. This is the belief of the author. Strümpell-Marie arthritis is so named because it was first described as a clinical entity by Strümpell in 1897 and Marie in 1898. It is characterized by ossification of the ligaments of the spine and by involvement also of the shoulders and hips. The sacroiliac joints are nearly always affected very early in its course. It usually develops without a known etiologic factor; however, many observers are of the opinion that the endocrine glands play a part in its etiology, as it is much more common in men than in women. It is thought that direct trauma, strain, faulty body mechanics, and infection are contributing factors. The affection often appears, however, in the absence of these influences. It occurs most frequently between the ages of twenty and forty years.

Pathology.—In addition to the pathologic changes of rheumatoid arthritis, a fibrous and osseous ankylosis occurs, of which the most outstanding feature is an ossification of the spinal ligaments. The anterior longitudinal ligament is first affected; the posterior longitudinal ligament, the ligamenta subflava, the capsular ligaments of the articular processes, the ligaments connecting the ribs with the vertebrae, and the supraspinous and interspinous ligaments are then involved in this order. Usually there is little change in the intervertebral disks. The vertebral bodies show generalized atrophy but remain unchanged in shape. There may be irregular spur formation and lipping of the vertebrae in addition to the ossification of the ligaments. The spurring may give to the spine the characteristic contours of osteoarthritis. The typical gross specimen has an appearance suggesting that liquid bone has been poured upon the anterior surface of the vertebral column and has congealed as it flowed down (Fig. 86).

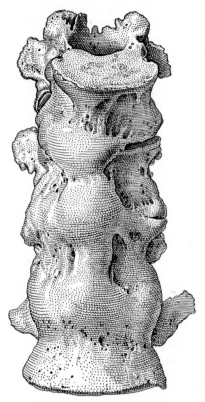

Fig. 86.—Specimen of advanced Strümpell-Marie arthritis of spine. (After Elizabeth H. Brödel.)

Clinical Picture.—The onset may be associated with acute pain, but, on the contrary, stiffness without pain is sometimes the first symptom. The pain often first appears in the hips or buttocks. Diminished chest expansion is one of the characteristic signs. As the disease progresses, kyphosis and flattening of the chest frequently develop unless preventive measures are taken. The pain and stiffening often progress very slowly from the low back farther and farther upward until finally the entire spine may become solidly ankylosed. The hips and shoulders may then become involved. If the hips become stiff, a characteristic gait develops in which the pelvis is rotated from side to side in order to compensate for lack of normal hip motion. In the typical case there is no involvement of the smaller joints.

Characteristic roentgenograms show in the lateral view a smooth, even ossification across the anterior surfaces of the vertebral bodies and intervertebral spaces. The anteroposterior view shows usually a thin line of ossification extending on either side of the midline of the vertebrae, corresponding to the position of the anterior spinal ligament. The sacroiliac joints show destructive changes in the early stages of the disease; later they appear fused.

Diagnosis.—The diagnostic criteria are similar to those of rheumatoid arthritis of the spine. Characteristic features, however, are the more commonly associated involvement of the shoulders and sacroiliac joints and the absence of changes in the smaller joints of the extremities.

Differential Diagnosis.—This is similar to that of rheumatoid arthritis.

Treatment.—The treatment is discussed at the end of the section.

2. OSTEOARTHRITIS

Incidence and Etiology.—Osteoarthritis of the spine is seen most often in stocky and obese persons over forty years of age and is more frequent in males than in females. It is approximately twice as common as rheumatoid arthritis of the spine and is most often observed in the lumbar spine. The repeated minor traumata of constant use of the back probably constitute the most important causative factor. Faulty body mechanics unquestionably play a part in putting an added strain upon the back, and focal infections may exert a predisposing influence. Disordered metabolism also is believed to be an important factor in the etiology.

Pathology.—In a large percentage of older people who have never been troubled by back pain, osteoarthritic changes in the spine can be demonstrated by roentgenographic examination. This is especially true in the case of heavy individuals. The pathologic changes discussed in Chapter X may be observed in osteoarthritis of the spine. Lipping and spur formation occur at the edges of the vertebrae, and there is considerable thinning of the intervertebral fibrocartilages. Marked eburnation of bone occurs about the articular facets.   In the later stages the vertebral body becomes flattened, and a tremendous amount of new bone may develop about its edges and produce the so-called "bridging" and "leaf formation" (Figs. 87A and 87B).

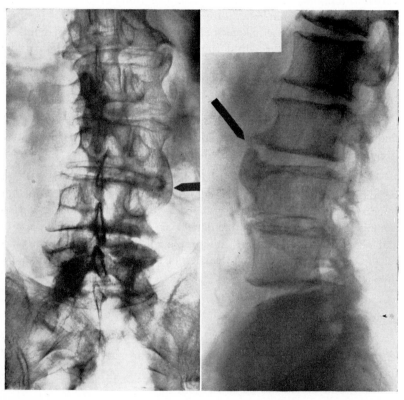

A.   *B.*

Fig. 87.—Osteoarthritis of the lumbar spine in a seventy-year-old man. *A,* Anteroposterior roentgenogram showing deformity of spine with spur formation and large bridge of new bone.

B, Lateral roentgenogram showing spur formation and almost complete bridging between second and third lumbar vertebrae.

Clinical Picture.—Following slight trauma or strain there may be complaint of pain in the lower part of the back, with considerable lameness and stiffness.   Associated with the restriction of motion there is muscle spasm.   Pain which radiates around toward the chest or abdomen or down the legs or arms is often present; this pain may be a result of compression of nerve trunks caused by small outgrowths of bone near the intervertebral foramina. Radiating pain is particularly common in involvement of the lumbosacral and sacroiliac joints and of the intervertebral foramina of the cervical spine. Deformity of the lumbar spine, often consisting of lateral curvature and a decrease of the normal lordosis, may develop. Complete ankylosis of some areas of the spine may follow. The lumbar and lower dorsal spine is more often involved than the middle and upper dorsal spine, and frequently is the first to become stiffened. There is often an associated disturbance of the gastrointestinal tract.

Diagnosis.—The diagnosis is made from the history, the physical findings, and the roentgenographic evidence of lipping, spurs, and irregular bone formation about the bone edges.

Differential Diagnosis.—Osteoarthritis of the spine must at times be differentiated from osteitis deformans and from rupture of an intervertebral disk in addition to the other affections mentioned. Occasionally it is necessary to differentiate *Von Bechterew's arthritis,* a rare and obscure type of osteoarthritis of the spine associated with a neurologic disorder manifested by weakness of the intercostal and abdominal muscles.

The Treatment of Chronic Arthritis of the Spine

Attempts should be made to eradicate all foci of infection which are suspected of being contributing factors. The surgical treatment of foci of infection may involve several successive operative procedures, however, and should not be carried out so long as the patient's general condition is poor. Faulty body mechanics should be corrected when possible. The treatment of constipation is important. Colonic irrigations may be indicated when intestinal stasis is persistent. In general, the diet should be rich in minerals, cellulose, and fatty foods but moderate in proteins and poor in starches and sugars. The caloric intake should be so regulated that the stout individual loses weight and the thin individual gains weight. Cod liver oil, viosterol, or a similar vitamin preparation should be prescribed to increase the patient's general resistance.

The local measures should first be directed toward the prevention of deformity. Throughout the painful stage of any form of chronic arthritis of the spine the patient should be kept in bed. If there is a tendency for kyphosis to develop, hyperextension exercises should be given and the position of hyperextension should be maintained. Hyperextension in recumbency can be obtained conveniently by using a hinged fracture board on a reversed Gatch bed. The support provided by a Whitman frame (Fig. 69) or a posterior plaster shell (Fig. 70) is a very satisfactory means of preventing and of correcting deformity. If bony fusion is already solid, attempts to produce hyperextension will be of no avail. When the patient begins to stand, the back should be supported by a strong belt, surgical corset, brace, or plaster jacket. For Strümpell-Marie arthritis the Baker or the Jewett three-point brace is particularly useful as it tends constantly to correct flexion. Massage and postural exercises, preceded by diathermy or other form of heat, should be given daily for a long period. Particular attention should be paid to increasing the chest expansion by means of deep breathing exercises. In arthritis of the cervical spine it may be necessary to use head traction to correct a flexion deformity of the neck, after which a Thomas collar or a Schanz cotton collar may be applied.

For persistent localized pain associated with arthritis of the spine, absolute rest in bed is indicated; the mattress should be firm and supported by a fracture board. For pain radiating down the leg it may be advisable to apply traction to the extremity. Heat and massage should be employed as auxiliary measures. Stretching of the hamstring muscles under spinal or general anesthesia will often relieve the acute radiating pain. It is sometimes advisable to follow the manipulation with immobilization of the hip and back in a spica cast for three to six weeks. Acute pain which radiates into the lower extremities may often be relieved by the injection of dilute procaine or salt solution into the sacral epidural space.

The pain of Strümpell-Marie arthritis can often be relieved effectively by roentgen therapy. In mild cases roentgen therapy may also check the disease process. This type of treatment has generally proved unsuccessful, however, in other forms of chronic arthritis. ACTH and cortisone have proved of little value in treating this type of arthritis.

Operative treatment is seldom indicated. When there is localized pain with roentgenographic evidence of bone changes over a small area of the spine, a fusion operation may be indicated for permanent relief of the discomfort. Only in rare instances, however, is spinal fusion advisable. To correct the marked flexion deformity of the back in Strümpell-Marie arthritis, an osteotomy of the spine may occasionally be indicated.

Chronic Arthritis of the Hip

The hip joint may be involved primarily in either rheumatoid arthritis or osteoarthritis. In the rheumatoid type the hip affection is often a part of a widespread arthritic process; this is sometimes true also in osteoarthritis. Rheumatoid arthritis of the hip is not unlike the same type of arthritis in other joints; an identical group of symptoms, signs, and pathologic changes is observed. Osteoarthritis limited to the hip, however, forms a clinical picture somewhat different from that of osteoarthritis of other joints. It is a degenerative lesion occurring usually after the middle period of life and is frequently spoken of as *malum coxae senilis.*

MALUM COXAE SENILIS

Etiology.—Trauma is believed to be an important factor in the etiology. The disease may not follow immediately after the accident, however, but may develop insidiously years later. The rôle of infection is not believed to be important, but that of metabolic changes is probably more significant. The disease often appears many years following an adolescent epiphyseal disturbance, such as coxa plana or slipping of the upper femoral epiphysis, a congenital subluxation, a reduced congenital dislocation or a traumatic dislocation. Some authors feel that a congenital dysplasia of the acetabulum precedes a majority of the cases of malum coxae senilis. Certain European authors have postulated the formation in early life of a second acetabulum situated slightly above the original acetabulum and developed as a result of laxity about the hip joint.

It is thought that the incongruity of the joint surfaces is the most important factor in causing progression of the disease.

Pathology.—In the early stages there are a diminution of the joint space and a slight flattening of the head of the femur which is similar to that observed in coxa plana. Proliferation of new bone around the head takes place in the form of a collar. New bone is formed also around the margin of the acetabulum. The cartilage becomes irregularly worn away over the head and in the acetabulum and is replaced by hard, eburnated bone. The acetabulum grows larger as the head of the femur flattens. The femoral neck becomes short and broad. In addition to spurring and gross changes of contour, roentgenograms show irregular areas of increased bone density, mottling of the head and neck, and numerous small cystlike areas near the articular surfaces (Fig. 88). The synovial membrane usually becomes thick and fibrous. It may be completely replaced by fibrous connective tissue.

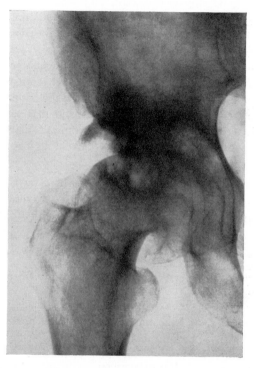

Fig. 88.—Anteroposterior roentgenogram showing osteoarthritis of hip in man fifty-eight years of age. Note large irregular, mushroom-shaped head of femur with areas of bone absorption and condensation. There is considerable sclerosis of bone immediately above the head, indicated by the dark undifferentiated area. The overlying ledge of bone from the superior acetabular margin is characteristic. The head has been displaced outward by new bone formation in the acetabulum. This is the so-called double acetabulum.

Clinical Picture.—The early symptoms may be aching in the hip region and slight stiffness or pain down the thigh to the knee following excessive exercise, which is completely relieved with rest. After standing or sitting there may be a slight catching sensation and pain in the hip on starting to walk. As the condition progresses, these symptoms appear most often in the morning and wear off during the day. After activity, however, the patient becomes easily fatigued. Gradually muscle spasm develops, causing flexion and adduction of the hip. Associated with the limitation of motion, there is usually pain upon pressure about the joint. Later slight shortening of the leg and a limp become noticeable. Creaking and grating develop in the joint, and the muscles atrophy. Later there is considerable pain on weight-bearing. Radiating pain often extends down the front of the thigh to the knee but is sometimes most marked on the posterior aspect. The leg gradually becomes externally rotated and the prominence of the greater trochanter increases. Abduction and internal rotation, as well as all other motions, are decreased in range. As the deformity of the hip increases, the added strain which is put upon the sacroiliac joint of the affected side may cause troublesome symptoms of sacroiliac arthritis. Arthritic symptoms may develop also in the lumbar spine as a result of strain. Recurrent attacks of extreme pain and disability are characteristic.

Diagnosis.—The diagnosis is not difficult. The roentgenographic changes, as well as the history and clinical signs, are quite characteristic.

Differential Diagnosis.—Subacute pyogenic infection, tuberculosis, and rheumatoid arthritis are most often confused with this monarticular hip affection.

Prognosis.—There is little possibility of complete restoration of function. If treatment is started early and is continued faithfully, however, the pain may be relieved. The hip usually becomes quite restricted in motion, and the limitation may even progress to complete ankylosis. When a flexion and adduction deformity develops, the disability is marked because of shortening of the leg.

Treatment.—The general treatment outlined for osteoarthritis should be used, with emphasis upon a diet low in proteins and carbohydrates if the patient is overweight, multi-vitamin capsules, thorough elimination, adequate rest, and in most instances a course of potassium iodide medication. ACTH and cortisone have proved to be of no permanent value.

Local.—In the early case diathermy, massage of the muscles, and gentle passive exercise of the joint may decrease the pain. These measures should be accompanied by efforts to relieve the trauma of weight-bearing; when the affected leg is shortened, a shoe with a heel elevation or high cork sole should be worn.

If the pain persists, a period of several weeks of recumbency with traction on the affected lower extremity and daily physical therapy is often most helpful. On returning to activity the patient can continue to use the traction at night. An alternative method of treatment is to immobilize the hip in abduction by means of a plaster spica cast for a period of six weeks. During this time partial ankylosis may occur. If ankylosis does not occur, the rest will relax the soft tissue structures, facilitate healing, and improve the range of motion. If deformity is present, the patient should be kept in bed and traction should be applied. It may be necessary to correct the deformity by cautious manipulation under anesthesia. Occasionally a walking hip spica cast or hip brace will relieve the pain by lessening the friction and strain upon the joint. At times a Thomas walking caliper splint with a high-sole shoe on the foot of the other leg is indicated to relieve the hip of weight-bearing. Often these conservative measures will result in complete relief of the pain, either with preservation of motion or with complete ankylosis.

Operative.—If severe pain persists despite conservative treatment, an operative procedure is indicated. The following measures should be considered:

1. *Manipulation.*—If the disease is not too far advanced, gentle manipulation will often release adhesions and may result in relief of the pain and increase of the range of motion. The improvement is usually not permanent. In occasional cases manipulation is followed by an increase of the pain and disability.

2. *Neurectomy.*—Section of the sensory nerve fibers supplying the hip joint will sometimes produce considerable relief of pain. This procedure is occasionally very helpful.

3. *Resection.*—In the most frequently employed type of resection the head of the femur is completely dislocated from the acetabulum and all irregular bony margins, or sometimes the entire head, are removed. The remaining head or the rounded neck is then replaced in the acetabulum, from which all projections and spurs have been removed *(cheilotomy).* In many cases the results of this operation have been satisfactory.

4. *Whitman Reconstruction Operation.*—The head of the femur is completely removed; the upper end of the neck is rounded and placed in the acetabulum; and the greater trochanter is transplanted down the shaft of the femur for a distance of about an inch and a half or two inches.

This procedure may result in considerable relief of pain and often provides a joint which, in addition to being stable, possesses a moderate range of motion.

5. *Arthroplasty.*—Occasionally an arthroplasty is indicated. The operative procedure includes complete remodeling of the head, shaping of a new acetabulum, and the placing of interposing material such as fascia lata or a Vitallium cup between the new head and the acetabulum (Fig. 63). In many clinics, especially in Europe, the application of a metal or plastic femoral head to the reshaped neck has replaced the cup arthroplasty (see p. 157). The results of these operative procedures to date have been encouraging.

6. *Arthrodesis.*—It is often advisable, especially in laborers, to fuse the hip. This is most effectively accomplished by a combination of the intra-articular and the so-called extra-articular methods, in which bone from the ilium or femur is placed along the neck from the upper end of the femur to the ilium after complete removal of the cartilage from the femoral head and acetabulum. Internal fixation can be effected with a long Smith-Petersen nail. When the ankylosis becomes firm, the hip pain is completely relieved. The author considers that in most cases arthrodesis is the operation of choice.

7. *Osteotomy.*—Occasionally the bifurcation operation of Lorenz, the subtrochanteric osteotomy of Schanz, or the transtrochanteric osteotomy of McMurray is indicated for the relief of pain.

The choice of operative procedure is largely dependent upon the physical condition of the individual. Most patients with malum coxae senilis are old and in such poor condition that extensive surgical procedures are extremely risky.

Chronic Arthritis of the Knee

The knee may be affected in both types of arthritis. It is the most frequent large joint to be involved by osteoarthritis.

The etiology and pathology are essentially the same as those discussed in the preceding chapter. Strain and trauma play a large part in the pathogenesis. Most of the affected individuals are heavy, and the increased weight is an important predisposing factor.

Clinical Picture.—Chronic arthritis of the knee often starts with slight stiffness in the joint after sitting or a tightness in the back of the knee associated with creaking. It becomes difficult to walk up stairs.

There may be swelling, tenderness, and increase of joint fluid, which together with the muscle atrophy give to the knee a spindle-shaped contour. A flexion deformity may develop, and pain may be caused by attempts to straighten the knee. Occasionally in chronic cases the tibia

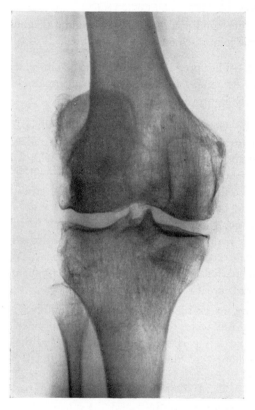

Fig. 89.—Anteroposterior roentgenogram showing osteoarthritis of the knee in a patient aged sixty-seven years. Note spurs about the tibial spines and femoral intercondylar notch, the medial and lateral tibial margins and patella, and irregular bone formation about external condyle of femur. This patient was entirely asymptomatic and seldom had had disability of the knee.

may become subluxated backward; this occurs more often in rheumatoid arthritis than in osteoarthritis. Chronic arthritis of the knee is most often bilateral.

The roentgenographic appearance of the knee in osteoarthritis is typical, spurs and lipping appearing about the margins of the femur and tibia as well as around the articular surface of the patella. Within the joint are often found loose bodies which have broken off from the small marginal projections of bone (Fig. 89).

Diagnosis.—The diagnosis is made from the clinical findings and the roentgenograms. The picture is typical and is not often confused with that of other conditions. In the differential diagnosis, tuberculosis and neuropathic joint disease must be considered.

Prognosis.—The prognosis is quite good in early osteoarthritis precipitated by trauma. In the advanced rheumatoid type, however, the prognosis for improvement is poor.

Treatment.—General treatment has been outlined in the previous chapter. The strain of weight-bearing should be relieved at once. If the pain is severe, the knee should be protected with a brace or a cast and crutches should be used. These measures will also prevent the development of a flexion deformity. Correction of an established flexion deformity should be carried out by means of traction or wedged casts. Exercise of the quadriceps and hamstring muscles is useful in stimulating circulation and maintaining muscle tone. In osteoarthritis moderate protection of the knees by bandaging or laced elastic kneecaps, when combined with partial or complete rest and the frequent application of heat, often affords great relief of the symptoms.

Synovectomy, or excision of the synovial membrane, is indicated in rheumatoid arthritis when the process has become quiescent throughout the body but has left persistent pain, thickening of the synovium, and limitation of motion of the knee. In osteoarthritis which has not responded to conservative therapy and which presents pain and stiffness about the anterior aspect of the knee, excision of the patella may be followed by a painless movable joint. In selected cases it may be advisable to combine thorough synovectomy and excision of the patella with removal of all degenerated cartilages, hypertrophic spurs, and pannus. After this relatively extensive surgical procedure, several weeks of traction and physical therapy are essential. When the arthritic changes are advanced, with roentgenographic evidence of destruction of the joint surfaces, arthrodesis of the knee may be indicated for the relief of pain. Knee flexion contracture due to rheumatoid arthritis is sometimes very difficult to correct. When such knees retain a fair range of flexion, straightening the leg by means of supracondylar osteotomy of the femur will correct the unsightly deformity and at the same time preserve the range of motion. In other cases posterior capsuloplasty may be indicated for the release of flexion contracture of long standing. Complete ankylosis of the knee in a young individual with good musculature may warrant arthroplasty, provided that no active inflammatory process is present in other joints of the body. While the results of arthroplasty are not always satisfactory, occasionally a movable and painless joint is obtained, and in recent years a number of successful arthroplasties have been reported with the use of a thin but tough sheet of nylon as an interposed material.

CHAPTER XII

NEUROMUSCULAR DISABILITIES: INFANTILE PARALYSIS

Infantile paralysis is an acute infectious disease caused by a filtrable virus which attacks the nervous system and possesses an especial tendency to affect the anterior horns of the gray matter of the spinal cord; hence the disease is often called *anterior poliomyelitis.* The infection is often accompanied by a paralysis which is entirely incidental and is not essential to the diagnosis. The disease occurs most often in early childhood, hence the term *infantile;* yet it is seen also in adults. Statistics in recent years have shown that the older age groups are being affected more often than in the past. The incidence is higher in boys than in girls, but in adults there is no sex variation. Infantile paralysis may appear in either sporadic or epidemic form. The greatest number of cases occurs in midsummer and early fall.

Etiology.—It has been rather conclusively proved that the infection is due to one of the filtrable viruses and that there are three principal strains of virus which cause the disease. Virus isolated from human cases has been proved to be the infecting agent of anterior poliomyelitis, as evidenced by the results of inoculating monkeys and certain rodents, notably the Eastern cotton rat. Poliomyelitis has developed in the inoculated animals and has been transmitted from animal to animal.

The virus can be isolated from the feces of patients and of persons in contact with them. It is frequently isolated from the oral secretion. During epidemics it has also been isolated from flies. At the present time the alimentary tract is considered to be the chief pathway for entry of the virus and spread of the disease. The susceptibility of different individuals varies and is thought by some observers to be increased by recent tonsillectomy, inoculations, and pregnancy. It has been shown that one attack confers absolute immunity against only one strain of the virus.

There are four distinct clinical types of the disease: (1) the abortive or nonparalytic; (2) the ataxic, in which there are pathologic changes in Clarke's columns, the cerebellum, or the basal ganglia with an accompanying nystagmus; (3) the cortical, in which the lesion is in the upper motor neurone with resulting spastic paralysis and hyperactive reflexes; and (4) the common spinal or subcortical, in which the lesion is in the lower motor neurone and results in a flaccid paralysis. The last type is recognized much more commonly than any of the others. Recent statistics indicate that the incidence of the upper spinal or bulbar type is relatively high in children who have had a tonsillectomy.

Pathology.—In the acute stage of the disease the virus has been found chiefly in parts of the central nervous system and in the alimentary tract. It is thought to spread from the alimentary tract by way of the peripheral nerve trunks to the central nervous system. The virus has a peculiar affinity for neuronal tissue, especially the motor portion, rather than for the supporting glial tissue of the central nervous system. After entering the central nervous system the virus diffuses in all directions, usually traversing the short chain pathways. By the time the disease is manifest clinically, evidence of widespread focal involvement of the brain, the spinal cord, and sometimes the meninges may be noted. The clinical findings, however, are never an accurate index of the extent to which the central nervous system has been involved.

The greatest changes appear in the anterior horn cells of the gray matter, especially those in the lumbar enlargement of the cord. These changes result in a motor paralysis. Occasionally the posterior horn cells or root ganglia or the higher sensory centers may be involved in the acute stage with the production of sensory disturbances. The cell bodies of these areas of the cord show evidence of atrophy and disintegration and may be replaced by scar tissue. The damaging effects upon the nerve cells may come (1) from direct toxic action by the virus; (2) from anemia through the constriction of local blood vessels; or (3) from direct pressure as the result of hemorrhage, exudate, or edema. There are also changes within the lymphatic system, such as swollen mesenteric glands, congested Peyer's patches, and enlargement of the spleen. In the chronic stage, when the motor cells have been replaced by scar tissue, degeneration of the peripheral nerves occurs and is accompanied by muscle and tendon atrophy and rarefaction of bone. In the chronic stage, microscopic examination of affected muscles shows areas of atrophy, fatty or fibrous replacement, and hypertrophy of the undamaged cells.

Clinical Picture.—The average incubation period is from seven to fourteen days, although it may be as long as thirty-five days. Clinically, the disease may be abortive (without involvement of the central nervous system); it may be nonparalytic (without gross evidence of flaccid paralysis); or it may be paralytic (with varying degrees of muscle weakness or paralysis). The first type is of little clinical concern; the second type is characterized by muscle tightness, particularly of the neck, back, and hamstring muscle groups, which yields readily to active physical therapy. The third type forms the chief discussion of this chapter.

After the onset of the disease there are three distinct stages: (1) the acute stage or stage of onset, which lasts from one to four weeks; (2) the stage of convalescence and recovery, which lasts from six months to two years; and (3) the residual stage, during which little or no spontaneous improvement occurs.

Acute Stage.—The symptoms during the acute stage may be divided into three groups: (1) systemic, (2) meningitic, and (3) paralytic.

The most characteristic systemic symptom is fever, which may reach from 100° to 105° F. (38° to 41° C.), last from one to six days, and then subside either by lysis or crisis. The fever, however, after subsiding completely, may return in a day or two. In this stage intense headaches and marked gastrointestinal symptoms, such as vomiting, constipation, and abdominal distress, are often observed. There may be associated upper respiratory symptoms, as well as drowsiness and irritability when the patient is aroused. Urinary retention occurs frequently. The cervical lymph nodes may be enlarged. Pain may be present spontaneously in the muscles or may be felt only when they are subjected to pressure.

The meningitic symptoms may consist of hyperactive reflexes and muscular twitchings or convulsions. Stiffness of the back and neck, with inability to touch the chin to the knees, is usually present, and is a valuable diagnostic sign. Kernig's sign is usually positive but not so constantly as in bacterial meningitis. The spinal fluid is clear with a great increase in cells, polymorphonuclear in the early stages and later mostly mononuclear, and there may be slight increase of its globulin and albumin content.

The paralytic symptoms appear usually on the second day and seldom after the eighth day. With the development of flaccid paralysis the reflexes become hypoactive or absent. In the occasional instances of cortical involvement the paralysis may be spastic in type with hyperactive reflexes. Paralytic symptoms are much more common in the lower extremities than in the upper; asymmetrical involvement is characteristic. It has been said that in the lower extremities recovery is less likely to take place than in the upper extremities, but this statement is not accepted by all observers. The return of muscle power begins usually in the first two weeks but may not become obvious until later. The most serious cases are those with paralysis of the diaphragm and of other respiratory muscles, which constitute the bulbar type. These symptoms often follow paralysis of the upper extremity and particularly paralysis about the shoulder girdle.

Great care should be taken to recognize paralysis of the abdominal and spinal muscles, since such paralysis may later lead to curvature of the spine. After weakening or paralysis of any muscles becomes evident, it is most important to determine which groups are involved, since the affected muscles need immediate rest. Tenderness of the muscles may be slight or extreme; it is a most characteristic symptom and has been known to persist for as long as sixteen weeks, although the average duration is six weeks. Gentle active exercise diminishes muscle tenderness.

In an epidemic there may be patients who show all the neurologic, febrile, upper respiratory, and gastrointestinal symptoms without evidence of paralysis. Such patients are said to have the nonparalytic type of the disease.

Convalescent or Recovery Stage.—In the convalescent stage the muscle tenderness has subsided and there may be a progressive increase of muscle power. The improvement in muscle strength may continue for a period of eighteen months to two years.

Periodic examinations of the different muscle groups should be made in order to follow the degree of muscle improvement. Much important information can be gained from careful observation of the gait. The so-called *steppage* or *foot-drop gait,* in which the anterior portion of the foot strikes the floor first with each step, is an indication of paralysis of the anterior muscles of the leg. This paralysis is often associated with equinus deformity, and there may be accompanying genu recurvatum, especially when the flexors of the knee are paralyzed. In paralysis of the quadriceps the patient often inclines his body forward and places his hand on the front of the thigh. This braces the knee in extension and prevents sudden flexion on weight-bearing. In paralysis of the gluteus maximus muscle the trunk sways backward in walking to prevent a sudden flexion of the body on weight-bearing. In paralysis of the gluteus medius muscle the body sways toward the affected side, and on this side the pelvis is tilted upward.

Weakness of the abdominal muscles is considered by many to be the most common cause of scoliosis and lordosis after infantile paralysis. In paralytic scoliosis the patient usually cannot raise his trunk from a supine to a sitting position without the aid of his arms.

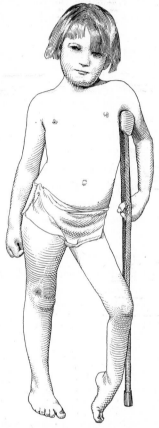

Fig. 90.—Deformities in infantile paralysis. Note flexion contracture of left hip and knee with equinovarus foot. (After Ombredanne and Mathieu.)

Residual Stage.—The paralytic symptoms and signs are now stationary or very slowly regressive. In this stage deformities may have begun to appear or already may be fully developed (Figs. 90-93). They will be described under the treatment of established deformity.

Diagnosis.—Except during epidemics the diagnosis is frequently not made until after the paralysis appears. It is usually based upon the history

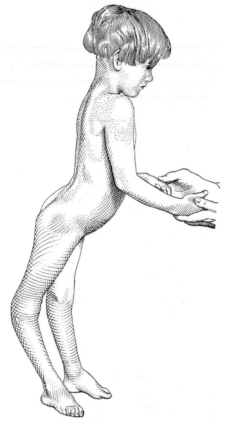

Fig. 91.—Deformities in infantile paralysis. Note bilateral genu recurvatum (back knee), equinus, hip flexion, and lumbar lordosis.

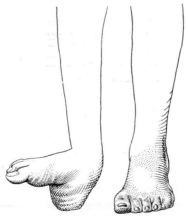

Fig. 92.—Deformities in infantile paralysis. Note marked calcaneo-cavus of right foot.

of slight systemic upset, the stiffness of the neck, the muscle tenderness, the paralysis, and the findings on examination of the spinal fluid.

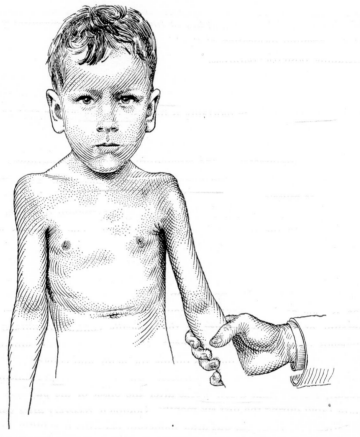

Fig. 93.—Deformities in infantile paralysis. Note atrophy and subluxation of left shoulder.

Differential Diagnosis.—Infantile paralysis is to be differentiated from (1) acute febrile affections usually not accompanied by paralysis, such as acute rheumatic fever, fever associated with upper respiratory infection, pyogenic arthritis, and osteomyelitis; (2) febrile affections which may be associated with paralysis, such as diphtheria, the Guillain-Barré syndrome, and other forms of polyneuritis; (3) primary affections of the central nervous system, such as encephalitis, meningitis, brain tumor, cerebral palsy, transverse myelitis, and amyotonia congenita; (4) diseases accompanied by pseudoparalysis or spasm, such as pseudohypertrophic muscular dystrophy, lead poisoning, lues, hypervitaminosis A, infantile cortical hyperostosis, scurvy, and rickets; (5) other conditions which present deformity and loss of function, such as congenital clubfoot and congenital dislocation of the hip; and (6) peripheral nerve injuries, including obstetric paralysis.

Prognosis.—The mortality rate is from 3 to 20 per cent during epidemics, increases with age, and is greater in males than in females. In the bulbar cases the mortality is highest, usually 50 per cent or more. Death is most often due to hypoxia from partial paralysis of the respiratory muscles with pooling of secretions in the throat, or from involvement of the respiratory or the circulatory center in the medulla.

The prognosis as to function is extremely uncertain. The extent of recovery of muscle power depends wholly upon the survival of the affected nerve cells. No method of determining the amount of power which will return to the paralyzed muscles is known. The prognosis is very favorable if there is a rapid return of power after the acute infection, and it is sometimes better for the upper extremities than for the lower. The prognosis is unfavorable in patients in whom muscle tenderness has been persistent. It is poor when the muscles have remained paralyzed for as long as three months without evidence of return of power. The amount of functional return in the tonically contracted muscle fibers depends largely upon the treatment. If sufficient rest and support can be given the paralyzed muscles during the acute and convalescent stage, the prognosis is relatively favorable. Spontaneous improvement, if it occurs, starts within a few weeks after the onset of the paralysis and is most rapid during the first six months. Complete recovery after extensive paralysis is uncommon, but after moderate paralysis it is quite common. An extremely high percentage of paralyzed patients in poliomyelitis epidemics either recover completely or are left with a very slight residual paralysis. In a careful two-year follow-up of 673 cases with paralysis in two Maryland epidemics there were found to be 55 per cent with complete recoveries, and 81 per cent with good recoveries. Retardation of the growth of the affected extremity may occur as a result of disuse.

Treatment.—*Prophylactic.*—Great care should be taken in isolating the patient, especially as regards contact with the nasal secretions and disposal of the feces. This strict isolation should be maintained from the onset to forty-eight hours after the temperature becomes normal. Infantile paralysis is thought to be most contagious during the first two weeks of the infection. During epidemics it is most important that children avoid fatigue, crowds, swimming pools, and contact with other children. Every effort should be made to exterminate all flies as it has been shown that they are sometimes carriers of the virus.

Acute Stage.—In the acute stage absolute rest in bed is essential. It relieves the pain, helps to reduce the inflammatory reaction, and aids thereby in the restoration of the injured neurones. During this time the bowels should not be allowed to become constipated. Inflammation of the nose and throat should be treated symptomatically. Convalescent serum has proved of little value. Transfusions of whole blood are often helpful. Lumbar puncture and intravenous injections of hypertonic glucose during the acute stage reduce the cerebrospinal fluid pressure and are of value in treating the meningismus. The hot moist packs which form a part of the Kenny method of treatment are extremely useful in relieving pain and spasm in the affected muscles and should be continued as long as these symptoms persist. In some clinics good results in relieving sustained muscle contraction by the use of curare, Myanesin or Tolserol, Priscoline, and neostigmine have been reported, but the use of these drugs is by no means an accepted procedure. The weakened muscles should be maintained in an attitude free from strain, and any affected joints should be held in the position of maximum functional utility. This part of the treatment is most important and is the best means of preventing the development of deformity.

If there is paralysis of the respiratory muscles, which is most common in the bulbar type, the patient should be kept quiet with his head down. The administration of oxygen may be helpful. If the respirations become difficult and extremely labored from paralysis of the primary respiratory muscles, he should be placed in a respirator and kept there until recovery of muscle power is sufficient to permit maintenance of normal respiration. He should not be left in the respirator longer than is necessary. If the pharyngeal muscles are paralyzed, care should be taken to forestall choking attacks and the aspiration of mucus. Occasionally tracheotomy becomes necessary. The patient should be fed parenterally and kept at complete rest.

If a choice of the muscles to be protected in order to prevent deformity is necessary, those groups which maintain the erect position should be given first consideration, i.e., the hip extensors, the knee extensors, the abdominal and erector spinae muscles, and the dorsiflexors of the ankle. Next in importance are the abductors of the shoulder, the dorsiflexors of the wrist, and the adductors of the thumb.

Convalescent Stage.—The convalescent stage extends from the subsidence of muscle tenderness to the slowing of the process of recovery of muscle power. It may last over a period of two years or more. To prevent joint contracture in this stage it is usually advisable to move the joints passively through their full range of motion each day. How long the muscles should be kept at rest is a debatable point. Partial immobilization should always be continued until an end stage in the return of muscle power has become apparent. Muscle training consisting of gentle active exercises should be started early in the convalescent stage and gradually increased. Muscles should never be exercised, however, to the point of fatigue. Exercises which do not involve weightbearing will improve the strength of the weakened muscles; however, if too much strain is put upon these muscles, as in weight-bearing, recovery will be definitely retarded. The muscle-resisting exercises of DeLorme may be of great value at this stage.

Hydrogymnastics do not take the place of training the individual muscles, but often the support of the water allows muscles to be moved more effectively and provides a pleasant way of carrying out the exercises. The water itself has no intrinsic therapeutic value. It must be remembered that muscle fatigue can appear with less warning in underwater exercises than in exercises given out of water.

Massage improves the local nutrition of the muscles, and heat adds effectiveness to the massage. Electrical stimulation of muscles, if not too vigorously performed, undoubtedly helps to preserve their nutrition. Muscle training establishes better coordination between partially paralyzed and normal groups. It should include instruction and training in gait as the patient resumes walking. Great care should be taken to prevent the development of deformities by proper positioning of the joints and early active corrective exercises. If preventive measures are not taken, permanent bone deformities may later develop as the result of malpositions which have remained uncorrected for a long period of time.

In the convalescent stage, braces and other apparatus are often necessary (1) to enable the patient to stand and walk, (2) to prevent deformity and malposition, and (3) to help in stretching certain groups of muscles which have become contracted. In general, however, apparatus is undesirable and should be used only when absolutely necessary. A back brace (Fig. 73) or a removable plaster jacket may be used for

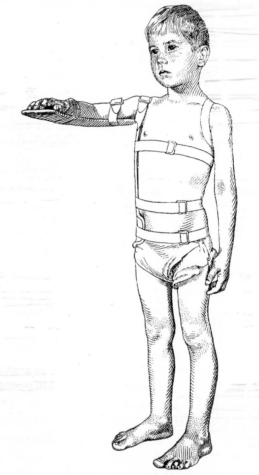

Fig. 94.—Abduction, platform, or airplane splint for paralysis of muscles about shoulder girdle.

paralysis of the back and abdominal muscles. An abduction arm splint is used for paralysis of the deltoid muscle (Fig. 94). A cock-up splint is used for paralysis of the extensor muscles of the wrist. A walking caliper brace with or without a joint at the knee is indicated in paralysis

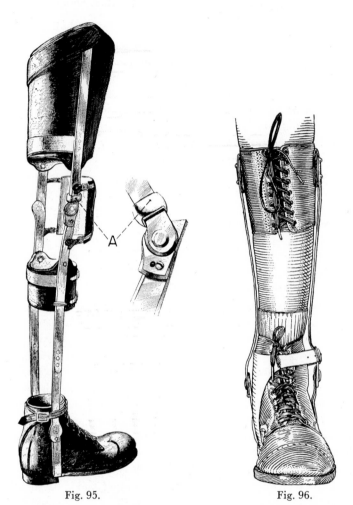

Fig. 95.　　　　　　　　　　　　　Fig. 96.

Fig. 95.—Long leg brace, with lock joint at knee (*A*) and right-angle stop joint and pull over strap at ankle. This type of brace is used for the weak lower extremity which has paralysis of the muscles of the thigh and leg with little or no stability of the knee.

Fig. 96.—Ankle brace with T-strap, for paralysis of muscles of the leg. The T-strap is used to prevent a deviation of the ankle toward the medial side.

involving the thigh muscles (Fig. 95) and this same type of brace with a waistband and a lock joint at the hip at times is used for paralysis of the extensors of the hip. An ankle brace may be used for paralysis of the dorsiflexor muscles of the ankle (Fig. 96). In paralysis of the gastrocnemius and soleus muscles either an ankle brace or a shoe with raised heel and stiff tongue may be used. In paralysis of the invertors or evertors of the foot a lateral iron and T-strap attached to the shoe may be used.

Residual Stage.—In the residual stage operations are performed to correct deformity, to improve muscle balance, and to secure the stability of joints. In general, procedures of the last two types should not be done until from eighteen months to two years have elapsed from the time of onset of the disease and procedures of the last type until the age of eight years has been reached in the normally developing child, or the age of ten years when the child is underdeveloped.

Operative Treatment.—The operative correction of deformities and disabilities of the joints following infantile paralysis forms a large part of the work of many orthopaedic surgeons. The procedures, when selected on the basis of sound indications, performed correctly, and followed by adequate after-care, are productive of most gratifying results. By operation a great many patients are enabled for the first time to walk, and others who have been in braces and on crutches are enabled to discard these supports. Great care must always be taken, however, that the operation do no harm. In every clinic, individual modifications of the accepted operative procedures have been adopted. There is no field of orthopaedic surgery in which mature judgment is more necessary for selection of the most beneficial operative procedures. Poor results are usually the consequence of (1) decisions made hastily on cases which have not been adequately studied or observed, or (2) operations which have not been followed by sufficient after-care and observation. Often more information can be gained, and the treatment can be more wisely selected, by watching the patient handle himself and walk than by performing tests of individual muscle function. Too much emphasis cannot be placed upon the necessity of waiting until the child is of adequate age, size, and bony development before proceeding with operations on bony structures which might later prove futile because of growth changes. Every operation for the correction of deformity or disability resulting from infantile paralysis should be followed by a long period of careful observation.

A. Operations for the Correction of Deformities of Long Standing

It often happens that the orthopaedic surgeon does not see the patient until months or years after the onset of the disease and that by this time the deformity has become firmly fixed.

The Hip.—It is not uncommon to observe a pathologic dislocation of the hip following paralysis of the gluteus maximus, and flexion-adduction deformity due to persistence of the function of hip flexors and adductors. A snapping sensation on motion of the hip may be associated with an incomplete dislocation. In the treatment of such a dislocation a two-stage shelf operation (Fig. 29) with reefing of the hip joint capsule may be performed. At the first operation the dislocation is reduced, the posterior portion of the capsule is plicated, and the leg is immobilized in a slightly abducted and hyperextended position. At the second operation an exaggerated acetabular shelf is created. At times paralytic dislocation of the hip is best treated by arthrodesis.

Hip flexion contracture usually results from allowing the patient to sit up during the convalescent stage and can be prevented by keeping the patient in the prone position for a few hours each day during this period. Hip flexion deformity is due to a contracture of the tensor fasciae latae, iliopsoas, sartorius and rectus femoris muscles together with weakness of the gluteus maximus muscle. The contracture may at times be gradually reduced by repeated stretching. Occasionally it may be necessary to carry out open division of the tensor fasciae latae muscle at the hip together with manipulation and stretching. A flexion deformity of the hip can usually be relieved completely by transverse section of the iliotibial band just above the knee (*Yount operation*) combined with a section of the tensor fascia latae just below the level of the greater trochanter, followed by adequate skeletal traction and plaster fixation. This procedure has been popularized by Irwin at Warm Springs. The operation of choice in more severe cases may consist of stripping the fascia lata and associated flexors of the hip subperiosteally from the anterior superior spine and crest of the ilium for a distance of about 1½ inches and of allowing them to slip down the side of the pelvis to become reattached at a more distal site (*Soutter operation*). This operation is followed by immobilization in a plaster cast for six to eight weeks with the hip in hyperextension. In the most severe cases the anterior superior spine and anterior portion of the crest of the ilium may be detached along with their muscle insertions, slipped down the side of the pelvis, and transplanted *en masse* into the bone at a lower level *(Campbell operation).* The hip is then immobilized in hyperextension in a plaster cast for eight weeks. The Soutter and Campbell operations have been far more popular in the past than they are at present.

The Knee.—Flexion deformity of the knee is extremely common. It is due to the contraction of strong hamstring muscles which are ineffectively opposed by a weakened quadriceps group. It is possible at times to reduce the deformity by applying traction to the leg. Wedged or turnbuckle plaster casts often serve very satisfactorily. Occasionally it may be necessary to lengthen the tendons behind the knee or to perform a *capsuloplasty* in which the posterior attachment of the joint capsule to the femur is released. It is often advisable to combine lengthening of the tendon of the biceps femoris with capsuloplasty. For persistent flexion contracture, a supracondylar osteotomy is sometimes indicated.

When a knock-knee deformity develops from quadriceps paralysis with a strong biceps femoris and a tight iliotibial band, it may be necessary to section the band, perform a supracondylar osteotomy of the femur, correct the deformity, and immobilize the extremity in a plaster cast for eight weeks.

When genu recurvatum has developed as a result of weakness of the hamstrings, or walking with an equinus contracture, a caliper brace with a posterior knee strap may stabilize the joint sufficiently to facilitate walking. In more marked cases the patella may be implanted into the upper end of the tibia to act as a bone block and to prevent the knee from undergoing hyperextension *(Campbell operation),* or a strong check ligament may be constructed posteriorly from the periosteum of the femur and the fascia lata *(Gill operation).* A wedge osteotomy of the upper two inches of the tibia with the base posteriorly and an osteotomy of the fibula, as described by Irwin, may also prove very useful in these cases.

Occasionally posterior subluxation and external rotation of the tibia may develop as a result of weakness of the quadriceps muscle while the hamstrings remain strong. For this deformity it is often advisable to carry out an arthrodesis of the knee; if this is not done, an accurately fitting brace should be applied.

The Ankle.—An equinus deformity or foot-drop may develop as a result of the persistent action of normal gastrocnemius and soleus muscles in opposition to weakened dorsiflexors of the foot. This is by far the commonest paralytic deformity of the ankle. An open lengthening of the Achilles tendon, followed by overcorrection in a plaster cast for six weeks, may be indicated. An ankle brace (Fig. 96) may then be necessary to prevent recurrence of the equinus. At times it is possible to stretch the Achilles tendon satisfactorily with wedged casts or a constant tension brace. When there is an external rotation deformity of the foot and lower part of the leg due to tibial torsion, correction may be effected by a rotation osteotomy of the tibia.

The Upper Extremities.—Contracture of the shoulder may develop as a result of paralysis of the abductors and persistence of the adductors. The deformity is one of adduction and internal rotation. It may be possible to overcome the contracture by manipulation. Otherwise the contracted structures should be exposed by open operation and incised. All early cases of deltoid paralysis should be treated with an *airplane* or *platform brace* (Fig. 94), or a *suspension splint* as described by Irwin, to forestall the development of adduction contracture.

Occasionally there may be a luxation of the head of the humerus due to stretching of the joint capsule following paralysis of the deltoid, triceps, and biceps muscles. When extreme relaxation is present in the chronic stage and is interfering with function, arthrodesis of the shoulder may be necessary (Fig. 99).

Deformities of the elbow, wrist, and hand, resulting from unbalanced muscular pull and the effects of gravity, may be of varied type. Operative correction of the deformity is occasionally indicated.

The Spine.—Great care should be taken to prevent the development of lateral curvature. When weakness of the muscles of the back or abdomen becomes evident, the use of a plaster cast or a brace is indicated; this support should be continued until there is a normal return of muscle power. Fascia lata transplants are occasionally used to reinforce partially paralyzed abdominal muscles *(Lowman operation)*, but on the whole their results in the hands of most orthopaedic surgeons have been disappointing. Incipient lateral curvature may be treated by recumbency with traction applied to the head and to the pelvis (Fig. 69), followed by the use of an accurately fitting back support. Correction of the curvature can usually be accomplished if treatment is started before secondary bone changes develop. In order to prevent the deformity from increasing, it is often necessary to stabilize the spine by operative fusion of the vertebrae (Fig. 74).

B. Muscle and Tendon Transplantations

In selected cases, improvement in muscle balance may be obtained by muscle and tendon transplantations. In tendon transplantation it is important (1) that any deformity of the joint should have been previously corrected, (2) that the tendon used should arise from a muscle with good power, preferably equal to that of the paralyzed muscle, (3) that the tendon should pass to its new insertion in a straight line through subcutaneous fat or through a tendon sheath, and (4) that the tendon should be inserted under slight tension directly into bone. Occasionally a portion of another or a transplant of fascia lata is used to supplement the tendon when its length is insufficient.

The Hip.—The unsightly gait caused by paralysis of the gluteus maximus or of the gluteus medius may often be much improved by one of the following operations.

For paralysis of the gluteus maximus muscle there are two useful operative procedures. In one the erector spinae muscles are freed from their lower attachments and a long strip of fascia lata is removed and sutured to them, passed over the paralyzed gluteus maximus muscle, and fixed into the femur at the insertion of the gluteus maximus (*Ober operation*). In the other, the origin of the tensor fasciae latae muscle with its bony attachment is transplanted into either the posterior superior spine or the adjacent posterior portion of the iliac crest (*Dickson operation*). After either of these operations a plaster spica cast applied with the hip in full abduction is to be worn for a period of from six to eight weeks.

For paralysis of the gluteus medius muscle the origin of the tensor fasciae latae may be transplanted posteriorly on the crest of the ilium to a point directly above the greater trochanter (*Legg operation*). This procedure tends to diminish the lateral sway of the body which is characteristic of abductor limp. An alternative procedure recently developed is transfer of the iliopsoas insertion to the greater trochanter.

The Knee.—Tendon transplantations about the knee frequently result in improvement of its function and stability. For quadriceps paralysis the most satisfactory operation, in the presence of strong hamstring muscles, is transplantation of the biceps femoris tendon, the iliotibial band, and one internal hamstring into the patella. If the hamstrings as well as the quadriceps are weak, the sartorius muscle and the iliotibial band may be transplanted into the patella.

The Foot.—Tendon transplantations combined with stabilizing operations on the joints often give very satisfactory results. For varus deformity the tibialis anticus muscle may be transplanted into the cuboid bone or into the base of the third or fourth metatarsal bone. For valgus deformity one of the peroneal tendons may be transplanted either into the scaphoid bone or into the base of the first metatarsal bone; however, these procedures are not so successful as the transplantations for varus deformity. For a calcaneus foot, transplantation of one or both peroneal tendons and the posterior tibial tendon into the os calcis may prove beneficial, but this procedure is successful only if some power is present in the calf muscles. The treatment of claw-foot deformity resulting from infantile paralysis is discussed on pages 479-480.

The Shoulder.—For paralysis of the deltoid muscle the acromial portion of the trapezius muscle may be transplanted into the upper part of the humerus *(Mayer operation)*, or the long head of the triceps and the short head of the biceps may be transplanted into the acromion process *(Ober operation)*. The arm is then held in an abduction spica cast for several weeks. Frequently the results of these operations are not so satisfactory as those usually obtained after tendon transplantations in the lower extremities.

The Elbow.—For incomplete paralysis of the flexors of the elbow the origin of the common flexor tendon, together with its bony attachment at the medial epicondyle, may be transplanted into the shaft of the humerus at a point about two inches proximal to its original site *(Steindler operation)*. This procedure often results in considerable improvement of the power of elbow flexion; it may even restore active flexion after this movement has been almost completely lost.

The Hand.—The indications for the transplantation of tendons in the hand are numerous, and many operations have been described. The most important mechanism in the hand is opposition of the thumb to the forefinger; operations to improve this function are performed most frequently. For paralysis of the opponens pollicis the palmaris longus or the flexor carpi ulnaris may be used as a motor, the tendon being transplanted into the extensor pollicis brevis tendon after having been looped to the ulnar side of the wrist *(Bunnell operation)*. An alternative procedure is to detach the tendon of the flexor sublimis of the fourth finger, loop it about the flexor carpi ulnaris, and fasten it into the base of the first phalanx of the thumb.

When no tendon is available for transfer, a bone graft placed between the first and second metacarpal bones will often make opposition of the thumb and fingers possible.

A most important part of tendon and muscle transplantation is the after-care. Exercise, supplemented by heat and massage, should be started as early as possible in order to lessen the likelihood of adhesions. Physical therapy should be continued as long as progressive improvement is demonstrable.

C. Operations to Increase the Stability of Joints

The most useful procedures in the surgical treatment of infantile paralysis are operations which restore stability to flail joints. Arthrodesis is the most important of these operative procedures. Bone block is an auxiliary measure which often results in marked improvement of function.

1. ARTHRODESIS

The Hip.—Arthrodesis of the hip after infantile paralysis is prone to be followed by incomplete fusion or by a poor functional result. It is wise therefore to denude the joint surfaces of cartilage very completely to place large extra-articular transplants of bone from the femur to the pelvis, and to fix these grafts securely at each end. Postoperative immobilization must be continued until firm union has taken place; this usually requires from twelve to twenty weeks. The return to activity must be gradual.

The Knee.—Arthrodesis of the knee is indicated only in selected cases. Many orthopaedic surgeons believe that a well-fitting brace with an adjustable lock at the knee is preferable to arthrodesis. In adults or in older children who wish to be free from the inconvenience of apparatus arthrodesis is to be advised.

The Ankle.—Arthrodesis of the ankle is occasionally indicated. It is seldom advisable in children because with subsequent growth late deformities are likely to develop. When arthrodesis is performed, the articular cartilage is usually removed through an anterior incision; it is wise to fuse the subastragalar and mediotarsal joints at the same time.

The Foot.—Arthrodesis of the subastragalar and mediotarsal joints is the most commonly performed operation in the entire surgical treatment of disability following infantile paralysis. The great value of stabilizing these joints was first shown by G. G. Davis in 1913.

The *Hoke operation* (Fig. 97), or one of its modifications, is the most popular type of arthrodesis in America at the present time. It may be used for varus, valgus, calcaneus, or equinus deformity. In this operation the head and the neck of the astragalus are taken out; the subastragalar joint surfaces are excised; the cartilage is removed from the posterior surface of the scaphoid bone; the denuded head of the astragalus is placed between the scaphoid and the body of the astragalus; and the foot is displaced backward upon the astragalus. Usually the calcaneo-cuboid joint surfaces are also removed. When this is done, the combined operation is sometimes known as a *triple arthrodesis*; this procedure was popularized by Hibbs and Ryerson.

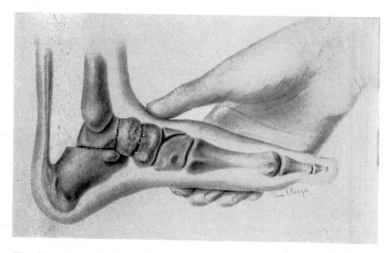

Fig. 97.—Operation for stabilization of the foot in infantile paralysis (medial view). The head of the astragalus has been removed, reshaped, and replaced; the articular surfaces have been removed from the subastragalar and the astragalo-scaphoid joints; and the foot has been displaced backward. (Hoke's original drawing.)

In England the *Dunn operation* is more popular than the Hoke. In this procedure the scaphoid bone is completely removed, the subastragalar and calcaneocuboid joint surfaces are excised, and the head of the astragalus and the posterior surface of the cuneiform bones are denuded of cartilage and approximated. Occasionally an arthrodesis of the ankle is performed at the same time. The Hoke and the Dunn operations are most used for the varus or valgus foot. In England and America the *Lambrinudi operation* is becoming more popular for the foot which needs a stabilization in the presence of weak dorsiflexors of the ankle and fairly strong plantar flexors. The operation consists of (1) removing the whole undersurface of the astragalus obliquely and the upper surface of the os calcis, (2) placing the astragalus in full plantar flexion, and (3) bringing up the forefoot at the mediotarsal joint so that the remainder of the head of the astragalus lies beneath a prepared bed in the undersurface of the scaphoid, while the astragalus and os calcis are approximated.

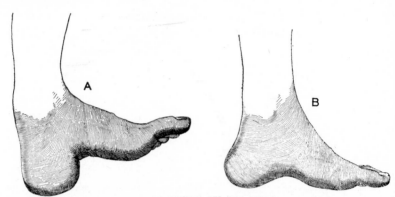

Fig. 98.—Calcaneocavus deformity in infantile paralysis (medial view). *A*, Before operation; *B*, after operative stabilization. Note posterior displacement of the foot and correction of the deformity.

For the calcaneal foot, many orthopaedic surgeons perform a triple arthrodesis and in some instances combine with it a fusion of the ankle joint. The Whitman astragalectomy has often been used in the past but is seldom done at this time. If an astragalectomy is performed, it is essential that the foot be displaced well backward upon the tibia.

The usual period of immobilization in plaster after arthrodesis of the tarsus is from eight to twelve weeks. It is frequently advisable to change the cast three weeks after operation; at this time, when necessary, manipulation can be carried out to improve the position of the foot.

The Shoulder.—Arthrodesis of the shoulder is not to be considered unless the muscles of the shoulder girdle are strong enough to permit shrugging of the shoulder and unless useful function of the hand has been retained. Satisfactory use of the fused shoulder is dependent upon power in the upper part of the trapezius muscle and the upper two-thirds of the serratus anterior muscle. A satisfactory method of arthrodesis is to denude the joint surfaces of cartilage, bevel the upper and lower flat surfaces of the acromion process, and then insert this beveled end into a prepared slot in the head of the humerus (Gill operation) (Fig. 99). Another method of obtaining fusion is to insert a massive bone graft into a hole drilled through the humeral head and into the scapula.

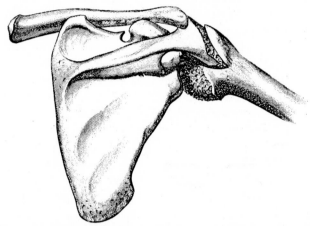

Fig. 99.—Arthrodesis of shoulder (Gill). The cartilage has been removed from the head of the humerus and the glenoid. The acromion has been denuded of periosteum, beveled on both of its flat surfaces, and placed in a slot prepared in the greater tuberosity of the humerus.

The Elbow.—Arthrodesis of the elbow is seldom necessary after infantile paralysis.

The Wrist.—Arthrodesis of the wrist is occasionally indicated. It may allow remaining flexors or extensors of the wrist to be transferred for use as motors of the fingers. The cartilaginous surfaces between the carpus and the lower end of the radius should be removed and the wrist immobilized in the position of 35 degrees of dorsiflexion. A popular technic for arthrodesis of the wrist is to use a cortical bone graft extending from the radius across the denuded dorsum of the carpal bones to the proximal end of the third metacarpal bone. If adequate power is present in the muscles of the fingers, the function of the hand is likely to be improved.

2. Extra-articular Check Operations About the Ankle

It is sometimes useful to abolish undesired ankle motion by creating surgically a bony block. This type of operation is often used to check plantar flexion in paralysis of the dorsiflexor muscles and occasionally to limit dorsiflexion when the plantar flexors are paralyzed. In either case the bone check operation is often preceded by a subastragalar arthrodesis.

To check the disabling equinus deformity of paralytic drop-foot, either of two procedures may be used. The posterior superior surface of the os calcis may be exposed and denuded and bone chips placed on the raw surface beneath the Achilles tendon. The mass of bone chips should extend up to the lower end of the tibia. When this transplanted bone becomes solid, there is a firm structure behind the ankle which prevents the foot from dropping beyond a right angle *(Campbell bone block operation)*. In the alternative procedure the posterior superior surface of the astragalus is split, elevated, and held in its new position by the insertion of a small wedge of bone *(Gill operation)*. This procedure is much easier to perform and is preferred by the author. Gill has also shown that the excessive dorsiflexion of paralytic calcaneus deformity can be limited by creating a bone block anteriorly; the anterior superior surface of the body of the astragalus is elevated by an analogous technic.

D. Leg Equalization Operations

Occasionally after infantile paralysis an extreme shortening of the affected leg is produced by the retardation of bone growth. It has been shown that this retardation of bone growth is dependent on the extent of the muscle paralysis. The asymmetry may be sufficiently deforming to indicate operative equalization of the length of the legs. The indication is sometimes provided by other causes of lateral asymmetry, such as developmental hemihypertrophy or retarded growth following epiphyseal injury. Equalization of leg length may be effected either by lengthening the shorter extremity or by shortening the longer one. Bone lengthening operations have been performed most often upon the tibia and fibula but have not yielded uniformly satisfactory results. The procedure is a gradual stretching of the soft tissues and lengthening of the bone after an osteotomy of special type. After the osteotomy it is necessary to maintain the fragments in satisfactory apposition and alignment, and for this purpose many types of apparatus have been devised. At times an increase in length of as much as 3 inches may be satisfactorily obtained. Great care and judgment are necessary in the selection of cases suitable for lengthening operations.

In most cases equalization of the length of the legs can be accomplished more satisfactorily by shortening the longer leg, since this involves no painful and hazardous stretching of the soft tissues. The shortening may be accomplished by performing a simple oblique osteotomy of the femur and allowing the fragments to override, or by removing a measured segment of the femur. In either case care must be taken to secure effective internal fixation of the fragments.

Gross inequality of leg length in children may often be treated satisfactorily by an operation to retard the growth of the longer leg. Local growth in length may be arrested permanently by fusing the epiphysis to the diaphysis. This operation, called epiphysiodesis, should not be done before ten years of age. In the selection of cases, a careful estimate of the relative rates of growth of the two legs and of the duration of further growth must be made. Since most of the growth in length of the leg occurs about the knee, the usual operative procedure is fusion of the lower femoral epiphysis or the upper tibial and fibular epiphyses, or all three, to the respective diaphyses. The operative technic must be careful and thorough to prevent later deformity of the knee from incomplete, asymmetrical arrest of growth. An alternative procedure, advocated in recent years by Blount, is to insert strong metal staples across the epiphyseal plate into epiphysis and diaphysis. Later, if resumption of growth is desired, the staples may be removed. The surgical technic of stapling must be meticulous. Long series of end-results are not yet available for evaluation.

CHAPTER XIII

NEUROMUSCULAR DISABILITIES (EXCLUSIVE OF INFANTILE PARALYSIS): INVOLVEMENT OF THE BRAIN AND SPINAL CORD

In addition to infantile paralysis, which has been described in the preceding chapter, the disease entities which may give rise to disability of the neuromuscular system are numerous and of diverse etiologic and clinical nature. They are perhaps most conveniently grouped according to the location of the basic pathologic changes. Entities characterized by involvement of the brain and spinal cord will be considered in the present chapter, while in the following one disorders of the peripheral nerves and of the muscles will be described.

PART I. INVOLVEMENT OF THE BRAIN

Cerebral Palsy (Spastic Paralysis, Little's Disease)

Definition.—Cerebral palsy is a common and extremely disabling affection seen most frequently in infants and children and characterized clinically by disturbance of voluntary motor function. The essential pathologic change is destruction or congenital absence of upper motor neurones. Mental impairment may be present. Involvement of a single extremity is termed *monoplegia*; involvement of arm and leg of the same side of the body is called *hemiplegia* (Fig. 100); involvement of both legs, *paraplegia*; and involvement of the four extremities, *quadriplegia* (Fig. 101). Statistics from a large series of cases showed quadriplegia in about 60 per cent, hemiplegia in 20 per cent, and paraplegia in 10 per cent.

Etiology.—The causes of cerebral palsy may be classified chronologically into three groups: (1) *antenatal,* consisting of congenital defects resulting from an arrested development of the cerebrum and pyramidal tracts in utero, metabolic disturbances due to endocrine imbalance, vitamin deficiencies, and incompatibilities of the Rh factors when an Rh-negative mother gives birth to an Rh-positive child in her second or third pregnancy; (2) *natal,* the most frequent type, consisting of nerve cell injury following cerebral hemorrhage due to trauma at birth, or anoxemia following winding of the umbilical cord around the baby's neck, too heavy sedation of the mother, or aspiration of mucus by the child; and (3) *postnatal,* consisting of infectious, vascular or traumatic lesions, such as those of encephalitis, meningitis, syphilis, cerebral poliomyelitis, and vascular accidents.

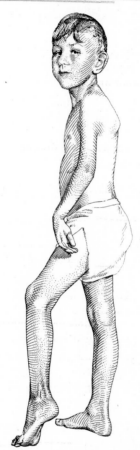

Fig. 100.—Spastic left hemiplegia in cerebral palsy.

The antenatal type is common in premature babies. Two-thirds of the patients of postnatal type are affected before the age of three years, and in 20 per cent of these children an infectious disease is the etiologic factor.

Pathology.—Although direct contusion and laceration of cortical tissue may be present, the factor of intracranial hemorrhage is believed to play a major rôle in the pathologic process. The hemorrhage may occur directly from a vessel ruptured when the dura mater is torn, or may

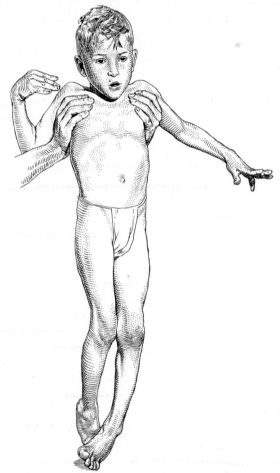

Fig. 101.—Spastic quadriplegia in cerebral palsy.

be of widespread petechial type resulting from increased tension when the venous circulation is temporarily obstructed. Degeneration of the injured nerve cells and fibers ensues and is followed by sclerosis. Grossly the affected areas may show atrophy and softening. The lesions may be more severe either in the cerebral cortex or in the basal ganglia. Degeneration of corresponding tracts in the spinal cord is a constant finding. A severe diffuse injury resulting in multiple hemorrhages through all parts of the brain may produce rigidity with mental retardation. A single hemorrhage or infarct involving the motor cortex may cause spastic hemiplegia or quadriplegia. Jaundice in the fetus due to incompatible Rh factors affects the basal ganglia and produces athetosis. Injury of the cerebellum produces ataxia.

Pathologic changes may occur in the spinal cord as the result of injury below the level of the brain. Traction applied during delivery is believed to be a frequent cause of such injuries. The clinical picture is in many respects similar to that of birth injury of the cerebrum or basal ganglia, and it is therefore convenient to consider cases of primary cord involvement together with those resulting from intracranial lesions.

Clinical Picture.—Intracranial hemorrhage in the newborn infant may be evidenced by severe asphyxia, bulging fontanels, refusal to nurse, spasticity or flaccidity, and convulsions. Lumbar puncture shows the spinal fluid to be bloody and under increased pressure. Many of these infants die shortly after birth. In milder cases the child may be considered normal until unusual delay in holding up the head, sitting, or standing becomes obvious.

Cases of cerebral palsy in older infants and children may be divided into several major groups according to the location of the lesion within the central nervous system. Each of these groups is characterized by outstanding clinical manifestations. The most important of these are: (1) *spasticity,* (2) *athetosis,* and (3) *ataxia.* In many cases the lesions are widespread, however, and the symptoms are of mixed type. Other forms of motor disturbances may also be present. Outstanding among these are *tension,* or widespread muscular hypertonicity; *tremor,* or rhythmic involuntary contractions limited to certain muscle groups; and *overflow,* an example of which is involuntary motion of the facial muscles during voluntary movement of the arm.

Spasticity.—Approximately 50 per cent of the cases of cerebral palsy fall into this group. In spasticity the lesion is cortical and the pyramidal tracts are involved. The evidences of spasticity are characteristic. The involved muscles are hyperirritable and contract on the slightest stimulation. The tendon reflexes are hyperactive, the Babinski reflex is positive, and clonus usually is easily elicited. Antagonistic muscle groups, hypersensitive to the stimulus of stretching, contract simultaneously with the protagonists; this results in difficult and inaccurate voluntary movements and in an increased muscular resistance to passive manipulation. The involuntary contraction of a spastic muscle when it is suddenly stretched is a useful diagnostic sign; it is called the *stretch reflex.*

An equinus limp is a frequent finding. The equinus deformity may be due not to weakness of the dorsiflexors but to simultaneous contraction of the normally more powerful plantar flexors and to the effect of gravity. In hemiplegia the patient can usually walk, but the affected lower extremity trails and is of little use.

In paraplegia and quadriplegia occurs the so-called *scissors gait* or *cross-legged progression,* characterized by disabling adduction of the hips which is a result of the greater strength of the adductors over the abductor groups and is augmented by the force of gravity.

Characteristic deformities develop as a result of the continued contraction of antagonistic muscles of unequal power. The hips may become flexed, adducted, and internally rotated. The knees are flexed. The feet usually assume an equinus or equinovarus position. The shoulders tend to become internally rotated and adducted and the elbows flexed. The forearm is pronated, while the wrist and fingers become flexed and the thumb is adducted. When the patient attempts to sit erect, unsightly bowing of the spine and forward protrusion of the head may take place.

Muscle atrophy is usually not conspicuous. Asymmetry of the extremities sometimes becomes marked, however, from retardation of growth of the affected limb due to trophic disturbances.

Athetosis.—Athetoid patients make up about 40 per cent of the cases of cerebral palsy, and according to Phelps can be grouped into twelve types. The lesion is subcortical, the basal ganglia and extrapyramidal tracts being affected. Athetosis is a more or less constant involuntary contraction of successive muscles. These arrhythmic, purposeless contractions become superimposed upon voluntary movements and result in marked incoordination. The reflexes are normal and the stretch reflex is absent.

Ataxia.—Cases of ataxia, or primary incoordination, are much less numerous than those of spasticity or of athetosis. The lesion is subcortical, and probably cerebellar in most instances. Characteristic clinical manifestations are incoordinated movements, impaired balance, and nystagmus. The reflexes are normal.

Mental Status.—Some degree of mental impairment, which may be either true deficiency or simply retardation, is usually present. Approximately 30 per cent of all cerebral palsy cases are mentally deficient, and by far the largest number of these are in the spastic group. Cerebral palsy with spasticity and mental deficiency, of which the ill-tempered, feebleminded, drooling child with scissors gait is the classical example, was described by Little in 1843 and is sometimes called *Little's disease.* Mental deficiency is more marked in quadriplegic and paraplegic patients than in hemiplegic ones. Some patients present obvious idiocy, with characteristically stupid facies and thick, unintelligible speech. In other cases, however, the appearance of subnormal mental endowment is unquestionably exaggerated by inability to control the facial or speech musculature, or by the deficient education which has resulted from absence of the normal locomotor activities of the growing child. Estimation of the mental capacity of the individual case is essential, since it is of primary importance in determining prognosis and treatment.

Diagnosis.—Accurate diagnosis is important in order to rule out certain progressive diseases in which the prognosis is hopeless and treatment is futile. History of difficult, prolonged, or instrumental delivery or of a definite episode of infectious disease during early childhood, although often not obtainable, may be useful auxiliary evidence. The spinal fluid should be examined when congenital syphilis is suspected. Developmental arrest of the central nervous system, hydrocephalus, brain tumor, atypical forms of infantile paralysis, and degenerative diseases of the central nervous system should be considered and excluded. Observation over a period of several months is often useful in ruling out the possibility of a disease process of progressive nature. For proper planning of treatment for the individual patient, an accurate differentiation of the type of cerebral palsy also is necessary.

Prognosis.—In untreated cases slow spontaneous improvement in the use of the extremities often takes place as motor experience and better control are acquired during the years of childhood. Well ordered treatment always results, however, in more rapid and more extensive improvement. Since the ability to cooperate and to learn is essential to effective treatment, the degree of improvement will depend to a large extent upon the mental capacity of the individual patient. Thus patients with paraplegia due to spinal lesions without cerebral involvement may regain considerable muscle function under treatment, while patients exhibiting marked mental deficiency improve little, form difficult nursing problems, and often succumb early to intercurrent infection. The prognosis of the patient with frequent convulsive seizures is unfavorable.

Treatment.—The treatment of cerebral palsy is essentially a process of rehabilitation, and of necessity embraces a long program of muscle training during which resort to operation is made only as an auxiliary measure. Treatment should begin as soon as the diagnosis is suspected, since otherwise valuable time may be lost. Subsequent therapy is governed largely by the patient's response. Since continued good hygiene, discipline, and freedom from excitement and worry must accompany the specialized muscle training, therapy is more often successful when given in an institution than when carried on in the home.

Nonoperative Treatment.—Motor re-education is the most important part of the treatment of most cases of cerebral palsy. The first step is to teach the child how to relax voluntarily; this is particularly important for the athetoid patient. When muscular relaxation can be initiated at will and maintained for as long as several minutes, training in the performance of simple movements is begun. In infants and in severe older cases attention is concentrated first upon learning to sit or to stand. A Thomas collar is sometimes provided to afford helpful support and prevent stretching of the neck muscles. A light corset is sometimes indicated. Braces and plaster shells, worn a part of each day or during the night, are often helpful in the treatment of mild spastic deformities. Daily massage is used for weakened muscle groups. The most important element of the treatment, however, is a program of exercises selected for the individual patient and carried out daily over a long period of time. Simple reciprocal motions of the extremities are started, at first passive and later active, and finally the patient is taught gradually to combine these simple movements into composite ones such as those of walking. Many aids to activity have been developed in recent years, such as ski shoes which allow the patient to stand and shuffle along without fear of falling. Neostigmine, Myanesin or Tolserol, and curare are being used in many clinics to relax spasticity, prior to motor re-education and other physical therapy. The therapeutic value of these drugs has not yet been fully agreed upon. Daily speech training is important in many cases. During the long period of training, the details of treatment must be adjusted to the needs of the individual patient, and experience, judgment, and patience on the part of the physical therapist are of the utmost importance. Occupational therapy forms an important part of the treatment of older patients, especially in motor re-education of the upper extremity.

Operative Treatment.—As a rule, orthopaedic operations for cerebral palsy are applicable chiefly to cases characterized by spasticity. In many such cases operative measures serve as a useful adjunct to motor re-education. Operation cannot be regarded as adequate treatment unless accompanied by conservative measures, however, and is unquestionably contraindicated when the disorder is a rapidly progressive one or when the patient possesses too little mental capacity to cooperate in the necessary postoperative training.

The object of operative treatment in cerebral palsy is to diminish muscle spasm, equalize the power of opposing muscles, and correct deformity. Of the great variety of procedures which have been devised and employed, many have proved with further experience to be unsatisfactory. In a series of approximately 2,500 cases operated upon in many different clinics, there were 50 per cent successful results and 50 per cent failures. In this series practically all of the operations upon athetoid patients were failures. The procedures now in common use may be classified as: (1) operations upon motor nerves, (2) operations upon muscles and tendons, and (3) operations upon bone.

1. *Operations Upon Motor Nerves (Neurectomy; Stoffel Operation).* —Division or partial excision of the motor nerves of spastic muscles is a valuable and commonly used procedure. Attempt is made not to paralyze a muscle group and so abolish its entire function, but to produce in the stronger muscles a loss of power sufficient to result in improved balance and hence increased capability for muscle training. This type of operation has produced better results in treatment of the lower extremity than of the upper. It has proved particularly suitable when applied to the branches of the obturator nerve for adductor spasm, the sciatic branches for hamstring spasm, and the internal popliteal branches for spasm of the plantar flexors. In selected cases of spastic pronation of the forearm and flexion of the wrist, section of appropriate branches of the median nerve is a helpful procedure.

2. *Operations Upon Muscles and Tendons.*—Procedures of this type include tendon transplantation, tendon lengthening, tenotomy and myotomy. They are often combined advantageously with section of motor nerves to the spastic muscle group. In each case adequate preliminary correction of the deformity must be carried out, care being

taken in the release of fibrous contractures of all involved periarticular structures. After operation the immobilization in corrected position and the subsequent physical therapy must be meticulously carried out.

The type of operation must be carefully chosen with regard to the nature and location of deformity in the individual case. Among the more commonly used procedures are the following:

a. *At the Hip.*—In cases of severe adduction deformity, tenotomy of a portion of the adductor muscles, followed by immobilization of the thighs for a period of about six weeks in wide abduction, often results in gratifying improvement of the gait.

b. *At the Knee.*—In persistent knee flexion, transplantation of the biceps femoris tendon into the patella is sometimes employed to improve the muscle balance. Occasionally it is sufficient to lengthen or simply to section one or more of the hamstring tendons. When in persistent knee flexion the patella is found to occupy an abnormally high position, transplantation of a small block of bone including the tibial attachment of the patellar ligament to a more distal position on the tibia occasionally produces marked improvement.

c. *At the Foot.*—Transplantation of the anterior tibial tendon to the lateral side of the dorsum of the foot may be used to improve spastic varus deformity. Lengthening of the Achilles tendon for talipes equinus is indicated only when there is unquestionable structural shortening, since spastic equinus would be all too easily converted into the more disabling deformity of calcaneus type. After lengthening of the Achilles tendon the ankle should be immobilized in a plaster cast in 90 degrees of dorsiflexion.

d. *At the Shoulder.*—For severe adduction and internal rotation deformity, the tendons of the pectoralis major and subscapularis muscles may be sectioned or lengthened.

e. *At the Forearm.*—Pronation contractures of spastic origin may be relieved by suitable transplantation of the tendon of the pronator radii teres muscle.

f. *At the Wrist.*—Tendon transplantation suited to the individual case is occasionally indicated.

3. *Operations Upon Bone.*—Only in carefully selected cases are bone operations indicated. In persistent varus or valgus deformity of the foot, subastragalar arthrodesis greatly improves stability and gait. When the wrist is flexed and cannot be held voluntarily in a neutral position,

radiocarpal arthrodesis in a position of 35 degrees of hyperextension produces great improvement in the appearance and function of the hand.

Joint Disabilities of Cerebral Origin (Hysterical Paralysis)

Cases of joint disability due partially or entirely to psychosomatic or psychogenic causes are encountered with considerable frequency. Often a part in the causation is played by the element of financial compensation or the desire to be relieved of some unpleasant duty. Functional or hysterical paralysis and deformity may simulate a variety of primary osteoarticular or neuromuscular diseases. Hence these disorders, although primarily of psychiatric interest, are of importance in the differential diagnosis of orthopaedic affections.

Clinical Picture.—Hysterical paralysis may occur in either sex and at any age. The history is likely to include discrepancies which suggest the diagnosis. The joint symptoms are varied, may be out of all proportion to the inciting trauma, and may change unnaturally from day to day. The physical findings also are inconsistent. Spasm and tenderness may be excessive while heat, redness, and swelling are completely absent, and the signs may change as soon as the patient's attention is diverted.

Diagnosis.—In diagnosis it must be remembered that organic and functional elements sometimes coexist and that in late hysterical cases a secondary structural element of circulatory changes and of contractures is almost always present. Examination under an anesthetic and roentgenographic visualization of the structures involved are of help. The diagnosis of hysteria should never be made until every effort to establish the presence of an organic lesion has been exhausted. The patient should be kept under observation for a considerable period, and repeated diagnostic examinations should be done.

Treatment.—The treatment of functional paralysis and deformity should be largely psychiatric. It is of fundamental importance that the confidence and active interest of the patient be secured. After this has been done it is usually advisable to place the patient upon a regime of gradually increasing corrective physical therapy. Emphasis should be placed upon active motion and active correction. Occupational therapy will often prove of value. When the element of compensation or disability insurance is present, termination of the payments and closure of the case is often followed quickly by relief of the disability.

PART II. INVOLVEMENT OF THE SPINAL CORD

Progressive Muscular Atrophy (Aran-Duchenne Type)

Progressive muscular atrophy is a primary disease of the spinal cord characterized by a slow degeneration of the anterior horn cells which produces muscular wasting without sensory losses. Although not of inflammatory nature, it has sometimes been called chronic anterior poliomyelitis. It is found most often in adults between twenty-five and forty-five years of age and is not hereditary or familial.

Clinical Picture.—The first evidence of the disorder is usually atrophy of the intrinsic muscles of the hand. The thenar eminence becomes flattened; the interosseous areas deepen; and with progression of the disease a claw hand (Fig. 109) develops. Gradually the paralysis extends to the muscles of the arms, shoulders, back, hips, and thighs. Other cases may first show atrophy and weakness in the shoulders, and rarely the legs are first involved. As the condition progresses, the deep reflexes may become hypoactive or absent. Fibrillation of the muscles is a constant finding and is of diagnostic importance.

When the disease has partially destroyed the pyramidal tracts, as evidenced by spasticity of the legs, hyperactive reflexes, and a positive Babinski sign, it is called *amyotrophic lateral sclerosis*.

Treatment.—The orthopaedic treatment is conservative, consisting of massage, exercises, and braces.

Friedreich's Ataxia

Friedreich's ataxia is a progressive disease, usually hereditary or familial, which often affects several children of the same family. It develops in early childhood, about 90 per cent of the cases appearing before the fifteenth year. The essential pathologic change is an extensive degeneration or sclerosis of the nerve fibers in the dorsal and lateral tracts of the spinal cord.

Clinical Picture.—The affection is characterized by weakness of the legs, ataxia, and a swaying, irregular gait with the feet placed widely apart. Nystagmus is characteristically present. The speech is usually thick. Equinovarus deformity of the feet is almost always present, and lateral curvature of the spine is often associated. Early in the disorder the deep reflexes are decreased, but the Babinski sign is present. Later there is often a loss of position and vibratory sense in the lower limbs, and disturbances of other types of sensation are sometimes observed.

Treatment.—At the present time no curative treatment is known. Muscle re-education and massage may be of help if carried out thoroughly each day. Braces are sometimes indicated. Occasionally when the disease is no longer progressive, operative stabilization of the feet is useful to improve the gait.

Subacute Combined Sclerosis

In pernicious anemia and deficiency diseases such as pellagra, the development of numbness and tingling in the hands and feet may be followed by the gradual onset of weakness. Later a well-marked flaccid or spastic paralysis of the legs may be present, and secondary deformities are likely to appear.

Treatment.—The use of physical therapy and of braces may be of benefit. Rarely is lengthening of the Achilles tendons or stabilization of the feet indicated in an effort to improve the gait.

Paralysis Following the Injection of Serum

A rare form of toxic paralysis, presumably of spinal cord rather than peripheral origin and of particular interest because it is a result of treatment itself, is that which sometimes develops after the use of prophylactic or therapeutic sera. The injection of the ordinary prophylactic dose of 1,500 units of tetanus antitoxin is sometimes followed by this complication, as is the injection of diphtheria antitoxin.

Clinical Picture.—Usually the patient develops an intense serum reaction several days following the injection. A few days later severe pain is experienced in the arms and other parts of the body, and after several more days weakness may become noticeable. The paralysis is almost invariably located about the shoulder girdle without relationship to the site of serum injection.

Treatment.—The treatment is rest and protection for the weakened muscles by means of braces and, in the convalescent stage, daily physical therapy. Thiamine chloride may be of some help. The prognosis for recovery of muscle power is only fair, particularly if muscle atrophy has occurred. A small percentage of these cases eventually require reconstructive surgery.

Neuropathic (Neurotrophic) Disease of the Bones and Joints

Etiology.—Chronic disease of the spinal cord may cause extensive trophic changes in the bones and joints. Such osteoarticular lesions are seen most frequently in association with the spinal cord involvement of *tabes dorsalis* and of *syringomyelia*. Statistics show that joint symptoms occur in from 3 to 4 per cent of patients with tabes and in from 10 to 40 per cent of those with syringomyelia. Similar joint changes occur less commonly with other affections of the spinal cord, including traumatic conditions, congenital malformations such as spina bifida with a myelomeningocele, tumor, tuberculosis, acute myelitis, poliomyelitis, and progressive muscular atrophy. They have been reported rarely after involvement of the peripheral nerves by trauma, toxic neuritis, or leprosy, or in association with the cerebral changes of dementia paralytica and of cerebral hemorrhage with hemiplegia.

Pathology.—The bone changes in neuropathic osteopathy include a thinning of the cortical bone and a diminution in lime salts, which may lead to spontaneous, painless fracture. Healing of such fractures occasionally takes place with the formation of an enormous amount of callus, which, however, may never become firm and may show degenerative changes leading to a second fracture.

The neuropathic arthropathies, often called *Charcot's joints* because they were first described by Jean Martin Charcot in 1866, are most frequently encountered in tabes. The articular cartilages and adjacent bone surfaces become worn away while at the same time hypertrophic changes take place at the joint edges, and loose bodies of irregular shape and size appear (Fig. 102). Marked deformity and instability result from mushrooming of the bone, relaxation of the ligaments, and accumulation of intra-articular fluid. The roentgenographic picture of fully developed cases is striking (Figs. 103*A*, 103*B*, and 103*C*). Both atrophic and hypertrophic bone changes are present. The joint surfaces appear extensively eroded and deformed. The bone margins are jagged, blurred, and sclerotic, and there may be many irregular islands of detached bone.

Clinical Picture.—In neuropathic arthropathy the early signs are insecurity, false motion, and swelling of the affected joint. These may increase rapidly or slowly, but pain is notably absent. Examination shows a tense or boggy nontender swelling, not uniform but containing indurated masses. As a rule the range of joint motion is increased. While most frequently only a single joint is involved, bilateral sym-

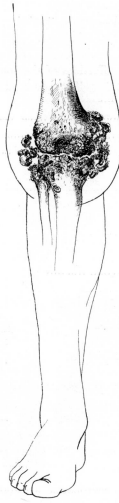

Fig. 102.—Neuropathic disease of the knee joint (Charcot joint). Note disintegration of articular surfaces with numerous detached fragments of bone.

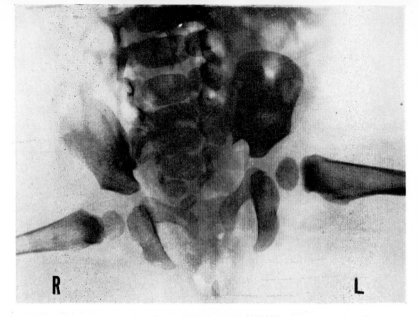

Fig. 103A.—Roentgenogram of lower spine, pelvis, and hips of infant, nine months of age, with spina bifida vera. Note large defects in lumbar vertebrae and sacrum, normal acetabula, and decalcification and underdevelopment of right femur.

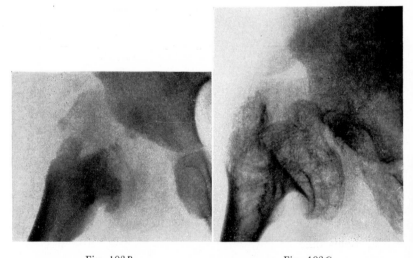

Fig. 103B.   Fig. 103C.

Fig. 103B.—Roentgenogram of right hip joint (same case as Fig. 103A), four years later, showing disintegration of joint. Note saucer-shaped acetabulum, projection of bony mass at upper acetabular margin, increased space between acetabulum and head of femur, and mushrooming of epiphysis and neck with decalcification.

Fig. 103C.—Roentgenogram of right hip joint (same case as Fig. 103A), eight and one-half years after first roentgenogram. Note almost complete disappearance of cup-shaped acetabulum, and mushrooming, decalcification, and cystic areas in head and neck of femur. The left hip developed normally during the eight and one-half years between Fig. 103A and this figure.

metrical lesions are occasionally seen and rarely a large number of joints may be affected. The knee, hip, shoulder, tarsus, elbow, wrist, and ankle are most frequently involved, in this order. Lesions of the spine are also encountered. Seventy-five per cent of the tabetic arthropathies occur in the lower extremity, while 80 per cent of the joints involved in syringomyelia are those of the upper extremity.

Diagnosis.—In advanced cases the diagnosis is often obvious, but in the early stages it may be difficult. In neuropathic arthropathy the local triad of swelling, instability and absence of severe pain should always suggest the diagnosis, and the roentgenographic evidence is most helpful. The findings of the general history and physical examination are of confirmatory value.

Treatment.—In tabes, antisyphilitic treatment is a major consideration. In neuropathic arthropathy protection for the affected joint is afforded by means of a brace, such as a walking caliper splint for the knee. Crutches may be necessary. With conservative treatment the progress of the disease may sometimes be retarded to a gratifying degree. Arthrodesis of the affected joint is not always successful but in some cases has given excellent results. Rarely, in extreme involvement of the knee or ankle, the impossibility of securing adequate stability either by apparatus or by arthrodesis may make amputation the procedure of choice.

Spina Bifida

Spina bifida is a congenital anomaly consisting of a developmental gap or defect in one or more of the vertebral arches (Figs. 103A and 105), through which the contents of the spinal canal may protrude and with which partial paralysis of the legs is sometimes associated. Spina bifida sufficiently marked to produce clinical deformity is present in about 1 in 1,000 births. Of these infants 80 per cent die within the first year. The projecting meningeal sac occasionally extends forward into the pelvis, abdomen, or thorax and is then called an *anterior spina bifida*. Spina bifida is most often found in the lumbar vertebrae but is occasionally observed at other levels of the spine.

Pathology.—The essential pathologic characteristic of spina bifida is incomplete development of the roof of the neural arch due to failure of complete fusion of the embryonic neural canal.

Each vertebra has three centers of ossification: one for the body and one for each half of the neural arch. The neural arch is formed by the posterior, midline fusion of the two laminae arising from their separate centers of ossification. Union of the laminae begins in the thoracic region and extends in both directions along the length of the developing spine. The lumbosacral and cervical regions are the last to unite, and in these two areas, particularly the former, faulty closure, resulting in spina bifida, is seen most frequently.

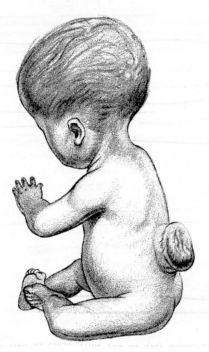

Fig. 104.—Spina bifida with myelomeningocele and hydrocephalus.

In the normal human embryo the entire neural tube is closed at the end of the third week, and by the eleventh week the partially ossified neural arches of the vertebrae are closed from the first cervical to the third or fourth sacral segments. The spinal cord and the vertebral column, are of equal length until the twelfth week. With further growth of the fetus, however, the vertebral canal becomes proportionately longer, so that in the adult the conus is at the level of the twelfth thoracic or first lumbar vertebra. When the nerve roots or the spinal cord are involved in a spina bifida, the upward migration of the cord is prevented. The defect may be large enough to allow the meninges or the spinal cord to form a protruding soft tissue tumor. According to the extent of the pathologic changes spina bifida has been classified into five types:

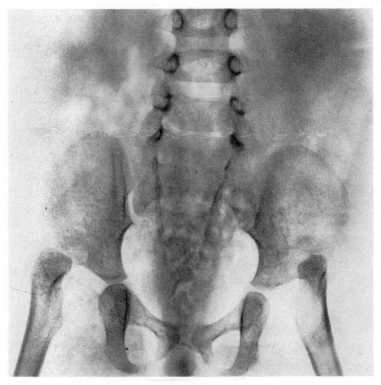

Fig. 105.—Spina bifida vera in boy three years of age. Note wide defect in laminal arches of lower three lumbar vertebrae and sacrum, and bilateral dislocation of hips. This patient had a myelomeningocele which was removed at one month of age.

1. *Spina Bifida Occulta.*—A defect is present in the spinous process and laminae of one or more vertebrae (Figs. 144 and 146). Herniation of the spinal contents may not be present or may be of insufficient size to be noticeable. If the herniation is of posterior type, which is most common, the skin may remain attached to the membranes, nerve roots, or cord itself by fibrous tissue called the *membrana reuniens*. These subjacent anatomic changes may be suggested by alterations of the skin such as indentations, pigmentations, telangiectasis, or hairy patches

(hypertrichosis). There may also be associated tumors inside or outside the vertebral canal, among them lipomas, angiomas, and dermoid cysts. As the growth of the spinal column later exceeds that of the spinal cord, adherence of the overlying structures to the cord may impede its normal ascent. In this manner, as well as through compression of the nerve roots by soft tissue at the site of the laminal defect, paralysis of gradual onset and incomplete type may result at a later age, particularly at a time of rapid growth.

2. *Spina Bifida With Meningocele.*—Through the defect of the incompletely closed arch of one or more vertebrae the meninges herniate and are covered by only a thin, parchment-like layer of skin. The hernial sac contains only cerebrospinal fluid; transillumination will reveal no nerve tissue.

3. *Spina Bifida With Myelomeningocele.*—With the bony defect is associated a hernial sac which contains spinal cord, nerve roots, or both, either free or attached to the walls of the sac. This type of developmental anomaly is usually much greater in extent, is more subject to ulceration if untreated, is usually associated with more neurological deficit in the lower extremities as well as bowel and bladder incontinence, and is more frequently associated with hydrocephalus (Fig. 104), particularly after surgical repair of the hernial sac, than is spina bifida with meningocele.

4. *Spina Bifida With Syringomyelocele.*—This is a severe type of myelomeningocele in which the herniated spinal cord contains a central canal greatly dilated and distended with cerebrospinal fluid.

5. *Spina Bifida With Myelocele.*—This condition is also known as *rachischisis.* It includes the more severe forms of spina bifida. As a result of the absence of laminae and pedicles, the wide bone defect forms an open groove, partially lined by imperfectly formed spinal cord tissue through which cerebrospinal fluid drains. As a consequence, infection quickly takes place and the infant succumbs early.

Of these five types, the last four are characterized by the presence of a soft tissue tumor due to herniation of the meninges and have been called *spina bifida manifesta* or *vera* (Fig. 104). The involvement of nervous tissue in these cases makes them primarily of neurosurgical interest. In the first type, spina bifida occulta, changes in the vertebral arch are of chief interest.

Clinical Picture.—The clinical picture may be characterized by any one or all of three features: (1) the tumor, or protruding soft tissue mass, (2) the neurological manifestations, and (3) the associated deformities.

The hernial protrusion is located in the midline, most commonly in the lumbar or lumbosacral region. It may vary greatly in size, and may increase with violent expiration as in crying. It is usually transparent on transillumination. A defect in the underlying bony structure is apparent on roentgen examination.

The neurological manifestations vary with the severity of the spinal defect and the amount of nerve tissue involved in the hernial mass. They may be absent in a spina bifida occulta and absent or minimal in a meningocele. In myelomeningocele they may consist of severe motor involvement or complete paraplegia with bowel and bladder incontinence, together with extensive sensory disturbance resulting in trophic ulcerations.

The associated deformities include most frequently clawfoot, clubfoot, contractures of the knees, flaccid or spastic paralysis of the lower extremities, malformations of the spine with varying degrees of scoliosis, kyphosis or lordosis, congenital dislocation of one or both hips (Fig. 105), and hydrocephalus.

Diagnosis.—The diagnosis is obvious in cases with a protruding hernial mass in the lumbar region. Among conditions to be excluded are lipomas and neurofibromas. Spina bifida of the occult type may be diagnosed as an incidental finding in roentgenograms made for other purposes; however, palpation of the area will sometimes demonstrate changes as compared with the normal findings at higher levels of the spine.

Treatment.—The hernial mass is best treated by a neurosurgeon. Considerable evidence has indicated that the meningeal portion of the sac should be retained after decompression and covered over by fascial and skin flaps obtained by rotation. It appears that the retained tissue aids in reabsorption of the cerebrospinal fluid and that hydrocephalus is less likely to appear than when the entire mass is amputated and a plastic closure performed. Drainage of cerebrospinal fluid, ulceration of the surface or nearby areas, paraplegia, absence of the anal reflex, constant dribbling of urine, poor general health, and an already existing hydrocephalus are believed by many to contraindicate operation.

Spina bifida occulta may require operation only in later childhood when neurological signs secondary to involvement of the cord by traction or compression may develop. Surgery then consists of careful excision of the membrana reuniens which unites the cord to the overlying structures. The prognosis following this procedure is usually good.

Orthopaedic treatment consists of the prevention or correction of deformities by casts, splints, or operations. These procedures should be carried out in a manner similar to that described in Chapter XII for corresponding deformities and disabilities following infantile paralysis. Care must be taken to avoid pressure ulcers. Training of the patient with severe involvement to walk with the aid of crutches and braces by a three- or four-point gait in the manner of a traumatic or poliomyelitic paraplegic may greatly facilitate his treatment and decrease his invalidism.

Transplantation of the gracilis muscle has been used successfully in some cases to provide sphincter control to patients with incontinence of bladder or bowel.

Psychotherapy is indicated in certain older patients to help them to become adjusted to their disability.

CHAPTER XIV

NEUROMUSCULAR DISABILITIES (EXCLUSIVE OF INFANTILE PARALYSIS): INVOLVEMENT OF PERIPHERAL NERVES AND OF MUSCLES

PART 1. INVOLVEMENT OF THE PERIPHERAL NERVES

Peripheral Nerve Injuries

Introduction.—Injury of the peripheral nerves is a frequent and serious complication of traumatic lesions of the bones and joints. Every injured extremity must be examined for the possibility of nerve damage, and in a considerable proportion of cases the neurologic lesion will prove of far greater significance than the osteoarticular. It is essential, therefore, that the orthopaedic surgeon become acquainted with that portion of neurology which deals with injuries of the peripheral nerves. The present description can include only a brief introduction to this branch of neurology, however, and for detailed information reference to the bibliography is suggested.

A brief review of the reactions of nerve trunks to injury forms a convenient preliminary to a consideration of lesions of the individual nerves.

Mechanism of Injury.—Traumatization of an extremity may involve the nerves in any of several types of injury. These may be classified according to the time of their occurrence with relation to that of the original injury.

1. *At the Time of the Original Injury.*—The nerve may be directly bruised, lacerated, or completely severed by the rough edge of a fractured bone or by a sharp object from without, such as the blade of a knife or a piece of glass. A portion of the nerve may be actually torn away; this happens not infrequently in severe gunshot wounds. An additional type of immediate injury is the severe stretching, tear, or even complete rupture of the nerve trunk from strong traction upon the extremity; this type of injury occurs, for instance, in *obstetric paralysis.*

281

2. *Several Hours Following the Original Injury.*—Temporary loss of nerve function may be occasioned by compression of the nerve trunk from edema or hemorrhage of gradual development.

3. *At the Time of Treatment of the Original Injury.*—Nerve damage is sometimes a result of excessive traumatization during the transportation of the patient when a splint has not been applied or during the reduction of a dislocation or fracture.

4. *Several Weeks or More Following the Original Injury.*—The nerve trunk may undergo gradual compression from cicatricial fibrous tissue or rarely from bony callus.

5. *Several Months or More Following the Original Injury.*—Friction or stretching of the nerve trunk is sometimes the result of a deformity caused by the original injury, as in late traumatic ulnar neuritis.

Gross Pathology of the Injured Nerve Trunk.—Following an old injury the damaged nerve is often recognizable only with difficulty because of extensive scarring of its sheath and the adjacent connective tissue. In infected wounds the adhesions are often particularly extensive, and in the proximal segment an ascending neuritis sometimes develops, causing widespread degenerative changes which are followed later by fibrosis. The appearance of the injured nerve varies especially with the degree of completeness of the tear. After complete division the nerve ends retract; a neuroma, or small bulblike growth of nerve fibers and connective tissue, forms at the end of the proximal segment; and the end of the distal segment may become narrowed and atrophic or may enlarge to form a pseudoneuroma, which is composed of connective tissue only. After incomplete laceration the injured trunk may show a fusiform enlargement, or nerve spindle, formed by the proliferation of fibrous tissue. In some cases there will be found a markedly thin segment which may suggest an incomplete division but which represents essentially a complete one, since all nerve fibers have ruptured and retracted while only the connective tissue sheaths remain intact. In other cases long segments of the nerve fibers may degenerate from friction or stretching while no macroscopic changes of any kind are apparent.

Degeneration and Regeneration of Nerves After Section.—The broad outlines of this fundamental and complex subject may be sketched briefly. According to the generally accepted *neurone doctrine,* when a peripheral nerve fiber has been sectioned that part of the fiber which is separated from the cell of origin will degenerate and that part which remains attached to the cell body will show attempts to regenerate. Degeneration of the axis cylinder and myelin sheath of the distal segment leaves an empty neurilemma within about two weeks after division. In the process of regeneration the axis cylinder of the proximal segment, still under the trophic influence of the nerve cell itself, gradually grows across the gap, enters the empty neurilemmal sheath, and continues to grow distally toward the end-organ while gradual restoration of the myelin sheath takes place. The rate of growth of the axis cylinder, under favorable circumstances, is said to be about 1 or 2 mm. per day.

Since anatomic and functional recovery of the injured nerve is directly dependent upon reestablishment of the pathway from nerve cell to end-organ by means of the regenerating axis cylinder, it is evident that the degree of recovery after any nerve injury will depend largely upon the ability of the axis cylinders to traverse the gap successfully and to find suitable waiting neurilemmas. Hence recovery will not take place if the defect is too extensive or if too much scar tissue is present. It has been shown that the optimal time for suture of a nerve is on the tenth day after injury. Some, however, believe this time should be longer. Even under the most favorable circumstances complete restoration of nerve function after division is scarcely to be expected.

Clinical Syndromes.—According to their clinical manifestations, it is possible to classify cases of peripheral nerve injury into four arbitrary groups. This classification is to some extent artificial and is not always appropriate, but it has been much used in the past and aids in formulating the therapeutic indications of the individual case.

1. *Syndrome of Complete Interruption.*—When a nerve has been completely divided, the muscles which it supplied show immediate and complete paralysis, loss of reflexes, and rapidly increasing flaccidity and wasting. After two weeks the characteristic complete *reaction of degeneration* appears; this is a qualitative and roughly quantitative muscular response to percutaneous electrical stimulation, dependent upon alterations in the excitability of the affected nerve and muscle to faradic and galvanic currents. There is absolute loss of cutaneous sensation over an area supplied exclusively by the nerve in question, and a relative loss over a larger area supplied only partially by the injured nerve. Vasomotor, trophic, and secretory changes are prominent; trophic ulceration may occur. There is usually no tenderness over the nerve trunk.

2. *Syndrome of Incomplete Interruption.*—The findings here depend upon the proportion of nerve fibers interrupted. Shortly after the injury there may be rapid changes in the extent of the paralysis as local edema and hemorrhage develop or regress. Muscle atrophy may be rapid although some tone is preserved, and the reaction of degeneration is incomplete. Anesthesia varies in extent and degree; trophic disturbances are more likely to be present than absent. The nerve trunk is not tender.

3. *Syndrome of Irritation (Traumatic Neuritis).*—The findings here also vary somewhat, depending upon the degree of nerve irritation. In mild types there are pain, hyperesthesia, tenderness along the nerve trunk, and trophic changes, such as cyanosis, glistening skin, and thickened nails. Reflex spasm sometimes occurs.

The most severe type of the irritation syndrome is known as *causalgia* and occurs most commonly after gunshot injury of the median or the internal popliteal nerve. Signs of incomplete nerve block coexist with sensory and trophic phenomena of extreme severity. The hand or foot may be the seat of a constant intense burning pain with frequent exacerbations of even greater severity, and the secondary lack of sleep may manifest itself in serious loss of strength and weight. The pain of causalgia is often most severe four or five months after the injury and in untreated cases may persist indefinitely.

4. *Syndrome of Recovery.*—As regeneration of the severed nerve fibers gradually takes place, a characteristic train of clinical symptoms and signs appears. Careful observation and record of these signs is important in determining prognosis and further treatment. Signs of recovery of nerve function after complete interruption may begin as early as five months following suture. A sensation of tingling produced distally by pressure or tapping over the nerve *(Tinel's sign)* is an early evidence of returning function. Deep and then superficial sensation is restored. Tone appears in the wasted muscles, and they become tender and less atrophic. Finally voluntary power and electrical excitability return.

Treatment of Peripheral Nerve Injuries.—The treatment of nerve injuries is either nonoperative or operative, and every case involves a decision as to whether spontaneous recovery can reasonably be expected or whether surgical exploration is the wiser course. A detailed history of the injury and a thorough neurological examination are essential. Of all the factors involved in the therapy of these cases, perhaps the most important are (1) surgical judgment in deciding when operation is indicated and (2) surgical technic in carrying out the procedure with a minimum of trauma and hemorrhage. The immense value of physical therapy in nonoperative and in postoperative treatment, however, is not to be underrated.

Nonoperative Treatment.—Nonoperative treatment is always indicated when there is evidence of progressive spontaneous improvement of nerve function, and is to be employed tentatively when such improvement may be expected following a probably incomplete division of the nerve. It should be explained to the patient at the outset that the course of treatment will be prolonged and that utmost cooperation with the surgeon will be obligatory.

The essentials of nonoperative treatment are two: (1) rest of the paralyzed muscles and (2) physical therapy. The affected muscles must be kept constantly in a position of relaxation; they must not be stretched by normal opponents. To this end, light retentive apparatus suited to the particular case is to be worn day and night. *Cock-up splints* in radial paralysis and *foot-drop braces* in peroneal paralysis are common examples. After a short initial period of rest, physical therapy should be used daily in an attempt to preserve muscle nutrition until regeneration occurs and to prevent the development of adhesions and contractures. It consists at first of heat and massage, passive exercises, and electrical stimulation; later, as recovery begins, muscle re-education and active exercises are added. The progressive restoration of power to paralyzed muscles usually observed in these cases is a source of gratification which makes the extended course of treatment well worth while.

Operative Treatment.—Operations for exploration or repair of a damaged nerve may be (1) *primary,* that is, performed immediately after a lacerating injury while the original wound is still unhealed, or (2) *secondary,* performed after the original wound has healed or when progress in the gradual recovery of nerve function has been unsatisfactory.

It is sometimes possible at the primary operation, as during the débridement of a compound fracture, to look for the injured nerve trunk, identify its cut ends, trim the uneven edges, and secure end-to-end approximation of the fibers by suturing together corresponding sides of the nerve sheath. If the wound does not become infected, good results are likely to follow such *primary nerve suture.* In the presence of uncontrollable oozing or of frank infection, however, primary nerve suture is useless except as a means of reducing the retraction of the cut ends. In such cases a *secondary nerve suture* should be performed after an ample period has been allowed for subsidence of the infection; it is best to delay such a secondary operation for at least eight to twelve weeks following healing of the original wound. During this interval the muscles and joints should be kept in as good condition as possible by means of daily physical therapy.

A nerve graft or transplant may be used to replace a defective or missing segment of a nerve trunk. Successful results have been reported in using nerve grafts from nerve banks. Some operators use a portion of the sural nerve as a nerve transplant. A sural transplant is more often successful than a graft from a nerve bank.

The indications for exploratory or secondary operation vary within certain recognized limits. When complete nerve division is suggested by the history and by extensive and persistent sensory and motor losses, exploration should be performed at once since, if actual separation has occurred, satisfactory regeneration will not take place without approximation of the nerve ends by suture. The time of appearance of the nerve signs with relation to the time of injury is sometimes of value in differentiating actual rupture from a temporary interruption of function by edema or hemorrhage. When the signs of incomplete interruption are present, nonoperative treatment should be adopted tentatively, but exploration should usually be carried out if definite improvement has not been shown after three or four months. The syndrome of nerve irritation and particularly of its more severe type, causalgia, indicates exploration and removal of the irritating factor. Procaine injections of the sympathetic ganglia or removal of the ganglia may completely relieve the pain and disability.

In operations upon peripheral nerve trunks scrupulous precautions to preserve asepsis and hemostasis and to avoid traumatization are essential. *Neurolysis,* or freeing of the nerve trunk from cicatricial adhesions and constrictions, is a common and often very beneficial procedure. It is sometimes necessary to compensate for shortening of a divided nerve trunk by fixing the adjacent joint temporarily in a suitable position or by transplanting the nerve to a shorter course. Postoperatively braces and physical therapy are used just as in the nonoperative treatment. Postoperative recovery of nerve function is slow and, as a rule, never quite complete, depending upon many factors, such as the duration of the paralysis, the age of the patient, the type of nerve involved, the level at which it is injured, and the degree of secondary change in muscles, tendons, and joints. Often with careful protection and physical therapy, however, progressive improvement can be expected to continue for as long as two or three years.

Injuries of Individual Nerves

Theoretically every peripheral nerve is susceptible to mechanical injury. Practically, however, and particularly in civil life, the frequent and important lesions are limited to a few of the major trunks. Nerve injury occurs far more commonly in the upper extremity than in the lower. In the upper extremity, lesions of the radial, ulnar, and median nerves are of major significance, while in the lower extremity injuries of the sciatic and peroneal nerves are most important. Lesions of other trunks occur less frequently but are of great interest in the individual case.

The Spinal Accessory Nerve (11th Cranial Nerve)

Etiology.—This nerve is sometimes divided by lacerating or perforating wounds of the neck or during neck dissections for cervical rib, tuberculous lymphadenitis, or tumor of the lymph nodes.

Clinical Picture.—If the nerve is divided in the posterior triangle after emerging from the sternocleidomastoid, only the trapezius muscle is paralyzed. This produces an unsightly deformity consisting of change in the contour of the neck, drooping of the shoulder, and occasionally slight winging of the scapula. Abduction of the arm is at first impaired but later may be partially restored by the action of other muscles of the shoulder girdle. If the nerve is divided in the anterior triangle of the neck, the sternocleidomastoid muscle also is paralyzed, which results in little loss of power but in a noticeable asymmetry.

Treatment.—Unless primary suture can be accomplished, the nerve lesion is as a rule irreparable. If winging of the scapula is conspicuous, the deformity may be lessened by operative measures to limit its displacement.

The Brachial Plexus

Etiology.—The nerves of the brachial plexus are subject to the following types of injury:

1. *Traction Lesions.*—If the head is laterally flexed while the opposite shoulder is fixed, or if the shoulder is violently depressed while the

head is fixed, the trunks of the brachial plexus become taut and, if the force increases, may be stretched, torn, or even completely ruptured. Such injury occurring during birth causes the common and important *obstetric paralysis* or *birth palsy*. Similar lesions in adults may result from severe stretching of the brachial plexus incident to the trauma of falls or heavy blows upon the shoulder.

2. *Friction, Contusion, or Compression Lesions.*—Nerve injuries of this type are of particular interest in connection with two clinical entities: (a) *cervical rib* or spasm of the scalenus anticus muscle, which may cause chronic friction or compression (see page 501); and (b) *dislocations or fractures at the shoulder joint,* including displaced fractures of the clavicle, in which the nerves may be injured by the original trauma, by secondary edema or hemorrhage following the original trauma, or by manipulation during reduction of the original displacement.

3. *Penetrating Lesions.*—Gunshot wounds form the commonest cause of this type of nerve injury. In the early treatment of these cases hemorrhage from associated injury of the great vessels is often an important factor.

Clinical Picture.—The symptoms and signs of lesions of the brachial plexus are complex and vary widely with the type of trauma. It is therefore convenient to consider the more important clinical entities separately.

The Root Syndrome

The nerve roots from which the brachial plexus is derived are subject to (1) *acute traumatic lesions,* such as gunshot injuries, and to (2) *chronic irritative lesions,* such as those occurring in osteoarthritis.

Acute traumatic lesions of the nerve roots cause a segmental type of anesthesia and paralysis. Exact diagnostic localization of the injury is often rendered exceedingly difficult by associated injury of the spinal cord or of the primary divisions of the plexus, and for detailed analysis of the lesion a thorough knowledge of the local neurologic anatomy is essential. Careful diagnosis is extremely important in determining surgical treatment, as most injuries of the roots and primary divisions of the plexus are irreparable.

Chronic irritative lesions of the nerve roots cause a distressing clinical syndrome which is seen with unfortunate frequency. These patients, usually past middle life, complain of severe burning pain, with frequent exacerbations of even greater intensity, occurring sometimes in a segmental distribution but often felt throughout the forearm and hand. There may be associated sensory losses or hyperesthesia and more or less muscular weakness. Stiffness of the neck is always present to some degree although the patient may complain little of neck pain. Because of intractable pain in the arm the patient's general health suffers; he may become a morphine addict or when first examined may show the clinical and laboratory findings of bromidism. Roentgenograms show arthritic changes in the lower cervical vertebrae and suggest encroachment of bone upon the intervertebral foramina; it is uncertain whether involvement of the nerve roots is a result of actual mechanical compression or low-grade inflammatory changes in the contiguous soft tissues. In the differential diagnosis, rupture of an intervertebral disk of the cervical spine must be considered. The treatment is often difficult and includes prolonged local heat, traction, salicylates and barbiturates, and general antiarthritic measures. In addition, it is sometimes advisable to provide absolute rest by recumbency in a plaster jacket or shell.

Obstetric Paralysis

Obstetric paralysis, or *birth palsy,* is a paralysis of the muscles of the upper extremity resulting from mechanical injury of the nerve roots of the brachial plexus during birth, and is most commonly seen in infants born after a prolonged and difficult labor. The actual nerve injury may vary from slight stretching to complete rupture of one or more of the nerve trunks. Edema and hemorrhage follow, and later cicatricial fibrosis occurs. Some observers believe that the primary lesion is a tear of the shoulder capsule and that the nerve involvement is secondary. Clinically the newborn infant may present, in addition to paralysis of the arm, transient spasticity of the other arm and the legs as a result of the hematomyelia accompanying avulsion of the nerve roots. Inequality of the pupils may be present from stretching or tearing of the cervical sympathetic nerves. Three main types of paralysis are encountered, depending upon the location of the injury:

1. *The Erb-Duchenne* or *upper arm paralysis* is by far the most common type and is due to injury of the fifth and sixth cervical trunks. Because of the distribution of the paralysis, the extremity occupies a typical position, with the shoulder internally rotated and adducted and

the forearm pronated. Movements of the wrist and of the fingers are not affected. There may be slight sensory changes which in the infant cannot be evaluated.

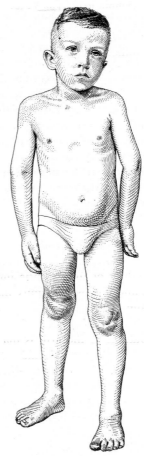

Fig. 106.—Obstetric paralysis, whole arm type. Note the characteristic deformity and atrophy.

2. *The Klumpke* or *lower arm paralysis* is much less common; it is due to injury of the first dorsal and the eighth cervical trunks. While the upper arm is not involved, the intrinsic muscles of the hand and sometimes the long flexors of the fingers are paralyzed. A homolateral *Horner'*

syndrome is often present because of involvement of the cervical sympathetic fibers in the first dorsal root; it is characterized by slight ptosis of the eyelid, enophthalmos, and miosis.

3. In paralysis of the *whole arm type* (Fig. 106), which in frequency occupies a position between the other two varieties, the extremity is often completely flaccid and powerless. Extensive sensory losses occur which in the infant are difficult to demonstrate.

Differential Diagnosis.—It must be remembered that at birth any of several injuries about the shoulder can cause a flail arm. Separation of the upper humeral epiphysis, fracture of the humerus, and fracture of the clavicle are of fairly common occurrence. Dislocation of the shoulder may be a true congenital luxation or a traumatic displacement due to injury during birth; each is extremely rare. In the infant, cerebral palsy must also be excluded, while in older patients it is necessary to consider the possibility of an old unrecognized infantile paralysis.

Prognosis.—In properly treated cases improvement usually takes place during the months following birth; however, the prognosis varies with the type of paralysis, and perfect recovery is exceptional. In the upper arm paralysis considerable return of power is to be expected; the lower arm type with paralysis of the intrinsic muscles of the hand has a relatively poor prognosis and a claw deformity may develop; the palsy of the whole arm is especially likely to show only incomplete recovery. The paralysis is followed by the development of contractures. The typical deformity of internal rotation of the arm is maintained by firm fibrous contractures of the muscles about the shoulder. In extensive late cases the entire arm and shoulder girdle are underdeveloped, and secondary growth changes, such as abnormal prolongation of the acromion and of the coracoid process, take place. In such cases the functional loss is great.

Treatment.—The early treatment of obstetric paralysis is conservative. As soon as the diagnosis is made, the extremity should be held by means of a brace in a position combining abduction and external rotation of the shoulder, flexion of the elbow, supination of the forearm, and slight dorsiflexion of the wrist (Fig. 107). The brace should be removed for care of the infant's skin and after the first few days for gentle massage and manipulation to prevent the development of contractures. While the brace is not being used, the general position of

correction should be maintained. When recovery of muscle power has
taken place, the brace may be removed very gradually. Active and
passive corrective exercises should, however, be continued for a long
while, and the child should be kept under periodic observation for signs
of developing contractures.

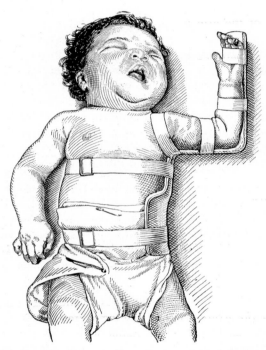

Fig. 107.—Obstetric paralysis. Brace for maintaining abduction and external
rotation of the shoulder.

When satisfactory recovery has not taken place after three to six
months of nonoperative treatment, neurosurgical exploration should
be considered; although most cases cannot be helped by operation,
neurolysis or end-to-end suture can occasionally be accomplished with
benefit. Contractures may be treated in the infant by manipulation under
anesthesia, but in all patients over the age of two years an open operation
is preferable. The procedure described by Sever, comprising section of
the contracted pectoralis major and subscapularis muscles near their
insertion into the humerus, is often useful. It may be necessary also to

section the coracobrachialis and short head of the biceps at this point. If the elongated acromion process is limiting abduction, it should be osteotomized at its base and bent upward. Late cases of internal rotation deformity may be treated by rotation osteotomy of the humerus or by forward transplantation of the insertions of the external rotators. These operations, while producing no direct increase of muscle power, may make motion of the arm less awkward. Occasionally in late cases with pronation deformity, tendon transplantation in the forearm or rotation osteotomy of the radius may be indicated. After any of these operative procedures the arm must be adequately supported in the appropriate position, and physical therapy must be careful and prolonged.

Paralysis Following Dislocation of the Shoulder

Paralyses complicating shoulder dislocations are not uncommon and are often of medicolegal as well as surgical interest. They fall into two major groups: (1) *supraclavicular traction injuries* of the plexus, produced by the original trauma and independent of the dislocation, and (2) *infraclavicular nerve trunk lesions* resulting from displacement of the humeral head at the time of the original trauma or during its manipulative reposition. Supraclavicular traction injuries are treated by measures similar to those used for the analogous obstetric paralysis. It is advisable, however, to resort to exploratory operation somewhat more freely than in birth palsy.

Infraclavicular nerve trunk lesions complicating dislocation may involve chiefly *the axillary nerve,* causing deltoid paralysis and epaulet hypesthesia; *the axillary and the radial nerves,* causing in addition a widespread extensor paralysis; *the inner cord* with paralysis of the intrinsic muscles of the hand and anesthesia in the ulnar distribution; or *the outer cord* with paralysis of the biceps, coracobrachialis, and the flexors of the fingers supplied by the median nerve. The extent of the paralysis depends in large degree upon the length of time during which the humeral head is allowed to remain displaced and in late cases may be extreme. The treatment of these cases is immediate reduction, which can usually be accomplished by a closed procedure, followed within a few days by splinting of the shoulder in moderate abduction and external rotation and of the wrist in dorsiflexion. Daily physical therapy, including electrical stimulation of the muscles and motion of the involved joints, is essential. Recovery is sometimes very slow and may continue for many months. Open operation for reduction of the dislocation, excision of the humeral head, or exploration of the nerves is occasionally indicated.

THE AXILLARY NERVE

Etiology.—The usual cause of injury is subcoracoid dislocation of the head of the humerus, but rarely the paralysis may follow fracture of the surgical neck of the humerus, the incorrect use of an axillary crutch, or traction injuries of the neck and shoulder.

Clinical Picture.—The deltoid muscle is paralyzed, causing a loss of true abduction of the shoulder and subsequently an unsightly muscle atrophy, prominence of the acromion, and instability of the shoulder joint. The paralysis of the teres minor muscle is unimportant. There is a loss of sensation over the lateral aspect of the shoulder and upper arm.

Treatment.—Nonoperative treatment is usually adequate. Surgical repair is difficult because of the short course of the nerve. After irreparable injury a muscle transplantation to provide abduction of the arm is sometimes done (see page 253), or the shoulder may be arthrodesed in 50 to 75 degrees of abduction.

THE LONG THORACIC NERVE

Etiology.—The long thoracic nerve, supplying the serratus anterior muscle, may be injured by (1) the carrying of excessively heavy burdens upon the shoulder or (2) accidental division at operation.

Clinical Picture.—Paralysis of the serratus anterior muscle results in an inability to raise the arm above the shoulder level in front of the body, loss of forward pushing movements of the shoulder, and winging of the scapula. The deformity and disability are sometimes severe.

Treatment.—Rest of the shoulder in an abduction brace and physical therapy are indicated. If recovery does not occur, excessive mobility of the scapula may be corrected by any of several operative methods involving anchorage of its lower angle to the wall of the thorax.

THE RADIAL (MUSCULOSPIRAL) NERVE

Etiology.—The radial nerve with its long and exposed course about the humeral shaft is the most frequently injured nerve in the body. It is particularly liable to two types of mechanical injury: (1) laceration by the sharp edge of a bone fragment in fractures of the humeral shaft or in supracondylar fractures, or involvement secondarily in a fibrous scar or in callus; and (2) compression from external objects, as in *crutch palsy,* or when the arm is allowed to hang for a long time against an object causing local pressure.   Even trivial injuries result usually in a complete motor paralysis rather than in a partial involvement.

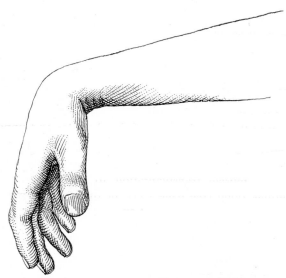

Fig. 108.—Wrist-drop in complete paralysis of radial nerve.

Clinical Picture.—Radial palsy involves the extensors of the elbow, wrist, and fingers and causes the characteristic sign of *wrist-drop* (Fig. 108). If the lesion is in or below the middle third of the upper arm, paralysis of the triceps is absent as its nerve supply is separated from the main trunk at a higher level.   The sensory loss is not so extensive as the wide distribution of the radial nerve would suggest; it consists usually of a small zone of anesthesia on the dorsal surface of the thumb and the adjoining portion of the hand.   The posterior interosseous branch of the radial nerve is occasionally injured in wounds of the elbow, with resulting paralysis of the extensor carpi ulnaris and the extensors of the fingers and the thumb.

Treatment.—Nonoperative treatment of radial paralysis consists in the use of cock-up splints and of prolonged physical therapy.   Operative procedures upon the nerve itself, of which neurolysis, end-to-end suture, and transplantation to the anterior aspect of the arm are the most common, are often successful since the radial nerve is peculiarly capable of functional recovery. When the lesion is irreparable, however, tendon transplantations about the wrist to supplement the weakened muscles can do much to relieve the disability.

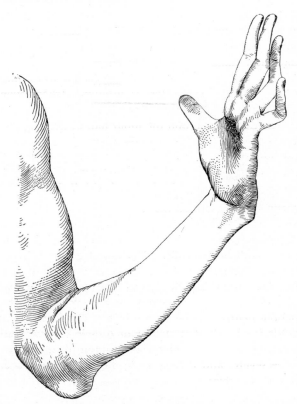

Fig. 109.—Claw hand in paralysis of ulnar nerve.

THE ULNAR NERVE

Etiology.—The ulnar nerve is frequently divided in lacerated wounds and may be injured by fractures in the region of the medial condyle and epicondyle, by dislocation of the elbow, and by secondary inclusion in scar tissue after elbow injury. It may be affected by postural pressure during a prolonged anesthesia. In addition the ulnar nerve is subject to *delayed* *traumatic neuritis* from stretching or from friction against the posterior surface of the medial humeral condyle in valgus deformity of the elbow secondary to old fracture.

Clinical Picture.—Lesions in the upper arm cause paralysis of the flexor carpi ulnaris, the medial half of the flexor digitorum profundus, the hypothenar muscles, interossei, two medial lumbricals, adductors of the thumb and the deep head of the flexor pollicis brevis. In cases of long standing the flattening of the hypothenar eminence, interosseous atrophy, and claw hand deformity are characteristic (Fig. 109). A dry and atrophied appearance of the skin and nails due to vasomotor disturbances may be present. Sensory loss is usually marked, even in incomplete division of the nerve, and is located over the ulnar border of the hand, the entire little finger, and the ulnar half of the ring finger. Lesions in the forearm cause the typical losses in the hand, but power in the flexor carpi ulnaris and the flexor digitorum profundus is retained. Lesions at the wrist, below the origin of the large dorsal cutaneous branch, cause the usual motor changes in the hand with little sensory impairment.

Late traumatic ulnar neuritis or delayed ulnar palsy is seen not infrequently in association with (1) recurrent dislocation of the nerve at the postcondylar groove and (2) old fracture of the lateral condyle with a cubitus valgus deformity. Various degrees of hypermobility of the nerve may occur developmentally or as the result of trauma, and occasionally there is actual slipping of the nerve trunk anterior to the medial epicondyle with each flexion of the elbow, which produces a typical friction neuritis. The nerve injury after old fractures of the lateral condyle is a result of stretching or friction due to the development of cubitus valgus (Figs. 131*A* and 132*A*). Pain in the ulnar distribution is likely to be severe, and there may be sensory changes and atrophy of the interosseous muscles.

Treatment.—Nonoperative treatment consists in the use of splints and of physical therapy. Primary nerve suture is sometimes indicated. When the nerve is shortened, it may with advantage be transposed to a position anterior to the epicondyle. The results of nerve suture are imperfect, since, as a rule, neither motor nor sensory losses are completely restored. In late traumatic neuritis immobilization may produce satisfactory temporary improvement, but for permanent cure it is often necessary to perform an anterior transposition of the ulnar nerve at the elbow. The results of this operation are excellent in most cases.

The Median Nerve

Etiology.—The commonest causes of median nerve paralysis are injuries from penetrating or lacerating wounds and primary or secondary involvement in association with supracondylar fractures of the humerus. At the wrist a median paralysis sometimes follows traumatic lesions such as transverse laceration of the soft tissues or anterior dislocation of the semilunar bone.

Clinical Picture.—Lesions in the arm or at the elbow cause paralysis of most of the flexors of the wrist and fingers, of the pronators of the forearm, the adductor-opponens group of the thumb, and the two lateral lumbrical muscles. Flattening of the thenar eminence is a conspicuous sign. The little and ring fingers can be flexed through the ulnar supply, but the patient cannot make a tight fist or pronate the forearm (Fig. 110). Power in the opponens pollicis muscle, which must be carefully differentiated from the adductor pollicis, is lost. In lesions at the wrist this loss of the opponens is the most valuable diagnostic feature. The sensory loss is the same at whatever level the nerve is divided; it may involve the thumb, the index, and the middle fingers and the lateral half of the ring finger. The nails may be atrophic and the skin shiny and dry. Incomplete division of the median nerve frequently results in causalgia.

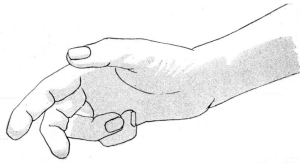

Fig. 110.—Paralysis of median nerve showing inability to flex fully the index and middle fingers.

Treatment.—After lacerating wounds it is often possible to perform a primary nerve suture. The technic must be scrupulous, owing to the likelihood of the development of causalgia. For traumatic neuritis, neurolysis is often sufficient. Splinting, to prevent stretching of the weakened muscles, and physical therapy are important parts of the treatment. The results of suture of the median nerve are more favorable than in the case of the ulnar nerve; however, the recovery is usually incomplete. In irreparable lesions tendon transplantations may be of benefit.

THE LUMBOSACRAL PLEXUS AND THE CAUDA EQUINA

Lumbosacral Plexus.—The trunks of the lumbosacral plexus may be injured by penetrating wounds, fractures, inflammatory conditions, and tumors of the pelvic wall or viscera. The management of these conditions consists primarily of treatment of the causative lesions. Rarely compression by the fetal head is said to cause plexus symptoms. More common is the entity of *maternal obstetric palsy,* in which sciatic pain and sometimes peroneal paralysis and sensory changes are the result presumably of stretching of the lumbosacral trunks during a difficult labor. The prognosis for spontaneous recovery is good. Nonoperative treatment, consisting of a foot-drop brace and physical therapy, should be employed. Very rarely, after a difficult birth, the infant may show temporary signs of a traction injury of the lumbosacral plexus analogous to the familiar stretching of the brachial plexus which produces obstetric paralysis of the upper extremity.

Cauda Equina and Conus Medullaris.—These structures may be injured in penetrating wounds or by severe trauma with or without fracture of the lumbar vertebrae or sacrum. Motor and sensory losses may be slight or very extensive, depending upon the extent of the trauma and the level involved. The complete *cauda syndrome* includes a total flaccid paralysis of both lower extremities, paralysis of the sphincters of rectum and bladder and anesthesia of the buttocks, the perineum, the entire posterior aspect of the legs, and the feet. The complete *conus syndrome,* resulting from involvement of the five fused sacral segments of the spinal cord, consists of paralysis of the sphincters and anesthesia in a saddle-shaped area of the buttocks and perineum. In most of the cases the only practicable therapy is nonoperative. Rarely an exploratory laminectomy is indicated.

THE SCIATIC NERVE

Etiology.—The sciatic nerve is involved commonly in gunshot wounds, and occasionally in displaced fractures of the pelvis or femur and dislocations of the hip. It is sometimes injured during a closed reduction of a traumatically or congenitally dislocated hip or during a manipulation of the hip and low back for sciatic pain.

Clinical Picture.—Complete division causes a total paralysis of all muscles below the knee, and of the hamstrings also if the lesion is above the middle third of the thigh. In partial division the external popliteal fibers are most often injured. The outstanding motor sign of sciatic paralysis is *foot-drop* or inability to carry out active dorsiflexion of the ankle. Also lost is active dorsiflexion of the toes. The *steppage gait* of foot-drop is characteristic. The paralyzed muscles develop severe atrophy. Sensation is lost in the foot and the lateral aspect of the leg. Trophic ulcers are very likely to develop at points of pressure on the sole and may extend deeply to involve the bones. After incomplete division the sciatic nerve is prone to develop the syndrome of causalgia.

Treatment.—Conservative treatment consists of physical therapy and of braces to prevent foot-drop and contractures, such as the Cabot splint for use at night and an ankle brace, fitted with right angle stop, for use when walking. Operative exploration and repair must sometimes be undertaken if satisfactory return of nerve function does not take place, but recovery is always slow and the results are usually not encouraging. During and after operation the optimal position for relief of tension upon the nerve, viz., hyperextension of the hip and flexion of the knee, should be preserved. At times advanced trophic changes and ulceration may make amputation of the extremity necessary.

THE EXTERNAL POPLITEAL (COMMON PERONEAL) NERVE

Etiology.—As the external popliteal nerve winds superficially about the neck of the fibula it may be injured by (1) lacerating wounds, (2) sudden compression from a blow, (3) gradual compression from an ill-fitting cast, (4) laceration, edema, or cicatricial involvement associated with fracture of the upper end of the fibula, or (5) stretching associated with the correction of a knee flexion contracture of long standing.

Clinical Picture.—The motor signs consist of paralysis of the anterior tibial, peroneal, and long extensor muscle groups with resulting foot-drop. As in the case of the radial nerve, the usual result of trivial as well as of major injuries is complete motor paralysis. In high lesions sensation is lost over an area situated on the lateral aspect of the leg and the dorsum of the foot.

Treatment.—Especial attention should be paid to the prevention of foot-drop. In most cases there is no indication for operation. When the syndrome of complete interruption is present after severe injuries, however, early exploration and suture are indicated.

The Internal Popliteal (Tibial) Nerve

Injuries of the internal popliteal nerve are uncommon; they are caused usually by penetrating wounds. Division causes paralysis of the plantar flexors and of the intrinsic muscles of the foot and a loss of sensation over the sole, the lateral surface of the heel, and the plantar surface of the toes. Vasomotor disturbances and trophic ulcers, particularly in the sole of the foot, may form serious complications. The treatment is based upon the usual principles.

The Femoral Nerve and the Obturator Nerve

Division of either of these nerves is excessively rare. Section of the *femoral nerve* causes paralysis of the quadriceps muscle together with slight sensory losses in thigh and leg. The power of extending the knee may be partially restored by transplantation of one or two of the hamstring tendons and the tendon of the tensor fasciae latae into the patella. Division of the *obturator nerve* causes an adductor paralysis without sensory changes. Nerve suture is theoretically possible.

Neuritis

In addition to acute traumatic injuries, peripheral nerves are subject to a wide variety of chronic irritative disturbances. These disorders, while of interest to orthopaedic surgery, are primarily of neurologic character and can be mentioned here only briefly and in their relationship to disease of the bones and joints.

Chronic irritative disorders of the peripheral nerves may be grouped conveniently into two classes: (1) *traumatic neuritis,* in which the causative factor is chronic mechanical injury, and (2) *toxic neuritis,* in which the nerve is affected by the presence of some deleterious chemical agent or toxin. Since such toxic substances are usually of systemic distribution, toxic neuritis is likely to involve more than one nerve, in which case it is known as *multiple neuritis* or *polyneuritis.*

The symptoms of *traumatic neuritis* are those of the syndrome of irritation, which has been discussed. Well-recognized forms of traumatic neuritis are those from prolonged hanging of the arm over the back of a chair or the edge of a bed or from the continuous pressure of a cervical rib. *Crutch palsy,* a partial paralysis of the radial nerve from pressure of a crutch in the axilla, is a common example. The sciatic symptoms sometimes found in association with mechanical derangement in the low back can be interpreted on a similar basis. Paralysis of varying degree, resulting from pressure upon the external popliteal (common peroneal) nerve as it winds about the head of the fibula, sometimes follows the application of a poorly padded or tightly fitting leg cast. The treatment of these lesions consists in removing the offending mechanical factor, in protecting the weakened muscles with braces when necessary, and in using daily physical therapy to encourage the return of function and to prevent atrophy and contracture.

While the subject of *toxic neuritis* is primarily of medical interest, the orthopaedic surgeon is often called upon to aid in the prevention of deformity and the restoration of function. In most of these cases disturbances of sensation, tenderness along the nerve trunk, and motor losses are observed, and the distribution may be symmetrical in the two corresponding extremities. Pathologically the chief change is a degeneration of the neuraxons, and the prognosis for recovery, usually good with adequate treatment, depends upon the extent to which this degeneration is followed by interstitial fibrosis. A common cause of toxic neuritis is poisoning by metals, such as lead or arsenic, or by organic compounds, such as methyl alcohol or carbon monoxide. Other common causative agents are the toxins of infectious diseases, such as that of diphtheria; occasionally toxic absorption from a simple pyogenic focus is responsible. The treatment of toxic neuritis is primarily medical and preventive, but, when paralysis has developed, rest in supportive apparatus and subsequent physical therapy is indicated.

Neuralgia

Although the term neuralgia may be correctly used to denote the symptom of pain arising from any irritative lesion of a nerve, it is too often applied loosely in a quasidiagnostic sense to any painful lesion whatever. This practice cannot be too much condemned, since it tends to obscure the true diagnosis and to lead to inefficient treatment. While it cannot be proved as yet that pain never arises idiopathically in a nerve free from demonstrable organic lesion, it is far better in each case to avoid the use of the term neuralgia and to preserve an open mind for the consideration of better known and more effectively treated entities.

Hereditary Muscular Atrophy of Peroneal Type
(Charcot-Marie-Tooth Disease)

This type of progressive atrophy and paralysis, caused by degenerative changes in the peripheral nerves, begins clinically with involvement of the peroneal muscles. It usually makes its appearance between the ages of five and ten years, affects boys more commonly than girls, and shows a familial tendency. Often a slight shortening of the heel cord and equinovarus deformity are the first changes. Slight stumbling and unsteadiness of gait develop and become progressively worse. There may be cramps in the legs. The hands and forearms may become involved. A claw foot (Fig. 168) or claw hand (Fig. 109) often develops. The atrophy slowly progresses upward but never extends above the elbows or the middle of the thighs. The reflexes are hypoactive or absent, Babinski's sign is absent, and numbness is occasionally present.

Treatment.—Operative lengthening of the Achilles tendon may lessen the deformity of the ankle and foot and improve the gait for several years. The operation should be followed by systematic exercises. Occasionally it is advisable to support the feet and ankles with braces in order to prevent the development of extreme equinovarus deformity. For patients in whom the disease is advancing only slowly, subastragalar arthrodesis is sometimes indicated. With the arthrodesis it is sometimes advisable to transfer the anterior tibial tendon laterally on the dorsum of the foot.

PART II. INVOLVEMENT OF MUSCLES

Progressive Muscular Dystrophy (Primary Myopathy)

The term progressive muscular dystrophy is commonly used to include a number of neuromuscular disorders, the most common of which is pseudohypertrophic muscular paralysis.

This affection appears most frequently at about the age of five years and is seen almost exclusively in boys. Symmetrical progressive muscular atrophy is accompanied by apparent hypertrophy of the muscles; the enlargement is usually most noticeable in the legs and forearms and about the shoulder girdle. The increase in size is due to hypertrophy of the muscle fibers, which is quickly followed by swelling of the nuclei, splitting of the fibers, increase of connective tissue, and deposition of fat. The etiology is unknown; it may be an intrinsic nutritional defect of the muscles. In about 60 per cent of the cases the disease is hereditary.

Clinical Picture.—Often the first evidence of progressive muscular dystrophy is weakness of the legs and resultant fatigue. The child stands with an obvious increase of the lumbar lordosis, walks with a peculiar waddling gait, has difficulty in climbing steps, and falls frequently.

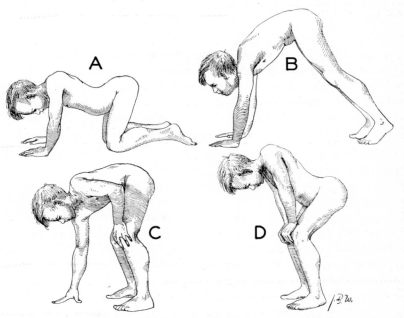

Fig. 111.—Progressive muscular dystrophy. Characteristic method of rising to a standing position, the arms being used to push the body erect. Note the increased lumbar lordosis, relaxed shoulder girdle, and enlarged calves.

Weakness of the extensor muscles of the legs and trunk is characteristic. On attempting to get up from the floor the patient usually climbs laboriously upon his legs and thighs (Gower's sign) (Fig. 111). Weakness about the shoulder girdle is characteristic also; when it is marked, the affection is sometimes spoken of as *facioscapulohumeral paralysis* (*Landouzy-Déjerine type of progressive muscular dystrophy*). The reflexes may be hypoactive. Sensation is usually unimpaired.

Diagnosis.—The diagnosis is made from the history, the characteristic clinical appearance, and the findings on physical examination. Because of the waddling gait progressive muscular dystrophy may be confused with bilateral congenital dislocation of the hip, excessive lumbar lordosis, or congenital coxa vara. Occasionally it is to be differentiated from infantile paralysis.

Prognosis.—The disease may progress slowly and result in total inability to walk. By the age of twelve years extreme disability is usually present, and later the patient dies of intercurrent infection. Occasionally, for no obvious reason, the disease is arrested before the disability becomes severe.

Treatment.—Systematic muscle training is indicated in all cases. If the Achilles tendons are contracted, operative lengthening will make walking easier. Braces are indicated when the ankles are weak and unstable. It may be necessary to support the back by means of a brace or corset.

The administration of vitamins, pilocarpine and epinephrine, glycine, or gelatin is of questionable therapeutic value. A few encouraging reports, however, have demonstrated temporary arrest of the disease following these types of medication.

Amyotonia Congenita

Amyotonia congenita is a disease of infancy present from birth and characterized by extreme muscular weakness and hypotonia. This entity and conditions closely related to it are seen frequently in crippled children's clinics. It is due to a developmental defect of the lower motor neurones and the voluntary muscles. If the weakness persists, it may be followed by postural deformities and a marked scoliosis. The affected child is excessively slow in developing sufficient muscle strength to enable him to sit or stand. There are no sensory symptoms or signs.

Treatment.—Massage and muscle training are of some benefit. Braces are sometimes indicated for support of the spine and legs. Treatment on the whole is discouraging.

CHAPTER XV

TUMORS

PART I. TUMORS OF BONE

Introduction and Classification.—Bone tumors theoretically may arise during any stage of cellular differentiation between that of the adult and highly specialized osteoblast and that of its remote and rapidly multiplying predecessor in the early mesoblastic tissue. It is not surprising, therefore, that the bone tumors show a wide range of histologic variation and that their clinical characteristics range from the extremely benign nature of osteoma to the highly malignant and rapidly fatal course of osteogenic sarcoma.

The importance of an accurate classification of these growths is obvious since it is a necessary preliminary to the accurate diagnosis upon which treatment and prognosis of the individual tumor must be based. Unfortunately, however, the subject of the classification of bone tumors has long been one of the most involved and unsettled fields of oncology. This confusion has been the result of a number of factors. Bone tumors, while not rare in the strict sense of the word, are yet sufficiently uncommon that a large or specialized experience is necessary to provide familiarity with the course of the various types encountered. The study of this group of tumors has been further encumbered by a complex and often contradictory terminology. Many designations appearing in the literature have possessed variations of meaning dependent upon the identity or the locality of the author. Confusion has arisen also from the fact that different portions of the same tumor may present dissimilar histologic pictures and that many cases, because of incomplete data, have been extremely difficult to classify with certainty. An additional confusing factor has been the difficulty of evaluating properly certain related pathologic entities, as, for example, localized bone cysts, which although in some respects very similar to tumors, are not primarily of neoplastic nature.

A rapid advance, however, was made in the study of bone tumors after the establishment in 1921 of the Registry of Bone Sarcoma by the American College of Surgeons. A nomenclature formulated by this agency was of great value in leading to a standard terminology. Statistical studies of the tumors reported to the Registry have led to an increased knowledge and to improved diagnosis and treatment.

For the present purpose the important bone tumors may be conveniently discussed according to the following outline.

A. Benign
    1. Osteoma, osteochondroma, chondroma, and osteoid-osteoma
    2. Benign giant cell tumor
    3. Bone cyst

B. Malignant
    1. Osteogenic sarcoma and chondrosarcoma
    2. Ewing's sarcoma
    3. Multiple myeloma
    4. Tumors metastasizing to bone

In addition to the important tumor entities enumerated in this simple classification, there are a number of less common new growths of bone which on occasion are of particular interest but because of infrequent occurrence are of less clinical importance. To this group belongs, according to Kolodny, the *periosteal fibrosarcoma* (also called *parosteal* or *extraperiosteal sarcoma),* a rare tumor of dense fibrous structure which is believed to arise from the peripheral layer of the periosteum and which pursues a course analogous to that of fibrosarcoma of the muscle sheath or fascia. Benign and malignant forms of *lipoma* and of *angioma* arise occasionally from the respective parent cells within bone; *hemangioma* occurs with considerable frequency in the vertebrae and in the skull but rarely gives rise to symptoms until its late stages. In recent years several instances of a localized tumor histologically resembling *myeloma* but of benign clinical course have been described. *Fibroxanthoma* appears near the end of a long bone as a benign lesion composed of whorled fibrous tissue and xanthoma cells. *Epiphyseal chondroblastoma* is a rare tumor, sometimes malignant, which arises in epiphyseal cartilage near the end of adolescence or shortly thereafter. *Extramaxillary adamantinoma,* a slowly growing tumor which does not metastasize but tends to recur locally unless completely excised, is found occasionally at the base of the skull and rarely in the tibia or ulna; prior to 1943 nineteen cases of extramaxillary adamantinoma had been reported. *Chordoma,* a rare malignant tumor arising from remnants of the embryonic notochord, occurs about the base of the skull or in the sacrococcygeal region and is characterized by extensive invasion of the surrounding tissues. Chordoma of the sacrococcygeal area must be distinguished from teratoma and from other tumors, primary or metastatic, which arise not infrequently in this location.

Benign Tumors of Bone

OSTEOMA, OSTEOCHONDROMA, AND CHONDROMA

It is convenient to consider these three tumors together since they possess an analogous histogenesis and exhibit an essentially identical clinical course. Certainly the great majority of these tumors are composed of both bony and cartilaginous elements and thus fall theoretically into the group of *osteochondromas.* Differentiation of this large group into a number of subdivisions is largely a matter of clinical usage and is not without clinical value.

Osteoma.—A benign tumor composed chiefly of bone is called an osteoma. The term *exostosis* is often used synonymously with osteoma but is better restricted to those instances of localized benign bony overgrowth which can be interpreted as the result of reaction to a local chronic irritation, such as calcaneal spurs or the multiple exostoses associated with osteoarthritis. Osteomas may be cancellous or compact and extremely hard. Microscopically tissue from an osteoma is often distinguished only with difficulty from normal bone. The bones of the skull are favorite sites for osteomas, which may form dense circular tumors of flat contour or may grow slowly to protrude into the orbits, paranasal sinuses, or mouth and cause symptoms from local pressure. The treatment of osteoma is excision, and, if the extirpation is complete, no recurrence need be anticipated.

Osteochondroma.—Osteochondromas constitute the most important group of benign tumors of bone. These neoplasms occur usually in persons between the ages of ten and twenty-five years and typically are situated near the ends of the long bones, where they form pedunculated bony overgrowths, the apices of which are covered by a layer of cartilage (Figs. 112*A* and 112*B*). The surface of this cartilage may be lobulated or roughened, and the protuberance is often covered, especially when in the vicinity of an overlying tendon, by a well-developed adventitious bursa

containing fluid of synovial type. The symptoms produced by these
growths are usually slight. Swelling is often the patient's only complaint,
although there may be discomfort in the adjacent joint. The duration of
symptoms is usually long, and the tumor may eventually reach enormous
dimensions. The commonest location for these growths is near the adjacent ends of the femur and tibia (Fig. 112A) or at the upper end of the

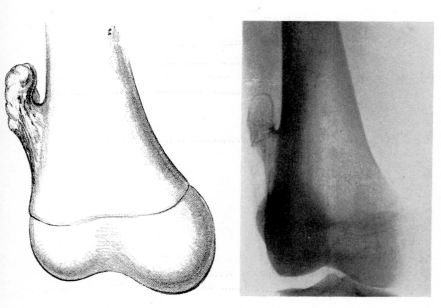

Fig. 112A.   Fig. 112B.

Fig. 112A.—Osteochondroma of lower end of femur in patient twelve years
of age.

Fig. 112B.—Roentgenogram of same case showing well-demarcated tumor
of broad pedicle.

humerus, although they are not uncommon in other sites. Of the flat
bones the scapula is most frequently involved. Roentgenograms show the
typical picture of an osseous base or pedicle of normal bone density,
springing directly from the cortex of the underlying bone and capped by
an expanded area showing irregular calcification (Fig. 112B). Microscopically the tumors present bone of normal appearance covered by a layer of
calcifying cartilage, which in turn may be bordered by a thin layer of fibrous tissue. The treatment is excision. Since osteochondromas rarely be-

come malignant, operation is not always necessary; however, any large osteochondroma in a location prone to traumatization should be removed. If excision is not done, periodic roentgenographic examination should be made, particularly in the older age groups.

Chondroma.—A benign tumor composed chiefly of cartilage is called a chondroma. This type of lesion often occurs within the shaft of a bone and is then sometimes termed an *enchondroma*; frequently several bones are involved simultaneously by *multiple enchondromas*. Chondromas are found most frequently in the small bones of the hands and feet, spine, wrist, sternum, scapula, and pelvis. Chondromas occur most often in patients between the ages of twenty and thirty years. The clinical picture is that of a slowly growing tumor, producing as a rule only slight discomfort. The characteristic roentgenograms show a rounded area of decreased density with a smooth outline, often expanding beneath a narrow shell of cortical bone. The treatment of chondroma is excision. This must be carried out with considerable care as regards completeness, as there is a tendency for recurrence and the recurrent tumor is likely to grow more rapidly than the original chondroma. After excision it is advisable to fill the cavity or space with cortical bone chips or cancellous grafts, especially when the bony continuity cannot be maintained by the remaining cortex.

Osteoid-Osteoma

Osteoid-osteoma is a benign osteogenic lesion which occurs in either cortical or spongy bone beneath the periosteum and usually near the articular portion. It has been found in persons between three and forty-six years of age, but most often between the ages of ten and twenty-five years. When arising in the shaft of a long bone it usually provokes a deposition of bone either beneath the periosteum or in the medulla.

Pathology.—In the early stage the lesion may consist largely of a vascular mesenchymal substratum, closely packed with osteoblasts and containing occasional osteoclasts. Later, intercellular substance develops between the osteoblasts, forming patches of osteoid tissue or numerous osteoid trabeculae, from which the name of the tumor is taken. This osteoid is gradually calcified, being converted into atypical hypercalcified bone which has the microscopic appearance of an osteoma rather than an osteoid tumor. Surrounding this lesion is always found a sclerotic

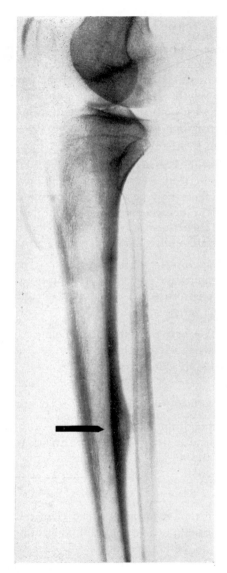

Fig. 113.—Lateral roentgenogram showing osteoid osteoma of tibia. Note the small rarefied area surrounded by osteosclerosis and periosteal new bone on posterior surface of middle third of shaft of tibia.

osseous zone which is slow in making its appearance and in which no microscopic evidence of inflammation has been observed.

Clinical Picture.—The principal complaint is pain which has been present for several months. The pain is mild at first and then increases in intensity until it is severe enough to wake the patient at night but is relieved usually by aspirin. There may be stiffness and weakness in the adjacent muscles, and a limp if the lesion is in a bone of the lower extremity. Localized swelling and tenderness may be present, but there is no elevation of body temperature.

Roentgenographic Picture.—The involved bone shows a small, rarefied, well-circumscribed area which is usually oval or round; in the center of this area there may be a minute shadow of increased density. This is surrounded by dense bone which, if the lesion is in the cortex, may extend several inches above or below the point of the original lesion (Fig. 113). Later, the entire lesion may become calcified.

Differential Diagnosis.—Osteoid-osteoma is most often confused with chronic nonsuppurative sclerosing osteomyelitis, osteitis of Garré, or Brodie's abscess. It is also to be differentiated from syphilis and from sclerosing osteogenic sarcoma.

Treatment.—The best treatment is complete excision of the lesion with all of the adjacent sclerotic bone. Roentgen therapy has been suggested, but its results are questionable.

Multiple Cartilaginous Exostoses (Dyschondroplasia)

Multiple osteochondromas, often associated with skeletal deformity, form a distinct clinical entity of hereditary nature which is discussed in Chapter IV under the subject of Affections of Growing Bone (page 76).

Benign Giant Cell Tumor

Benign giant cell tumor, formerly called giant cell sarcoma, is considered by most authorities a benign tumor of bone, although some observers do not believe it to be a true neoplasm. Gradations ranging from simple inflammatory giant-cell reactions all the way to outspoken malignant forms are encountered. The typical benign giant cell tumor (Fig. 114), however, is a slowly growing lesion beginning eccentrically in the epiphyseal end of a long bone in the young adult, causing obvious swelling with little pain, presenting on roentgenographic examination a circumscribed area of bone destruction with a trabeculated cystic appearance, and possessing no tendency to recur after complete surgical excision.

Pathology.—The benign giant cell tumor begins typically as a circumscribed growth occupying an eccentric position within the epiphyseal and retroepiphyseal region of a long bone. The lower end of the femur, lower end of the radius, and upper end of the tibia are most commonly involved, although the tumor is not infrequently seen in the femur at the hip, in the tibia or the fibula at the ankle, in the humerus at the shoulder, and in the mandible and vertebrae. As growth slowly advances, the overlying cortex is expanded and thinned. Lines of relative thickening of the involved cortical bone, often continuous with fibrous septums extending into the tumor, cause the characteristic roentgenographic appearance of trabeculation.

Grossly the tumor tissue is of friable, hemorrhagic, densely cellular appearance with areas of partial fibrous organization and of hemorrhagic softening. Microscopically a typical cellular stroma, consisting of small round cells and small fusiform cells, is interrupted by large thin-walled spaces containing red blood cells, by numerous areas of frank hemorrhage, and by the large multinucleated giant cells which give the tumor its name. The nuclei of these giant cells are well differentiated and stain lightly, in marked contrast to the pleomorphic and densely staining nuclei of true tumor giant cells. In these respects the giant cells of benign giant cell tumor resemble those found in association with foreign bodies. For this reason, benign giant cell tumor is considered by some observers not to be a true neoplasm but to represent the result of an abnormal process in the repair of a bone injury or the effect of a low-grade inflammatory process.

Clinical Picture.—The lesion occurs usually in persons between the ages of fifteen and thirty years. In the majority of cases a history of local trauma may be obtained, but trauma has no proved importance in the etiology. Pain of moderate severity is usual and may be associated with slight tenderness. Increase in size is very gradual and may go long unnoticed. Occasionally pathologic fracture occurs.

Roentgenographic Picture.—Characteristically the benign giant cell tumor presents the appearance of a multilocular bone cyst in the epiphysis of a long bone with expansion and thinning of the overlying cortex (Fig. 114). Cystic involvement often extends to, but does not invade, the articular cartilage of the adjacent joint.

Treatment and Prognosis.—The usual treatment for benign giant cell tumor is curettement and filling the resulting space with bone chips, preferably of cancellous bone; replacement of the tumor tissue with normal bone is particularly advisable if the loss of cortical bone is extensive. When the tumor occupies a favorable site, as in the proximal end of the fibula, resection is to be preferred; in some instances wide

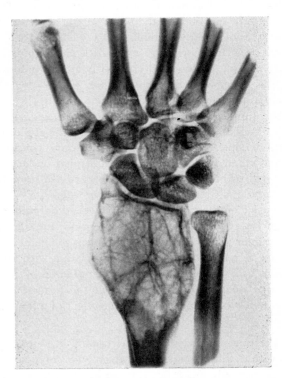

Fig. 114.—Benign giant cell tumor of the lower end of the radius. Note trabeculated cystic appearance and expansion of the cortex.

excision must be followed by a massive bone graft. In early cases deep roentgen therapy alone may be used if a careful follow-up can be made, but some forms do not respond to irradiation. Some workers advise against roentgen therapy because of the malignant changes which may follow. A combination of irradiation and surgery is sometimes considered to give better results than either alone. After incomplete excision recurrence is likely to take place, and such recurrent cases should be treated less conservatively than primary ones. In the majority of cases the prognosis with adequate treatment is excellent. Rare cases are on record, however, in which the tumor has become malignant and fatal metastases have occurred. A guarded prognosis should be made in the presence of rapid clinical growth, frequent recurrence, and the microscopic finding of a large proportion of spindle cells as compared with giant cells.

BONE CYST

The term *osteitis fibrosa cystica* has in the past been applied to two distinct disease entities between which no close relationship has been proved. Of these, the generalized form is a systemic disease exhibiting widespread skeletal changes and characterized by an excess of parathyroid hormone in the blood stream. It is discussed in Chapter V under the title of Hyperparathyroidism. The second, or localized, form of osteitis fibrosa cystica, appearing clinically as the *solitary bone cyst,* is a degenerative process rather than a neoplasm but is conveniently considered here because of its clinical similarity to true bone tumors and its consequent importance in differential diagnosis.

The typical bone cyst is a slowly growing, bone-destructive lesion occurring in childhood near one end of the diaphysis of a long bone, often first heralded by a pathologic fracture, and presenting on roentgenographic examination a characteristic unilocular cystic area with thinned overlying cortex.

Pathology.—Although other bones are not infrequently affected, a large majority of the cysts occur in the upper portion of the shaft of the femur, humerus, or tibia. Grossly there is often a connective tissue lining beneath the layer of thinned cortical bone, and the cyst contents may be serous fluid or degenerated grumous material. Microscopic sections of the cyst wall show fibrosis with secondary new bone formation in the cortex. No trabecular elements are found.

Clinical Picture.—Bone cyst is a disease of late childhood, the majority of cases occurring in children between the ages of ten and fifteen years although occasional ones are found even in individuals over twenty years of age. In approximately half the cases the first clinical symptoms

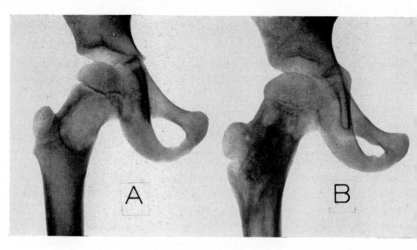

Fig. 115a.—Roentgenograms of solitary bone cyst in the neck of a femur of a child aged ten years. A, Before operation; B, six months after operation, which consisted of curetting the cyst and packing the cavity with bone chips taken from the crest of the ilium.

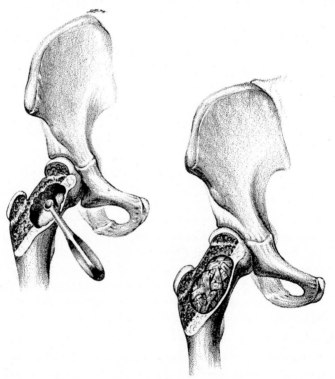

Fig. 115b.—Solitary bone cyst in neck of the femur. Sectional drawing to show appearance of cyst during curettement and after being packed with bone chips.

are occasioned by fracture, which takes place on slight traumatization of the thinned cortex.

Roentgenographic Picture.—The roentgenographic appearance of a single or, less typically, a multilocular central bone defect occurring in the diaphysis, with a smooth and intact outline formed by thinned and often slightly expanded cortical bone, is characteristic (Fig. 115).

Treatment and Prognosis.—When fracture has occurred through a bone cyst, the usual treatment of the fracture may be followed by obliteration of the cyst. When the diagnosis is made before fracture has occurred, or when the cyst persists after fracture, healing may be brought about by curettement and packing of the cavity with numerous small grafts of healthy bone preferably from the ilium (Figs. 115a and 115b). Irradiation may be tried as auxiliary therapy. With careful treatment the prognosis is excellent, and late complications are exceptional.

Malignant Tumors of Bone

Osteogenic Sarcoma

Osteogenic sarcoma is perhaps the most important member of the entire bone tumor group since it is the commonest primary malignant neoplasm of bone. Typically it occurs near the end of the diaphysis of a long bone in late childhood or early adult life. It is characterized clinically by early and severe pain, together with a rapidly increasing swelling. Radiographically both osteolysis and osteogenesis are usually present although occasionally either may occur alone; invasion of the soft tissues is conspicuous. Metastasis occurs early, and the prognosis for life, despite early and efficient treatment, is unfavorable.

From the group of osteogenic sarcomas, tumors consisting chiefly of cartilage may be separated as *chondrosarcomas*. These tumors are frequently recognizable in the roentgenogram by characteristic blotchy shadows cast by irregular strands and islands of calcification and ossification. Chondrosarcomas usually grow rapidly but metastasize less early than osteogenic sarcomas. In chondrosarcoma the prognosis is somewhat more favorable than in osteogenic sarcoma.

Pathology.—The upper tibia, lower femur, and upper humerus are the most common sites of osteogenic sarcoma although involvement of other bones, including those of the axial skeleton, is not infrequent. Pathologically there is wide variation among the individual tumors of this large group, and it has been the custom to subdivide it into a number of classes, varying from the more slowly growing, or *sclerosing* type, in which bone formation is prominent, to the rapidly advancing *telangiectatic* type, in which vascularity and osteolysis are conspicuous. Tumors of the latter group sometimes pulsate and hence have been

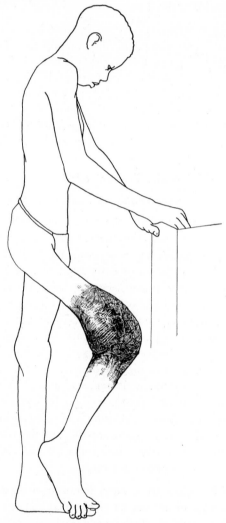

Fig. 116.—Osteogenic sarcoma of lower end of femur, advanced stage. Note the tense skin and distended veins.

called *bone aneurysms.* The typical cell of osteogenic sarcoma is spindle-shaped, and in the more malignant tumors hyperchromatism, pleomorphism, mitotic figures, and true tumor giant cells are frequent. Small islands of newly formed bone are common, together with irregular areas of cartilage in various stages of differentiation.

Clinical Picture.—Osteogenic sarcoma is commonest in children and young adults. It occasionally occurs in later adult years; in such cases an underlying osteitis deformans may be present. Pain is as a rule the first symptom, and a history of local trauma is usually obtained. Noticeable swelling and secondary limitation of motion in the adjacent joint soon follow. The more rapidly growing tumors are likely to show distended superficial veins (Fig. 116) and an increase in surface temperature. Other cases are less typical in onset and in their early stages are differentiated only with difficulty from other bone tumors and from low-grade inflammatory conditions.

Roentgenographic Picture.—Areas both of bone destruction and of new bone formation are usually visible. Small spicules of bone at right angles to the shaft, forming the characteristic "sun-ray appearance," are frequently conspicuous. In advanced cases there is evidence of irregular invasion of the surrounding soft tissues (Figs. 117*A* and 117*B*).

Prognosis and Treatment.—Early diagnosis and treatment are of the utmost importance. The prognosis is always unfavorable because of early metastasis to the lungs, but amputation of the extremity, if performed early, can be expected to result occasionally in cure. Ferguson believes that survival may be prolonged by delaying amputation until a preoperative course of roentgen therapy has been given; this method of treatment is employed in some clinics, but by most observers is not considered advisable. Even after the recognition of pulmonary metastases, amputation is often justifiable in order to remove a focus which is painful and which will ultimately ulcerate and bleed. In advanced cases roentgen therapy is usually advised but cannot be expected to accomplish more than a temporary retardation of the malignant process.

Ewing's Sarcoma

Ewing's sarcoma, called also *Ewing's tumor* and *endothelial myeloma,* often simulates a low-grade osteomyelitis, with an onset characterized by pain, tenderness, fever, and leucocytosis. It may occur in any bone of the body and is primarily bone-destructive, causing osteogenesis only

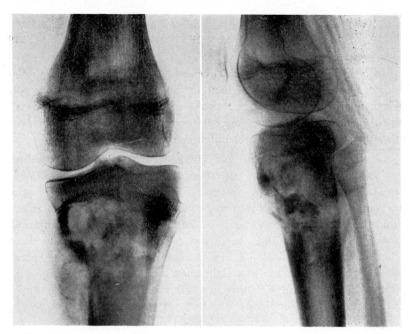

Fig. 117A.—Anteroposterior and lateral roentgenograms showing osteolytic type of osteogenic sarcoma of tibia with pathologic fracture, in patient thirteen years of age. Note areas of irregular destruction in upper tibia, new bone formation in the soft tissues, and slight angulation with break in the continuity of the cortex on the medial side of the tibia. Also note that the destructive process has not crossed the epiphyseal cartilage plate.

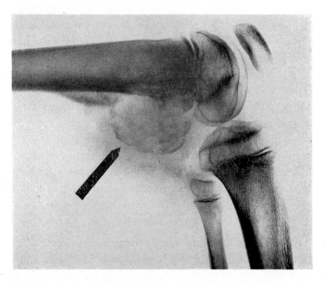

Fig. 117B.—Lateral roentgenogram showing osteogenic sarcoma of the femur in a girl seven years of age. Note large calcified mass posterior to lower end of diaphysis and the erosion of adjacent bone.

oy periosteal reaction and so producing a characteristic roentgenographic appearance of lamination. The tumor is at first most susceptible to irradiation, but usually this response is only temporary and metastasis and death soon supervene.

Pathology.—The typical site of origin of Ewing's sarcoma is near the middle of the shaft of a long bone. The tumor occurs in the femur more commonly than in any other bone. It also occurs in the flat bones. Grossly the main mass of the tumor often lies subperiosteally but outside the thickened cortex, which forms a reactive wall tending in the early stages to prevent invasion of the medullary cavity. Although the histogenesis of these tumors is obscure, the histologic structure is characteristic. The tumor tissue is made up of large areas of closely packed small polyhedral cells with scant cytoplasm and dense round or oval nuclei. There is no intercellular stroma. Connective tissue septums form a network dividing the tumor tissue into rounded areas, and many large vascular spaces containing blood and lined by tumor cells may be present.

Clinical Picture.—The tumor is most frequently met with in patients between the ages of ten and twenty-five years. A history of trauma can often be obtained. Pain is an early and distressing symptom although there may be periods of complete freedom from discomfort. There is often a constitutional reaction suggesting a low-grade inflammatory process. Palpation may reveal a smooth fusiform tumor continuous with the bone and of slight or extreme tenderness. Temporary subsidence of the pain and tenderness is believed to be due to relief of tension when the tumor has broken through the periosteum. In advanced cases there may be symptoms from metastases to the lungs or to bones, particularly the skull.

Roentgenographic Picture.—The roentgenographic appearance often is similar to that of a subacute or chronic osteomyelitis and must be carefully differentiated. In very early cases condensation of reacting bone about small areas of destruction may be visible. Many cases show widening of the shaft of the bone due to the formation of endosteal and subperiosteal bone in layers parallel to the long axis of the shaft; these layers sometimes produce an onion-peel appearance (Fig. 118). In late stages areas of bone destruction are evident.

Treatment and Prognosis.—Since Ewing's sarcoma is markedl
sensitive to irradiation, roentgen therapy is a useful first step in th
treatment as well as a therapeutic test of the diagnosis and a desirabl
preliminary to operation. Early radical operation offers a chance o
cure. A combination of radium therapy and surgery is considered b
many authorities to be the treatment of choice at the present tim
With any form of therapy, death is likely to occur not later than a ver
few years after the appearance of metastatic tumors.

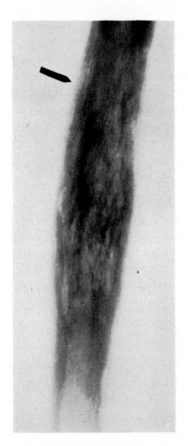

Fig. 118.—Lateral roentgenogram showing Ewing's sarcoma of femur. No
areas of rarefaction and increased density, absence of medullary cavity, and layin
down of thin sheets of bone on the outside of the cortex where the arrow
pointing. This is the so-called onionpeel appearance.

Multiple Myeloma

Multiple myeloma is a highly malignant tumor arising in middle adult life and most commonly affecting the bones of the axial skeleton. The lesions, which are entirely bone-destructive, present roentgenographically a characteristic punched-out appearance. Multiple myeloma is highly sensitive to irradiation, but the ultimate outcome is uniformly fatal.

Pathology.—Ribs, sternum, skull, and vertebrae are the most common sites of multiple myeloma. Many bones may be found to be involved simultaneously or in quick succession, and in advanced cases the distribution is widespread. The tumor begins in the marrow cavity and extends rapidly, replacing the normal bone marrow. The cortical bone is also invaded and usually shows many discrete areas of destruction. There is no bone formation other than a slight widening of the shaft from periosteal reaction. The process may extend to perforation of the periosteum and invasion of surrounding soft tissues. In the majority of cases the typical cell is identical in appearance with the plasma cell, and the differentiation of multiple myeloma from some types of endothelioma is difficult.

Clinical Picture.—Multiple myelomas are commonest among males in the age group of from forty to sixty years. In contrast to the other bone sarcomas, this tumor does not produce characteristic early symptoms. The onset is insidious, and vague pain, swelling, signs of local pressure, or pathologic fracture, commonly of a rib, may be the first manifestation. In later stages the pain may become more marked. Anemia resulting from invasion of the bone marrow, severe cachexia, and a slight febrile reaction are present in advanced cases. *Bence-Jones albuminuria* is a valuable confirmatory finding but is frequently absent. The serum protein may be high because of an excess of globulin. Kidney function is often impaired.

Roentgenographic Picture.—Multiple punched-out areas appearing in the bones of the axial skeleton are characteristic of multiple myeloma but must be differentiated from similar lesions produced by metastasis from osteolytic carcinoma of visceral origin (Figs. 119*A* and 19*B*).

Treatment and Prognosis.—As a rule, the central situation or the multiplicity of the bones involved contraindicates surgical treatment;

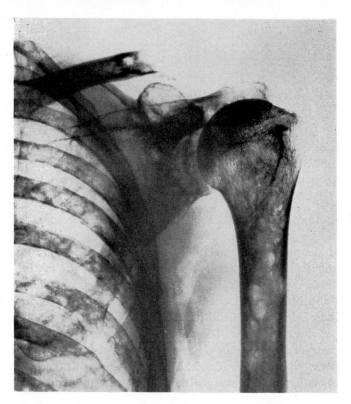

Fig. 119A.—Roentgenogram showing multiple myeloma. Note small punched out areas in ribs, scapula, and humerus with complete disappearance of the outer end of the clavicle.

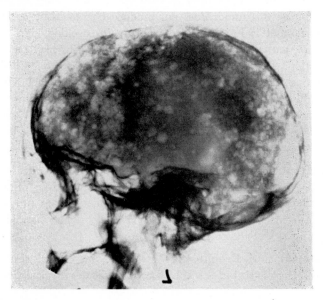

Fig. 119B.—Lateral roentgenogram showing multiple myeloma of the skull (same case as Fig. 119A). Note multiple small punched-out areas.

painful involvement of a long bone may occasionally make amputation the treatment of choice. Multiple myeloma is highly susceptible to irradiation, which should be employed to the limit determined by the resultant leucopenia. Stilbamidine, Pentamidine, urethane, or cortisone sometimes relieves the pain and inhibits the tumor process. Immobilization may be indicated to prevent pathologic fracture. The prognosis is uniformly unfavorable, the average duration of life being approximately three years although rare instances of survival for as long as ten years or more have been recorded.

Tumors Metastasizing to Bone

In the diagnosis of bone tumors the possibility of involvement of bone by metastasis or by direct extension from a tumor primary elsewhere is always to be kept in mind. Bone metastases are most common in carcinomas of the breast and of the prostate gland and in hypernephroma, but are also frequent in cancer of the thyroid gland, gastrointestinal tract, female genitalia, and lungs. Erosive changes in the bones may occur in the leucemias and in Hodgkin's disease.

Pathology.—The most common sites to be involved by metastatic tumors are the upper end of the femur, the pelvis, vertebrae, ribs, skull, and humerus. Metastatic tumors are rare below the elbows and the knees. Metastases from hypernephroma are usually osteolytic; those from the breast are predominantly osteolytic although they may present areas of bone formation as well. In cancer of the prostate gland, bone metastases of osteoplastic nature occurring in the pelvis and lumbar spine are typical. The histologic appearance of bone metastases depends upon the histogenesis of the primary tumor but is often not sufficiently characteristic to provide a basis for specific diagnosis.

Clinical Picture.—The clinical appearance of metastatic bone tumor is not uniform. The age of the patient is of aid in rendering primary bone sarcoma other than multiple myeloma unlikely. There is often a history of preceding operation upon breast or prostate gland. Pain may be an early symptom and often occurs before there is roentgenographic evidence of bone involvement. In some cases, on the other hand, pathologic fracture is the first clinical sign. The presence of lung metastases is to be suspected and may be a valuable point in ruling out multiple myeloma. The alkaline phosphatase may be elevated.

Roentgenographic Picture.—The areas of involvement are often multiple. The appearance of the bone varies with the type of the original tumor. Punched-out areas of bone destruction without new bone formation are frequent in the osteolytic tumors (Fig. 120), while in the case of metastases from the prostate gland a diffuse increase of density is the rule.

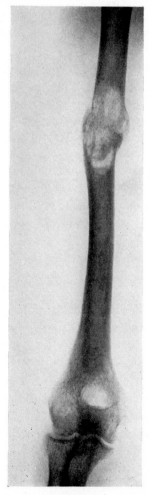

Fig. 120.—Roentgenogram showing pathologic fracture of humerus in metastatic lesion from carcinoma of the breast. Note localized well-demarcated area of bone destruction.

Treatment and Prognosis.—Biopsy should usually be performed f the diagnosis is uncertain. Irradiation can do much to relieve the pain caused by metastatic tumors and in the case of the more radiosensitive growths may prolong life. Cortisone sometimes affords relief of pain. Pain caused by bone metastases from carcinoma of the prostate gland can be relieved by orchidectomy and the administration of estrogen. Traction, intramedullary nailing, cast, or corset may be indicated for a pathologic fracture. While the prognosis is uniformly unfavorable, palliative treatment can do much to relieve the patient's discomfort.

PART II. TUMORS OF THE JOINTS, TENDONS, TENDON SHEATHS, AND BURSAE

Neoplasms of joint structures, of tendons and tendon sheaths, and of bursae form a small but interesting group of tumors about which little is known with certainty. The majority of these growths arise probably from derivatives of the early mesoblastic cells which are the predecessors of mature joint structures; hence these tumors possess the potentiality of forming cartilage and bone.

Within the joints occur benign osteochondromas and chondromas, sometimes diffusely involving the synovial membrane and giving rise to multiple loose bodies. *Osteochondromatosis* of the knee joint (see page 457) is the most common clinical example of this diffuse type of tumor although the process may be observed also in other joints. Fibroblastic tumors, with or without xanthoma cells and giant cells, may occur in the synovium and sometimes invade the surrounding structures. Tumors arising from the synovial membrane and hence called *synoviomas* have been described; in most instances they are highly malignant. From the articular cartilages may arise cysts and cartilaginous bodies of questionably neoplastic nature. Fibromas, fibrosarcomas, lipomas, and angiomas of joints have also been reported.

Tumors of the tendons themselves are rare. The tendon sheath is a more common site of tumor origin. Fibroma of the tendon sheath is frequently observed, particularly in the hand and foot. Tendon sheaths may also be the locus of giant cell tumor, benign osteochondroma, or myxofibroma, while involvement by embryoma or fibrosarcoma has occasionally been described. By some authorities the common ganglion of the wrist or ankle is believed to be the degenerated product of a low-grade neoplastic process.

SUMMARY OF THE CHIEF TYPES OF BENIGN BONE TUMOR

	APPROXIMATE AGE AT ONSET OF SYMPTOMS	OUTSTANDING EARLY SYMPTOMS	BONES MOST FREQUENTLY INVOLVED	LOCATION WITHIN INVOLVED BONE	OUTSTANDING X-RAY CHARACTERISTICS	OUTSTANDING HISTOLOGIC CHARACTERISTICS	RATE OF GROWTH	TREATMENT OF CHOICE	PROGNOSIS
Osteochondroma	Late childhood and early adult years	Swelling	Long bones	Diaphysis near epiphyseal line	Pedunculated outgrowth	Bone and cartilage cells of normal appearance	Slow	Excision	Excellent
Benign giant cell tumor	Early adult years	Swelling	Long bones	Epiphysis and adjacent diaphysis	Eccentric trabeculated cyst with expanded cortex	Giant cells in typical stroma	Slow	Excision and bone grafting; or curettement, cauterization, and irradiation	Excellent
Bone cyst	Late childhood	Slight discomfort, pathologic fracture	Long bones	Diaphysis near one end	Central cyst, often unilocular, with thinned cortex	No tumor cells	Slow	Excision or curettement, followed by bone grafting	Excellent

SUMMARY OF THE CHIEF TYPES OF MALIGNANT BONE TUMOR

	APPROXIMATE AGE AT ONSET OF SYMPTOMS	OUTSTANDING EARLY SYMPTOMS	BONES MOST FREQUENTLY INVOLVED	LOCATION WITHIN INVOLVED BONE	OUTSTANDING X-RAY CHARACTERISTICS	OUTSTANDING HISTOLOGIC CHARACTERISTICS	RATE OF GROWTH	TREATMENT OF CHOICE	PROGNOSIS
Osteogenic sarcoma	Late childhood and early adult years (rarely in later adult years)	Pain	Long bones	Diaphysis near one end	Bone destruction, bone formation, and invasion	Pleomorphic cells and disordered bone formation	Rapid	Amputation and irradiation	Unfavorable
Ewing's sarcoma	Late childhood and early adult years	Pain with periods of remission	Long bones	Diaphysis near mid-point	Laminated expansion early; bone destruction later	Characteristic small round cells not forming bone	Rapid	Amputation and irradiation	Unfavorable
Multiple myeloma	Middle adult years	Variable onset	Axial skeleton	Multiple areas	Multiple punched-out areas	Plasma cells	Rapid	Irradiation; supportive	Unfavorable
Metastatic tumors	Middle and late adult years	Pain	Variable distribution	Variable location	Osteolytic or osteosclerotic	Dependent upon primary tumor	Usually rapid	Irradiation; supportive	Unfavorable

Bursal tumors are rare. Chondromas and sarcomas have been most frequently reported, and their location is most often in the prepatellar bursa.

Diagnosis and Treatment.—Accurate diagnosis of tumors of the joints and tendons is often impossible prior to exploration. The treatment is surgical and varies with the clinical and microscopic characteristics of the individual tumor. Small circumscribed growths should be removed with a wide margin of surrounding tissue. Synovectomy is sometimes indicated for diffuse involvement. Every joint tumor case must be observed carefully for evidence of recurrence. When the diagnosis of malignancy is established, resort usually must be had to radical surgery combined with irradiation.

PART III. TUMORS OF MUSCLES AND FASCIAE

Although soft tissue tumors are encountered clinically with great frequency in muscular regions of the extremities and the trunk, these new growths arise almost invariably from mesoblastic derivatives other than muscle itself. While cases of *myoblastoma* and *rhabdomyoma,* tumors derived from voluntary striated muscle cells, have been reported, their excessive rarity makes them of little clinical importance. The great majority of the subcutaneous soft tissue tumors are derived from cells of connective tissue, of fatty, or of endothelial type. Of these, the benign varieties are *fibroma, lipoma,* and *angioma,* while the only malignant new growth of common occurrence is *fibrosarcoma.*

Fibroma, Lipoma, and Angioma

These tumors may arise at a subcutaneous level or deep within the musculature. They grow very slowly, cause few symptoms, and may be noted early as small nontender nodules or only much later after having attained considerable size. *Fibromas* are encapsulated and are palpable as firm circumscribed masses, often movable to some extent on the underlying tissue; they are particularly common in the hands and feet. *Lipomas* possess little or no capsule; they may be either circumscribed or diffuse and of irregular contour. *Angiomas* are of less frequent occurrence and have been described particularly as arising in the muscles of the arm or forearm. Unlike fibromas and lipomas, they may extend locally and involve the surrounding tissues.

In diagnosis these tumors must be differentiated from masses of similar clinical appearance which may occur at corresponding sites; for instance, lipoma of the popliteal fossa may be distinguished only with difficulty from distention of the gastrocnemio-semimembranosus bursa. Their differentiation from the malignant fibrosarcoma is occasionally difficult, and the diagnosis is sometimes established only by exploration.

The treatment of these benign tumors is excision. Recurrence need not be feared in the case of lipoma but must be kept in mind after the excision of fibromas. Any involvement of surrounding structures by an angioma necessitates wide excision and prolonged observation to rule out recurrence.

Fibrosarcoma

Pathologically the fibrosarcomas of nonvisceral origin can be divided into several varieties according to the cellular morphology, but clinically they form a single important group with well-marked characteristics.

Fibrosarcoma may occur at any age but is commonest in the fifth decade. It is particularly likely to occur in the lower third of the thigh, in the forearm, or in the abdominal wall. A history of suddenly increased rapidity of growth or of recurrence after surgical removal suggests the diagnosis of malignancy. Fibrosarcomas are typically of firm consistency and owing to the involvement of surrounding fascial structures are relatively immobile. Metastases may develop early, especially in the lungs, and in advanced stages are characteristically widespread.

When malignancy is suspected, biopsy is always warranted. The treatment should consist of early, wide, and thorough excision of the tumor. The usual tendency is toward a too conservative removal, which favors recurrence. Irradiation treatments should, as a rule, both precede and follow operative removal of the fibrosarcoma. When the tumor is situated in an extremity, amputation is often the best treatment.

PART IV. TUMORS OF NERVES

True *neuroma,* a tumor derived from nerve elements themselves rather than from their investing connective tissue sheaths, occurs so rarely as to be of little clinical importance. *Neurofibroma,* which arises in association with peripheral nerves and is composed of cells derived from some part of the nerve sheaths, is, however, very common. By special staining, many of these tumors may be shown to contain little or no tissue of true nerve origin, and failure to demonstrate the presence of nerve fibers or ganglion cells does not invalidate the diagnosis of neurofibroma. Indeed it is held by many well-informed oncologists that most of the fibromas and fibrosarcomas so commonly encountered are of neurogenic origin and are more properly termed *neurofibromas* and *neurofibrosarcomas*.

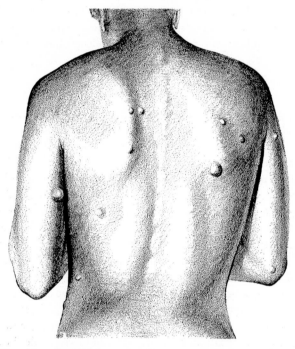

Fig. 121.—Von Recklinghausen's disease or neurofibromatosis. Note the multiple small tumor masses over the back and arms. These are pedunculated soft tissue tumors associated with scattered areas of skin pigmentation (café-au-lait spots) which are not shown on this drawing.

Of the tumors which tend to occur in close relationship to nerve trunks, two varieties may be distinguished: (1) *solitary neurofibroma* and (2) *multiple neurofibroma,* called also *neurofibromatosis* and *von Recklinghausen's disease.* Intermediate clinical types are common. While these conditions histogenetically are identical, it is convenient from the clinical standpoint to describe them separately.

A *solitary neurofibroma* is usually a firm, nontender, slowly growing mass attached to one of the larger nerves but not as a rule interfering with its function. When malignancy is present, growth is more rapid, the tumor mass becomes fixed, and nerve irritation or block may develop. Operative removal of the tumor is indicated. In the presence of malignant changes wide excision should be carried out, and preoperative and postoperative irradiation may be employed with advantage. In advanced cases of neurofibrosarcoma excision may be impossible, and amputation, as a palliative measure, may be indicated.

Neurofibromatosis, or *von Recklinghausen's disease,* which is sometimes of hereditary nature, is characterized by the gradual development of numerous pedunculated soft tissue tumors (Fig. 121), frequently associated with small scattered areas of skin pigmentation which are called café-au-lait spots. The tumors vary greatly in number and size and lie in the subcutaneous tissue or skin of any or all parts of the body. At times a large diffuse mass may develop about the head or neck and form an unsightly drooping fold of skin and soft tissue. Tumors attached to deeper nerve trunks, such as the sciatic nerve, as well as intraspinal tumors, are seen not infrequently. Bone changes secondary to involvement of the local nerves are often observed; they include cystic areas and irregularities of contour and length. Scoliosis is frequently an associated finding. An intraosseous neurofibroma may sometimes be the cause of a congenital pseudarthrosis (Fig. 125).

The tumors tend to progress slowly and to cause few symptoms except from local mechanical pressure. They possess, however, a definite tendency toward malignant change, and the ultimate outcome is often fatal. Excision of deforming or disabling growths must be done with the realization that removal is often followed by the appearance of recurrent tumors of heightened malignancy.

CHAPTER XVI

FRACTURE DEFORMITIES

Introduction.—In a short textbook of this type there is insufficient space for an adequate discussion of the methods of treating recent or fresh fractures. It is most important, however, that a brief synopsis be presented of the poor results which sometimes follow the treatment of fresh fractures, or *fracture deformities;* of what treatment should be employed to restore them to satisfactory structural and functional condition; and of what should be done to minimize the frequency of these unsatisfactory results.

This chapter includes a discussion of the following subjects: (1) the repair of fractures, (2) delayed union, (3) nonunion, and (4) malunion.

The Repair of Fractures

It is appropriate, before the abnormalities of bony union are considered, to discuss the basic physiologic and biochemical phenomena of osteogenesis and bone repair. Such a discussion may help to answer some of the following questions:

1. Why, under ideal conditions of early anatomic reduction and treatment by approved methods, are callus formation and bony union in certain fractures frequently very slow in taking place?

2. Why, with no evident reason, is there occasionally complete failure of callus and new bone formation at the site of fracture?

3. Why, with roentgenographic evidence of callus formation and early bony union, do a gradual absorption across the fracture line and a decalcification of the fragments on either side sometimes follow, resulting finally in fibrous union?

One should first appreciate the fact that there are two schools of thought regarding bone formation: one contends that fibroblasts change into osteoblasts or specific bone-forming cells which lay down the new bone; the other school maintains that bone is formed at the site of fracture by a chemical process in which deposition of calcium salts occurs in the presence of a suitable fibrous medium.

Following fracture, hemorrhage occurs immediately and invariably. The blood, together with a sterile inflammatory exudate, infiltrates all of the neighboring spaces, where it clots. These clots are quickly invaded by granulation tissue, which is a loose meshwork of capillaries and young fibroblasts. Three days after a fracture, small calcium deposits are visible microscopically in the form of a lacelike mesh in the tissues. This network is laid down in relatively avascular areas, and, as new bone forms, the deposits of calcium become more clearly outlined.

In the callus or preosseous substance which appears at the site of the fracture, cartilage-like cells can be demonstrated in addition to deposits of calcium. These cells are of extremely immature appearance and vary inversely in number with the amount of motion allowed at the site of fracture. They seem to arise by metaplasia of the connective tissue cells in the organized hematoma and aid in forming a temporary semirigid tissue which tends to immobilize the fracture fragments. The callus is later invaded by new connective tissue cells from the periosteum and also from the medullary cavity.

The first bone which is formed has coarse trabeculae and is comparable to cancellous or spongy bone. It is thought by some observers that true bone forms beneath the periosteum and endosteum near each end of the fractured bone and grows toward the fracture line, gradually replacing the callus. The new spongy bone is slowly converted into hard cortical bone while the excess callus is resorbed. From this point on, the structure of the new bone becomes adapted, according to *Wolff's law* (see page 76), to the stresses and strains to which it is subjected.

On the tenth day after fracture, microscopic bone granules are perceptible in the tissue about the fracture site. The fibroblasts flatten out, elongate, and become indistinguishable from similar cells seen in scar tissue.

On the twenty-fifth day of the healing of a diaphyseal fracture the callus is clinically firm, and on the thirtieth day it is quite compact. Osseous union is firm in from four to twelve weeks, depending upon the type of bone fractured. Complete bony union occurs in from four to six months, but it requires from nine to twelve months for the permanent architecture of the bone to be restored.

The exact source of the calcium salts which are used to form new bone has never been determined. Some authorities believe that they are derived locally from the bone fragments, as evidenced by the rarefaction and decalcification which can be demonstrated by roentgenographic examination. Others believe that the calcium salts come from the blood serum. It has been definitely proved that the two processes of calcium resorption and calcium deposition take place simultaneously. Adherents of the osteoblastic theory of bone formation believe that calcium salts exert on the connective tissue cells a specific influence which causes them to grow actively and to undergo metaplasia into osteoblasts.

It was shown in 1923 by Robison in England that a ferment or enzyme is present at the site of bone repair. This enzyme is called *phosphatase* because the phosphorus radicles are the hydrolyzable elements in the process of calcification. Phosphatase causes the precipitation of calcium from a mixture of calcium salts and organic matter in vitro. Phosphatase is normally present in the blood, and where there is tissue death, such as that at the site of fracture, phosphatase is liberated in great quantities. It has been proved that in order to function properly this enzyme requires a certain hydrogen ion concentration. It has also been shown experimentally that by decreasing or increasing the hydrogen ion concentration in the presence of phosphatase and calcium salts in vitro, i.e., by creating a more acid or more alkaline medium, the amount of calcium precipitation can be proportionately increased or decreased. With an increase of hydrogen ion concentration, the medium becomes more alkaline and the precipitation is decreased. The hydrogen ion concentration in the tissues depends largely upon the circulation. If the circulation at the site of fracture has been markedly impaired by injury of the blood vessels, there will be definite retardation of the new bone formation.

Delayed Union

Delayed union is said to be present when a fracture fails to consolidate in the time usually required for union to take place. In delayed union the processes of bone repair are retarded but are still going on and, with sufficient time, will produce firm union without surgical treatment.

The period required for bone consolidation after fracture varies considerably in different individuals and under different circumstances. Delayed union is said to be present in the tibia if the fracture does not become clinically firm in twelve weeks (Fig. 122); in the humerus in ten weeks; and in the femur, in twelve weeks. These are common sites of delayed union.

The causes of delayed union are:

1. Inaccurate reduction.

2. Inadequate or interrupted immobilization.

3. Severe local traumatization.

4. Impairment of circulation following open operation.

5. Infection, as in compound fractures.

6. Loss of bone substance, such as might occur in compound fractures after free excision of devitalized fragments.

7. Distraction or separation of fragments by excessive traction, a frequent sequel of too strong skeletal traction.

8. Advanced age.

9. Acute or chronic infectious disease, of which syphilis is an example.

10. Disturbance of the calcium-phosphorus metabolism.

Treatment.—Delayed union can best be avoided by (1) an early, accurate, and gentle reduction, uncomplicated by circulatory impairment from pressure of the splint or unnecessary surgical interference; (2) avoidance of the repeated traumatization of unnecessary attempts to perfect the alignment; (3) frequent observation of cases in skeletal traction to forestall separation of the fragments; and (4) protection against undue strain upon the fracture line, especially in the lower extremity.

The treatment of delayed union should be directed toward stimulating bone formation by increasing the volume of the local circulation. Diathermy has an important place in increasing circulation at the site of fracture. In delayed union of the femur or tibia, weight-bearing in a walking cast will help to accelerate the formation of bone. The cast should be applied with little padding and moulded snugly to the extremity. The operation of drilling many small holes through the ends of the fracture fragments may hasten union by opening new channels for circulation and bone formation. The value of parathyroid and other gland extracts is very doubtful. A diet rich in red meats, liver, green vegetables, and milk is thought by some authorities to be of benefit. Calcium and vitamin medication may be of value if the patient has a dietary deficiency.

Nonunion

Nonunion is present when the processes of bone repair, after having failed to produce firm union, have ceased completely. Unless this situation is changed radically by treatment, the nonunion will continue as a permanent and in most instances a severely disabling condition.

No fracture should be considered ununited until at least six months after the date of injury. Even after eight months or more have elapsed, firm union will occasionally take place without surgical aid.

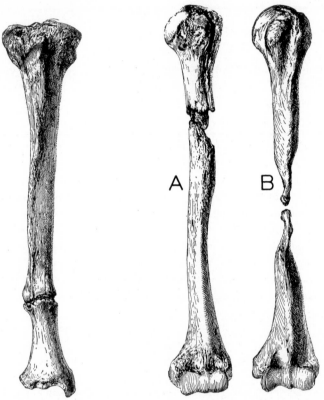

Fig. 122.   Fig. 123.

Fig. 122.—Delayed union of fracture of tibia. (Drawing from specimen.)

Fig. 123.—Nonunion of fracture of humerus. *A,* Common type with moderate bone absorption. *B,* Pencil-point type characterized by extreme absorption. (Drawing from specimens.)

Etiology.—The cause of nonunion may be of local or of constitutional nature. Probably the importance of the constitutional factors is frequently overestimated because of failure to discover the true local cause.

Local Causes.—Nonunion may result from (1) separation of the fragments, which is the most common cause; (2) loss of bone substance, resulting from extrusion or excision of small fragments in compound fractures; (3) inadequate fixation, allowing of excessive motion at the site of fracture; (4) repeated manipulation to improve the position, causing disturbances of the circulation; (5) interposition of soft parts such as muscle and fascia between the fragments; (6) infection which may develop following a compound fracture; (7) impairment of circulation by injury of the nutrient vessels or other sources of blood supply at the time of the original injury; (8) disturbance of circulation resulting from operative reduction; and (9) formation of scar tissue between the bone fragments before calcium deposition has taken place.

Constitutional Causes.—Nonunion may occur in association with: (1) a focus of infection, such as diseased teeth or tonsils, which lowers the general resistance and health of the patient; (2) hypothyroidism or hyperthyroidism; (3) debilitating disease, such as diabetes or malaria; (4) a disturbance of the calcium-phosphorus metabolism; (5) multiple fractures, in which the bone-forming capacity of the patient may be overtaxed; and (6) in some instances, syphilis.

Pathology.—Nonunion is characterized by several pathologic changes which should be remembered (Fig. 123). The fragments may be connected by a fibrous or fibrocartilaginous tissue, or there may be a pseudarthrosis between the fragments with the formation of a thick bursal sac containing synovial fluid in which rice bodies may be present. The ends of the fragments usually consist at this time of hard, sclerotic, eburnated bone; they may, on the other hand, become porous, atrophic, and cone shaped. Associated with the formation of new bone, there may be excessive callus limited entirely to one fragment, usually the proximal.

Clinical Picture.—Mobility at the site of fracture varies widely. In some cases it is slight and hardly demonstrable, while in others, and particularly in pseudarthrosis, there may be excessive movement in all directions. The pathologic mobility may be obvious when the patient attempts to move the extremity. Occasionally motion elicits pain, but usually little discomfort is associated with the motion of a pseudarthrosis. In cases of nonunion in the lower extremity there are often pain on weight-bearing and a slight amount of swelling following activity. Pain and swelling are more conspicuous when there is almost complete union of the fracture than when, as in pseudarthrosis, there is no union. Muscle atrophy is extreme and joint function may be limited. Especially great is the loss of mobility of the knee joint which may accompany an ununited fracture of the femur.

Treatment.—The treatment consists of constitutional and local measures. The constitutional treatment is of questionable value. In patients in whom there is a calcium-phosphorous imbalance, it may be wise to give a calcium salt preparation by mouth, a cod liver oil concentrate, lime and orange juices, and a diet rich in bone-producing elements and including red meats, liver, green vegetables, and milk. Calcium and phosphorus salts are of doubtful value when administered alone. Glandular extracts have been used but their value is questionable. Capsules containing all of the common vitamins may be helpful.

The local treatment consists of the use of braces or of surgery. Braces are entirely palliative and are used primarily to relieve strain and accompanying pain. In ununited fracture of the humerus, a firmly fitting laced leather cuff extending from the shoulder to the elbow will improve the function of the arm. A Thomas walking caliper splint fitted with a moulded leather cuff for the thigh will brace an ununited fracture of the femur sufficiently to permit the patient to walk. A similar brace may be used for ununited fracture of the tibia; it should be fitted with a leather cuff which has been moulded closely to the leg at the level of fracture.

The operation of perforating the fragment ends with many small drill holes, used frequently for delayed union, has been successful occasionally in the treatment of nonunion; however, the only highly effective treatment of ununited fractures is bone grafting.

When nonunion follows the frank infection of a compound fracture, operative treatment should usually be delayed three to six months following the healing of the wound, since the development of infection in a wound containing transplanted bone often means complete failure of the operative work. The use of chemotherapy and antibiotics, however, has made it possible to shorten the waiting period in some cases. It is often advisable to perform the operation of bone grafting in two stages. In the first stage the potentially infected scar tissue should be thoroughly excised and the hard, eburnated ends of the bone fragments removed. Infected, scarred, or poorly nourished skin areas should be removed and replaced preferably by a single skin graft of pedicle, flap, or split-thickness type. If healing takes place without signs of infection, the bone graft operation may be performed several weeks later.

Most ununited fractures require a bone transplant before union can be obtained. When the bed is being prepared for the graft, all surrounding scar tissue and sclerotic bone should be removed until healthy bleeding occurs from the bone ends and from the surrounding soft tissues. There is no accepted opinion as to what happens to the free autogenous bone transplant. Some investigators believe that it lives and adapts itself to its new environment. Others believe that it dies and remains only as a scaffold or framework into which the new bone grows. Still others believe that many of its cells die, but that substantial new bone is formed by proliferation of the surviving cells. Survival of the graft is probably dependent upon early reestablishment of its circulation. It is apparent that grafts which have an extensive area of contact with neighboring bone fragments are likely to live and form satisfactory bridges. Firm mechanical fixation and protection from excessive stress and strain are as essential to the success of the graft as extensive bony contact.

Several types of bone graft are in common use. Choice of the variety of graft for the individual case depends largely upon the site of nonunion, the condition of the bone fragment ends, and the training and experience of the operator. A description of the more important types of bone grafts follows.

1. *Massive Onlay Graft* (Fig. 124,*A*).—This type of graft is taken usually from the tibia. It may include the periosteum as well as the full thickness of the cortex. The bed is prepared across the fragment ends by removing the periosteum and outer cortex. No attempt is made to place the graft in contact with the endosteum or medullary cavity. As a rule, fixation is best secured by the use of Vitallium or stainless steel screws long enough to traverse both cortices. Onlay grafts produce very satisfactory results in the hands of operators who are accustomed to the special technic which their application requires.

The *dual graft,* described by Boyd, comprises two massive onlay grafts which span the defect on opposite surfaces of the fractured bone. They are fixed firmly by screws going through both grafts and both cortices. Dual grafts are particularly useful for the more difficult cases of nonunion.

2. *Inlay Graft* (Fig. 124,*B*).—This graft, popularized by Albee, includes periosteum, cortex, and endosteum, and is spoken of as a

full-thickness or cortical graft. The bed for the graft is usually prepared in the fragments with the same double-bladed motor saw which is used to cut the graft. The transplanted bone should be accurately fitted in its bed and firmly fixed with screws of Vitallium or stainless steel. In the past, chromic catgut, kangaroo tendon, heavy silk, and stainless steel wire have been used for fixation of the graft, but these materials have now been almost entirely discarded in favor of metallic screws which fix the graft more securely. In fracture of the lower third of the tibia, a sliding inlay graft may be most suitable; it is cut from the upper fragment, slid into a bed across the defect, and fixed in place with metal screws.

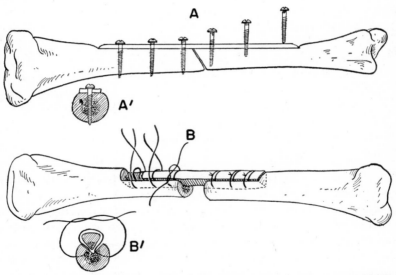

Fig. 124.—*A*, Onlay graft. The graft is fixed with metal screws. *A'*, Cross section to show method of fixation. *B*, Inlay graft. Fragments have been separated to show details of the graft insertion. Sutures are used to hold the graft in place. This graft can also be fixed with metal screws as in *A*. *B'*, Cross section to show a method of fixation.

3. *Osteoperiosteal Graft.*—This graft is usually taken from the anteromedial surface of the tibia in such manner as to include the periosteum and a thin layer of small adherent chips of cortical bone. The particular advantage of this graft is that it is pliable and can be moulded to fit the contour of the fragments and the defect.

4. *Cancellous Graft.*—This graft consists of spongy bone usually taken from the crest or wing of the ilium. The circulation is more readily reestablished through its cancellous structures than through the dense bone of a cortical graft, and union takes place in less time. It is the most useful type of non-rigid graft.

5. *Multiple Grafts.*—Occasionally it is wise to put many small splinters of bone in and about the main graft or across the fractured area. These should be cancellous in type when possible. They form a local depot for calcium and undoubtedly aid tremendously in the solidification of the fracture. These small multiple transplants are sometimes spoken of as rat, sliver, or chip grafts.

6. *Intramedullary Peg Graft.*—This form of graft has an occasional place in the treatment of ununited fractures. In many clinics, however, it is not used. In the past the argument against its use was that if the graft were properly applied it must fit tightly into the medullary cavity and thereby impair the circulation. However, since the widespread and successful use of snugly fitting intramedullary nails, the author doubts that this argument would be valid in the minds of many surgeons today. The intramedullary peg graft is sometimes a particularly convenient means of securing internal fixation in the femur, humerus, radius, and ulna. It should usually be supplemented with small sliver grafts.

After any bone transplant the fragments should be immobilized by means of ample and well-moulded plaster splints or cast. Bleeding from the denuded bone surfaces always occurs, and care must be taken postoperatively that this does not cause excessive pressure and ischemia. A properly padded cast which is elevated on pillows postoperatively does not usually require splitting; if it must be cut to relieve pressure, complete temporary bivalving is the safest method. After grafting of a major bone of an extremity the cast must usually be left in place for a period of at least twelve weeks. The plaster should then be bivalved and physical therapy instituted.

Congenital Fractures and Nonunion.—A defect in the bony continuity resembling an ununited fracture or pseudarthrosis is occasionally demonstrable in the bone of an infant immediately after birth. Lesions of this type can be differentiated by means of roentgenograms from fractures occurring during delivery; they must also be differentiated from bony defects caused by intraosseous nerve tumors in neurofibromatosis. They are thought to be due to a congenital deficiency of bone

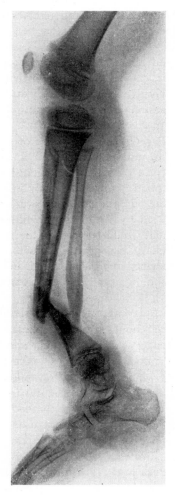

Fig. 125.—Lateral roentgenogram showing congenital pseudarthrosis of the tibia in a boy seven years of age. Two bone graft operations have been performed without union. Note tapered and thin bone ends with decalcification of all bony structures. (Courtesy of Dr. R. H. Hutchinson.)

production. These fractures are rare, are seen in the tibia much more often than in other bones (Fig. 125), and unfortunately are very resistant to treatment. Three types of poorly united congenital fractures have been recognized: (1) those which are quite unstable at birth; (2) those which present a feeble malunion and which later are very easily fractured; and (3) those with a feeble union in good position; these also are easily refractured.

Attempts to induce union of these fractures, especially of those of the first type, have often been unsuccessful. The living homogenous dual graft of Boyd, however, permits of early operation and occasionally has given good results. The grafts are best taken from a person closely related to the patient.

The Treatment of Massive Defects of the Long Bones.—Extensive loss of continuity in the shaft or at one end of a long bone is seen occasionally as the result of a severely comminuted gunshot fracture, radical resection of bone for a malignant tumor, failure of bone regeneration in osteomyelitis, or a congenital anomaly. The replacement of a large defect in the continuity of the bone or the creation of a new bony structure to replace the absent end of the bone constitutes a problem much more difficult than the ordinary bone grafting for nonunion. Such cases must be considered individually and great care must be exercised in selecting the operative procedure most suitable for improving the function of the disabled extremity.

It is essential that certain conditions be fulfilled before the reconstructive bone operation is performed. Any infection which may be present must first be eliminated. Poorly nourished skin and scars must be replaced with healthy tissues by means of plastic surgical procedures. The nutrition, mobility, and strength of the extremity must be restored as nearly as possible to normal by means of physical therapy, and the general physical condition of the patient must be good.

The technic of the reconstructive bone operation varies with details of the individual case. In the lower extremity extensive defects may often be successfully bridged by a massive sliding onlay or inlay graft, by a massive graft from the tibia of the opposite leg, or by use of the shaft of the fibula as a graft. A dual graft is often indicated. In most instances the cortical graft should be supplemented by the addition of a considerable amount of cancellous bone; this may be taken conveniently from the ilium. The ribs also form a useful source of grafts of high

osteogenic power. It is sometimes advisable to transfer the shaft of
the fibula into the ends of the tibia above and below (see page 350)
without exposing the tibial defect.

In the upper extremity length is not an essential consideration. It
is often advisable to approximate the fragment ends rather than attempt
the spanning of a large defect in the humerus. The entire upper part of
the fibula may be used to replace a lost portion of the humerus or
radius. In rare instances of extensive defect of the shaft of the radius
a transference of the distal end of the radius to the shaft of the ulna
may be indicated.

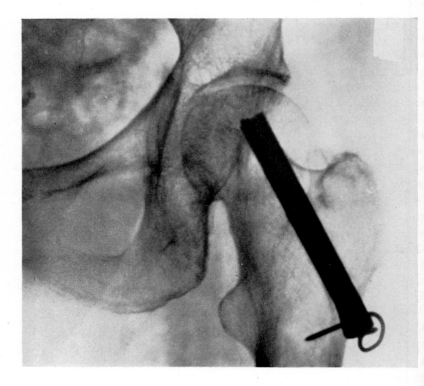

Fig. 126.—Roentgenogram showing solidly united fracture of neck of femur
fifteen years following successful nailing with Smith-Petersen triflange nail in
patient eighty years of age. Note the mechanically sound valgus position of head
and neck. Hip now has normal range of painless motion.

Nonunion of Individual Bones

NECK OF THE FEMUR

This is a common site for nonunion. It is considered to be present when no clinical evidence of union has appeared after six months. Statistics show that from 30 to 45 per cent of the patients treated for fracture of the neck of the femur suffered nonunion when the abduction method of reduction and immobilization, as first described by Whitman and later modified by Leadbetter, was employed. In cases in which the fragments have been fixed with three-flange nails (Fig. 126), special screws or multiple pins, the percentage of nonunion is reported to be much smaller. The reasons for nonunion of the neck of the femur are 1) an anatomically meager blood supply; (2) inability to secure perfect approximation and immobilization of the fragments; and (3) the presence of synovial fluid, which bathes the fractured surfaces and perhaps retards the process of bone formation.

The outstanding symptoms of nonunion of fracture of the neck of the femur are (1) pain in the hip on weight-bearing; (2) shortening and, as a rule, external rotation of the lower extremity; and (3) grating in the hip on motion. It is not uncommon for roentgenograms to demonstrate evidence of union soon after fracture and for absorption of bone to take place later across the fracture line, resulting in gradual separation of the fragments. Additional complicating factors which may be present include aseptic necrosis of the femoral head, which appears roentgenographically as changes in the density of the head, and osteoarthritis which may restrict the mobility of the head in the acetabulum (Figs. 127A and 127B).

Treatment.—Operation is required, but no one procedure is suitable for use in all cases. The patient's general condition and the details at the fracture site must be given careful consideration. In individuals under sixty years of age who are in good condition and who do not show marked absorption of either the distal fragment or the head of the femur, a *bone peg* operation may be followed by solid union. In the Albee type of bone peg operation the hip joint is opened, the fibrous tissue is removed, and the fragments are freshened on either side and approximated. A peg graft taken from the crest of the tibia is then inserted through the greater trochanter far into the neck and head. For additional strength a three-flange nail may be inserted alongside the graft. The results of this operation in selected cases have been satisfactory in leading to union and return of function.

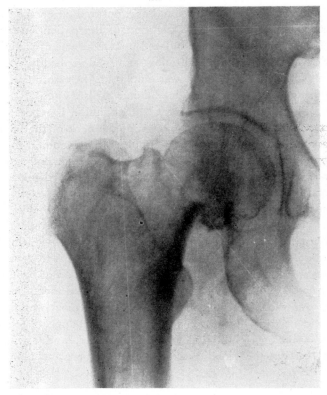

Fig. 127*A*.—Roentgenogram showing ununited fracture of the neck of the femur. Note upward displacement of neck and similar density of the head and neck indicating a viable head.

When the ununited fracture is more than a year old and a large amount of bone atrophy has taken place, a Whitman, Colonna, Albee, Moore, or Brackett reconstruction operation may be indicated. The Whitman reconstruction has been popular; however, at the present time, the operation of Dickson or McMurray, or one of their modifications such as the Leadbetter, which consists of a high osteotomy and shift of the femoral shaft medially under the head, is more widely used.

An acrylic or metal hip prosthesis may be inserted to replace the femoral head. Institution of early motion and activity should be insisted upon after the Whitman, Colonna, or Albee reconstruction, or after the application of a hip prosthesis, but not after the Brackett, the Moore, or the McMurray operation. A relatively painless hip, possessing good stability but some limitation of motion, is to be expected. If after several years of relief the pain recurs, an arthrodesis is indicated.

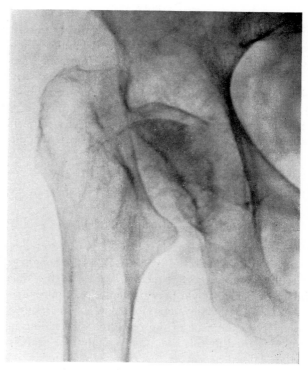

Fig. 127B.—Roentgenogram showing ununited fracture of the neck of the femur with marked upward displacement of the greater trochanter and shaft four years after unsuccessful open nailing, in patient eighty years of age. Neck of femur has completely disappeared. Relative increased density of head of femur indicates a nonviable head.

SHAFT OF THE FEMUR

Nonunion of the shaft of the femur is fairly common. If the fragments are overriding, it may be best to begin the treatment with a short period of skeletal traction. The operative treatment consists of the use of a bone graft of inlay or onlay type. It is necessary that the graft be ample in size and firmly fixed with metal screws and that a well-fitting double plaster spica cast, extending down to the knee of the well leg, be applied to insure adequate immobilization. An alternative method of fixation is the use of an intramedullary nail.

PATELLA

Nonunion of fractures of the patella is relatively uncommon when the fragments have been properly sutured. There is often little disturbance of knee function even when the fragments are definitely separated. Fibrous union may take place, and this type of healing allows fair extension and flexion of the knee. In diagnosis, a bipartite patella (page 46) must be excluded. The operative treatment of choice may be the use of an inlay graft fixed with sutures of heavy silk, or wire. It is sometimes necessary to lengthen the quadriceps tendon before the fragments can be approximated (see p. 151). Sometimes complete excision of the fragments and repair of the ligaments and joint capsule are followed by a good functional result.

TIBIA AND FIBULA

In the experience of many authors the lower third of the tibia is the most common site of nonunion (Fig. 128). This is thought to be due to the poor circulation over the flat medial surface of the tibia. In some cases the intact or healed fibula may prevent close approximation of the tibial fragments. Occasionally nonunion may be the result of injury of the nutrient artery at the time of the fracture. The sliding inlay type of graft is commonly used at this site. Occasionally the graft is placed on the posterior or lateral aspect of the tibia, which makes it possible to cover the transplant with healthy muscle tissue. Nonunion of the fibula rarely requires treatment with an inlay or onlay graft.

Surgical transference of the shaft of the fibula into the tibia above and below the level of the ununited fracture is sometimes preferable to the use of a free graft. This transference is particularly useful if the tibial defect is large or chronically infected as a sequel of compound fracture or osteomyelitis. The operation is usually carried out in two stages. The postoperative cast, which is worn for several months, must

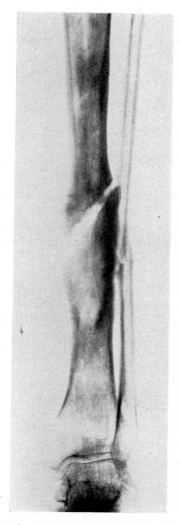

Fig. 128.—Anteroposterior roentgenogram showing ununited fracture of tibia. This patient had had a sliding bone graft operation without union. Note smoothness of ends of fracture fragments, wide gap between fragments, and decalcification of all bony structures. Fibular fracture has united.

often be followed by a brace to protect the fibular transplant until it has undergone sufficient hypertrophy to withstand the stresses normally placed upon the tibia.

Ununited fracture of the tibial malleolus should be treated surgically if causing symptoms. If the malleolar fragment is quite small it may be excised. If larger it should be replaced and fixed by a screw; the addition of a small bone graft is often helpful.

TARSUS AND METATARSUS

Ununited fractures of the tarsus and metatarsus are extremely uncommon.

HUMERUS

Ununited fractures of the middle third of the humerus have been common in the past; since the introduction of the "hanging cast" treatment of the fresh fractures by Caldwell in 1931, they are encountered much less frequently. This is a light arm cast which provides gravitational traction and coaptation splinting while leaving the shoulder free for active exercises.

Nonunion of the shaft of the humerus is often treated by the *step-cut operation,* a splicing of the refreshened and fitted ends of the fragments plus internal fixation by means of a screw, suture, or intramedullary nail. Some surgeons prefer simple oblique osteotomies and internal fixation. In difficult cases massive onlay grafts fixed by metal screws form an excellent means of inducing union.

Ununited fracture of the external condyle of the humerus, with resulting valgus deformity of the elbow, should be treated by replacing the condyle and fixing it with a screw, nail, or threaded Kirschner wire. Small osteoperiosteal grafts placed posteriorly are often advisable to facilitate bony union in this location. Small ununited fragments of the external or internal condyle which cause pain and grating in the elbow should be excised.

RADIUS AND ULNA

For nonunion of both bones of the forearm, the fixation of onlay grafts offers difficulties. It is usually best effected with Vitallium or stainless steel screws. Alignment of the fragments can often be maintained conveniently by the insertion of an intramedullary nail or pin. Ununited fracture of the radius or ulna alone, however, is more common. If the fracture is in the lower third of the radius, an inlay or onlay graft may be used, the distal end of the graft being sharpened and driven into the cancellous bone of the distal fragment. Ununited fracture of the lower third of the radius is often accompanied by an unsightly prominence of the lower end of the ulna. This prominence may necessitate resection of the protruding portion of the ulna. Ununited fracture of the ulna near the elbow is best treated by dual onlay grafts.

CARPUS AND METACARPUS

Ununited fracture of the scaphoid bone is not uncommon. The nonunion is presumably due to the poor blood supply; the scaphoid has three articulating surfaces bathed in synovial fluid and two small nonarticulating surfaces through which the blood vessels enter. A great many "sprained wrists" with prolonged disability will on roentgenographic study show an ununited fracture of the scaphoid. With several months of rigid immobilization by means of a plaster cast which includes the thumb and holds the wrist in slight dorsiflexion and radial deviation, many old fractures of the scaphoid bone will unite. Drilling small holes across the fracture surfaces previous to immobilization will open up new channels for circulation and may promote union. Satisfactory results have been reported following (1) the insertion of a small inlay bone graft into a prepared tunnel or trough, (2) removing the cancellous bone from both fragments and replacing it with chips of fresh cancellous bone, or (3) driving small slivers of bone across the fracture line. In some instances excision of one or both fragments or excision of the radial styloid process leads to improved function and less pain in the wrist. If a nonunion of long duration is attended by pain and arthritic changes in the adjacent bones, arthrodesis of the wrist may be indicated.

Ununited fractures of the metacarpal bones are uncommon. They may be treated by open reduction, temporary internal fixation with an intramedullary wire, and grafting with small strips of cancellous bone from the ilium.

Malunion

Union in poor position is usually caused by: (1) failure to secure accurate reduction or (2) failure to maintain effective immobilization for a sufficient length of time. Malunion is thus the outcome of inefficient treatment. The principal evidences of malunion are: (1) a shortening of the extremity due to overriding of the fragments (Fig. 129), (2) a deformity due to angulation of the fragments, (3) an abnormal rotation of the fragments with relation to each other, and (4) an abnormal limitation of joint motion due to a bone block.

Malunion of Individual Bones

Femur

Malunion of the neck of the femur is infrequent as compared with nonunion (Fig. 127B). Malunion may take place with the thigh externally rotated and adducted, with resultant coxa vara, retroversion of the femoral neck, and shortening. The deformity causes a limp and a tendency to tire quickly. Its correction may require an osteotomy of the outer portion of the neck of the femur or of the upper end of the femoral shaft.

At times fractures about the hip unite with irregularities which cause pain upon walking. For symptomatic relief such cases often require arthroplasty, reconstruction operation, or arthrodesis.

After fracture of the shaft of the femur, external angulation or rotation of the shaft may develop as a result of weight-bearing before the callus has become firm. It is sometimes possible to correct this type of deformity by manipulation. If the fracture has become solid an osteotomy is indicated. An intramedullary nail may be used to maintain the corrected alignment. It is advisable to mobilize the stiffened joints before operation by the use of physical therapy.

When overriding has caused appreciable shortening (Fig. 129), it may be necessary to separate the fragments and correct their alignment by means of an open operation. Following this procedure it is often necessary to apply skeletal traction just as in the treatment of a fresh fracture of the femoral shaft.

Following fracture of one of the condyles of the femur, a varus or valgus deformity of the knee may develop. In most instances this should be corrected by supracondylar osteotomy.

Patella

Occasionally a fractured patella unites with a rough articular surface which causes considerable pain and disability. The operative treatment consists of smoothing the posterior surface of the patella or excising the entire bone. If the quadriceps muscle has become contracted, excising

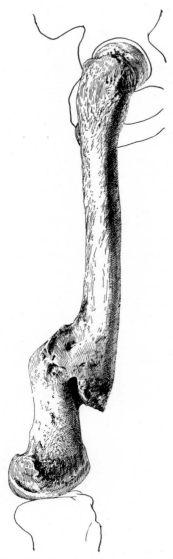

Fig. 129.—Malunited fracture of lower third of the femur. The overriding fragments have become firmly united. (Drawing from specimen.)

the surrounding scar tisue or lengthening the quadriceps tendon will improve the range of knee motion.

Tibia and Fibula

Occasionally a depressed fracture of the external or internal condyle of the tibia leaves irregular or displaced joint surfaces and abnormal weight-bearing lines which give rise to severe pain and disability. It may be possible to elevate and fix the depressed fragment and to remove the irregularities about the tibial plateau. In less favorable cases arthroplasty or arthrodesis of the knee joint is indicated. The type of operation will depend largely upon the age, physical condition, temperament, and occupation of the patient.

Fractures of the tibial and fibular shafts may unite with unsightly and disabling angulation. In order to correct the deformity, osteotomy may be performed through the site of angulation. After osteotomy of the middle or lower thirds it is advisable to fix the fragments with a graft, a plate, or both. With moderate angulation a supramalleolar osteotomy to correct the angle of the ankle joint surface to the weight-bearing axis of the leg is preferable. A rotation deformity of the foot and leg below the site of fracture sometimes follows failure to align the fragments accurately at the original reduction. Such rotation deformity can be completely corrected by osteotomy.

Ankle

Malunion of fractures of the lower end of the tibia and fibula results in severe disability. The foot usually becomes fixed in marked valgus with abnormal prominence of the medial malleolus (Fig. 130). The Achilles tendon may become contracted. Pain on weight-bearing is severe. At the original reduction of a fracture of the lower end of the tibia and fibula, the astragalus should be so placed against the medial malleolus that the longitudinal axis of the tibia bisects at a right angle the transverse diameter of the upper articular surface of the astragalus. If this anatomic relationship can be maintained and there is minimal injury of the articular surfaces, permanent disability seldom results. After adequate reduction of such a fracture, care must be taken that too early weight-bearing does not lead to the development of deformity. No weight-bearing should be permitted for at least eight weeks; thereafter it should be started in a closely fitting walking cast.

In cases of malunion with only slight displacement, the pain and disability may be relieved by a longitudinal arch support and ankle bandages. This treatment, however, is only palliative. In adults most malunited fractures involving the lower articular surfaces of the tibia and fibula require open operation.

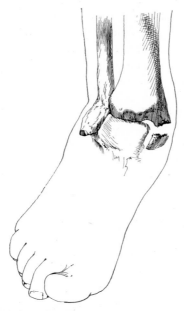

Fig. 130.—Malunited fracture-dislocation of ankle with abduction and lateral displacement of foot (malunited Pott's fracture).

In cases of only a few weeks' standing, it may be possible to break the beginning union by means of a Thomas wrench and to correct the deformity by manipulation. In cases of longer duration the fractured surfaces should be separated at open operation. Care must be taken to examine the posterior margin of the tibia ("posterior malleolus"), and if this is significantly displaced, its position should be corrected. It is usually necessary to retain the corrected position of the fragments by means of an autogenous bone peg, screw, or nail.

In old cases a reconstruction operation is sometimes indicated. It may be necessary to perform an osteotomy at the old fracture line in the fibula before the astragalus and foot can be mobilized and brought into alignment. In an eversion fracture of the lower end of the tibia and fibula it is sometimes advisable to place a bone graft across the defect between the fragments of the fibula. For associated nonunion of a fracture of the tibial malleolus, it may be necessary to excise the pseudarthrosis and fix the fragment to the tibia with a bone peg, screw, or nail. The Achilles tendon occasionally requires lengthening.

At times a wedge osteotomy of both the tibia and fibula is indicated. Bone chips or a cortical graft may be placed about the separated fragments of the osteotomized tibia and fibula.

The persistence of severe pain in a patient over forty-five years of age, due in large measure to traumatic arthritis, is an indication for arthrodesis of the ankle joint. After reconstruction operations there is always the danger of traumatic arthritis, particularly if the posterior margin of the tibia has been displaced, and an arthrodesis, producing a stiff but painless ankle, is in most instances the preferable procedure. Arthrodesis involves removal of all joint surfaces and stabilization of the ankle with the foot in a neutral position.

Following a displacement and reposition of the distal epiphysis of the tibia, the epiphysis may unite prematurely, resulting in the gradual development of a varus deformity of the foot and a marked prominence of the lower end of the fibula. The treatment is similar to that of malunited fracture.

ASTRAGALUS

Malunion of a fracture of the astragalus is likely to produce an equinus or equinovarus deformity. Persistent pain and disability following fracture of the head and neck of the astragalus are indications for a triple arthrodesis (see page 255). Disability due to malunion of a fracture of the body of the astragalus may be lessened by arthrodesis or astragalectomy.

OS CALCIS

Before the introduction of the methods of Cotton and, later, of Böhler for the treatment of fresh fractures of the os calcis, attempt was seldom made to correct the bone compression which often accompanies the fracture. Malunion of these fractures results in (1) broadening of the heel; (2) piling up of bone beneath both malleoli, particularly the lateral; (3) abduction deformity of the foot; and (4) in many instances, pes planus. The patient seldom if ever regains the normal range of inversion and eversion of the foot.

In the milder cases it is occasionally possible to correct some of the eversion deformity by means of forcible manipulation. This may result, however, in a chronically painful subastragalar joint. Longitudinal arch supports, Thomas heels elevated on the medial side, and ankle supports may afford partial symptomatic relief. Operative treatment is more effective. Arthrodesis of the subastragalar joint, removal of the excess bone beneath the malleoli, and smoothing of the bony projections on the inferior surface of the os calcis are to be advised. The results of this type of operation are quite satisfactory. Subastragalar motion is lost, but there is only slight deformity, and the patient walks with little or no pain.

Metatarsus

Occasionally following fracture of a metatarsal an irregular mass of bone may become prominent on the sole of the foot because of plantar angulation. For this type of lesion it is advisable to osteotomize the metatarsal, remove the excess bone with its projecting spurs, fix the fragments in accurate approximation with an intramedullary wire, add small cancellous grafts, and immobilize the foot in a plaster boot. When the patient starts walking, a pad should be fitted under the injured metatarsal bone to prevent recurrence of its plantar angulation.

Clavicle and Scapula

Malunion following fracture of the clavicle or scapula often results in limitation of motion of the shoulder. Little can be done to improve the deformity. Any sharp projecting spurs should be removed. Stiffness of the shoulder joint can be improved by physical therapy, traction, and gentle manipulation. Resection of the outer end of the clavicle (Mumford operation), for pain in the acromioclavicular joint following an old fracture or dislocation, may be followed by complete relief of the symptoms.

Humerus

Operation for malunited fracture of the upper end of the humerus is seldom indicated. Occasionally, however, the removal of sharp bony spurs and edges is necessary. Stiffness of the shoulder may be improved by physical therapy or gentle manipulation under anesthesia. Resection of the head of the humerus seldom results in a satisfactorily functioning shoulder. It is only occasionally necessary to perform an operation for malunion of the shaft of the humerus. An osteotomy may be indicated to correct an extreme angulation or rotation deformity.

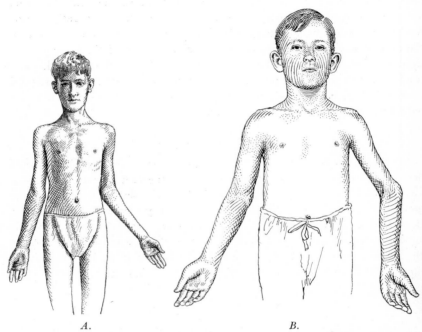

A.   *B.*

Fig. 131.—*A,* Malunited fracture of lower end of left humerus, showing cubitus valgus.

B, Malunited fracture of lower end of left humerus, showing cubitus varus.

The lower end of the humerus and the elbow are often involved in malunited fractures. Unreduced or incompletely reduced supracondylar fractures may cause limitation of joint motion. Bony spurs which project anteriorly into the joint and limit its range of motion may be resected. The operation should be followed by a program of supervised active exercise. The increase in range of motion is often slow.

In children unreduced fracture of the external condyle is always followed by the development of a marked valgus deformity of the elbow (Fig. 131,*A*). Delayed ulnar palsy or late traumatic ulnar neuritis from friction or stretching of the nerve trunk (see page 297) frequently accompanies a severe cubitus valgus. For correction of the deformity a supracondylar wedge osteotomy of the humerus with replacement or removal of the detached external condyle is often necessary (Fig. 132). Varus deformity of the elbow (Fig. 131,*B*), which most often follows an incompletely reduced supracondylar fracture, occasionally forms an indication for a similar type of osteotomy.

Occasionally following fracture about the elbow joint, a mass of new bone may form in the olecranon fossa and prevent normal extension of the elbow. Removal of the excess bone may be followed by improvement of mobility. Occasionally following a severely comminuted fracture involving the joint surfaces, complete or partial ankylosis develops. For this type of lesion a resection of the elbow, reconstruction operation, or arthroplasty may be indicated.

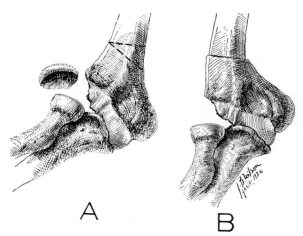

A   B

Fig. 132.—Ununited fracture of the external condyle of the humerus and valgus deformity resulting from an old malunited fracture of the lower end of the humerus. *A*, Before operation; *B*, after operation in which the detached external condyle was removed and a wedge osteotomy performed to correct the valgus deformity.

In association with fracture or dislocation about the elbow joint a mass of bone may form in the brachialis anticus muscle (*traumatic myositis ossificans,* see page 527). This bony mass may be directly connected with the periosteum of the lower end of the humerus. If spontaneous absorption fails to take place after prolonged rest and conservative therapy, the mass of new bone should be excised with as little traumatization of the surrounding tissues as possible. If the excess bone is removed too soon, it may recur; excision should not be attempted until at least six months after the injury.

After operations upon the elbow the recovery of joint motion is notably slow.

RADIUS AND ULNA

Malunited fracture of the head of the radius often causes severe disability. Rotation of the forearm is restricted and extension of the elbow may be impaired. In such cases the head and neck of the radius should be completely excised. Small comminuted fragments of the head of the radius may have become lodged in the joint and at operation must be carefully removed.

The combination of fracture of the upper third of the ulna and dislocation of the head of the radius, first described by Monteggia in 1814, is frequently seen. This type of injury may be followed by an unsightly deformity due to outward angulation of the upper third of the ulna. In these cases it is advisable to osteotomize the ulna, correct the alignment, and fix the fragments with a massive or dual onlay graft, an intramedullary pin, or a metal plate. The dislocation of the head of the radius should be reduced, especially if the patient is a child, and a new annular ligament should be constructed to maintain the reduction. When local conditions in the adult are unfavorable for the fashioning of such a ligament, the head of the radius may be excised.

Malunion or even nonunion of fractures of the olecranon process often results in little or no limitation of elbow function.

Fracture of both bones of the forearm may be followed by a radio-ulnar synostosis, which prevents rotation. In such cases the excess bone should be resected and fascia or fat placed between the radius and ulna. If the operation is indicated, it should be done promptly to minimize the accompanying muscle atrophy.

When fracture of both bones has been followed by severe angulation and overriding but firm union, osteotomies at the sites of angulation are indicated for correction of the deformity. It is usually necessary to hold the fragments in apposition by means of bone grafts, intramedullary pins, or metal plates.

Wrist

In the reduction of a Colles' fracture, whether recent or old, particular attention should be paid to the alignment of the joint surface of the radius. Normally a line drawn anteroposteriorly across the articular surface of the lower end of the radius forms anteriorly an angle of from 70 to 80 degrees with the longitudinal axis of the radius, and a line drawn laterally across the articular surface of the lower end of the radius forms radially an angle of from 105 to 110 degrees with the longitudinal axis of the radius. These relationships must be restored before a Colles' fracture can be considered adequately reduced.

Fibrosis and stiffness of the metacarpophalangeal and interphalangeal joints are occasionally observed after immobilization of the wrist for a fresh Colles' fracture and often cause greater disability than the fracture itself. This is especially true in older people. It is essential to start motion of the fingers and thumb soon after the injury. In fractures about the wrist joint, and especially in Colles' fracture, it is important that the splints should not be carried posteriorly beyond the knuckles or anteriorly beyond the middle of the palm. If the fracture has been properly reduced and immobilized, the danger of slipping is not significantly increased by movement of the fingers and thumb. Following Colles' fracture in old people, stiffness of the elbow and shoulder is also a common finding. During the course of treatment these joints should be put through their full range of motion actively once or twice a day.

Unreduced Colles' fracture or displacement of the distal radial epiphysis causes a very unsightly deformity. There is usually a "silver-fork deformity," marked prominence of the lower end of the ulna, and radial deviation of the wrist (Fig. 133). The deformity is accompanied by pain, restriction of wrist and finger motion and forearm rotation, and considerable disability of the hand.

In early cases it may be possible to reduce the deformity by the use of a Thomas wrench. This procedure should be carried out without the use of excessive force. When the deformity cannot be reduced easily by manipulation, a wedge of bone should be removed from the volar surface of the lower end of the radius and the alignment corrected. Internal fixation with wire or pin is useful to prevent postoperative slipping of the small distal fragment. When there is undue prominence of the lower end of the ulna, the projecting bone should be removed at the same operation. Occasionally when the prominent lower end of the ulna is extremely mobile, its removal together with a portion of the lower end of the shaft will result in improved function of the wrist.

Unreduced dislocation of the semilunar bone is frequently observed among old injuries of the wrist (see page 532). The semilunar should be excised.

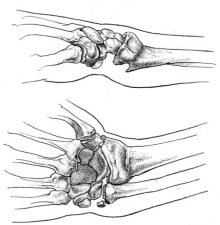

Fig. 133.—Malunited fracture of lower end of the radius (malunited Colles' fracture). Note dorsal displacement of distal fragment, posterior tilting of articular surface of radius, radial deviation of hand, prominence of lower end of ulna, and detached styloid process of ulna.

HAND

Angulation of a metacarpal shaft due to malunion is a common finding in pugilists. The deformity can be corrected by osteotomy. After osteotomy an intramedullary wire is useful for temporary immobilization of the fragments. As a rule little need be done for the "prize-fighter's knuckle," which is a malunited fracture of a metacarpal neck, since the disability is slight. Fractures about the phalangeal joints, such as are found in "baseball fingers" (see page 540), are seldom improved by operation. The fragments are often too small to be replaced accurately and fixed securely.

PELVIS

Occasionally stiffness and pain in the hip may persist following fracture of the pelvis, particularly if the acetabulum has been involved. Sometimes a gentle manipulation to break up adhesions will result in relief of the symptoms. If the pain persists, however, it is wise to consider a reconstruction operation with removal of the head of the femur, an arthroplasty, or an arthrodesis. The choice of these procedures depends chiefly upon the age and occupation of the individual.

SPINE

Following a severe injury of the back it is not uncommon for compression of one or more vertebral bodies to be discovered as a late manifestation. The lesion may evidence itself by kyphosis associated with considerable pain and disability in the back. The fracture is particularly likely to be overlooked unless good lateral roentgenograms are made following the injury. In rare cases, however, fracture may not be evident in films taken immediately after the injury but may appear several days later when postural stresses have increased the deformity of the weakened vertebral body. After any type of severe trauma, particularly that associated with an automobile or industrial accident, which is followed by any back pain whatever, anteroposterior and lateral roentgenograms should be made. Failure to diagnose these fractures may prove most embarrassing. Many malpractice suits are based on failure of the doctor to recognize injuries of this type in the beginning, even when no treatment would have been indicated had they been recognized.

When pain and disability are associated with an old compression fracture, treatment consisting of recumbency in a posterior plaster shell or on a Bradford frame for several weeks, followed by the use of a plaster jacket or brace for several months, may lead to symptomatic relief. In most cases with persistent pain, however, an operative fusion of the spine should be done, two vertebrae above and two below the site of injury being included in the arthrodesis.

In the case of an old injury of the cervical spine it may be necessary for the patient to remain recumbent with head traction, obtained with a halter or skull tongs, for several weeks and then to wear a plaster collar and later a Thomas leather collar. Rarely is arthrodesis of the cervical spine indicated unless a persistent or recurrent dislocation is associated with the fracture.

Comment.—In this chapter on fracture deformities an attempt has been made to point out common mistakes in the handling of recent fractures and to emphasize the occasional disastrous and disabling results of faulty treatment. These unfortunate results are of course not always avoidable, but certainly their number could be materially reduced if more effective initial measures were taken by the physician who bears the responsibility for the early treatment of these patients. The orthopaedic surgeon is often called upon to help his colleague out of trouble when the latter obtains an embarrassing result. The orthopaedist is often fully aware that had the doctor been more familiar with the proper method of handling the fracture in question the misfortune could have been avoided. In the mind of the patient a fear of permanent crippling is always present, and in his eyes anything short of perfect cosmetic and functional recovery is tragic. Full appreciation by the patient of a poor result may unfortunately embitter him and induce him to bring suit against the attending physician for malpractice. There should be closer cooperation between the orthopaedic surgeon, who is primarily interested in bone injury and the restoration of function, and the physician who is treating a broken bone along with innumerable conditions foreign to the management of fractures. The state industrial commissions and the insurance companies who reckon these injuries in dollars and cents have come to realize the difference in compensation benefits between fractures treated by the orthopaedic and trauma specialist and those treated by the general practitioner and general surgeon. The public is gradually recognizing it and in many sections is demanding the services and consultations of doctors who have been especially trained in fracture work. It is the duty of every medical student who is anticipating practice and of every practitioner of medicine to equip himself with a knowledge of the principles of fracture treatment in order that he may be competent to handle these problems intelligently. This is the day of preventive medicine, and it should be also the day of preventive fracture treatment, in order that the number of fracture deformities may be minimized.

CHAPTER XVII

BODY MECHANICS AND PHYSICAL THERAPY

PART I. BODY MECHANICS

Introduction.—Correct postural relationship of the various parts of the body when standing, sitting, lying, or moving is of fundamental significance to the physiology of the individual and forms an important basic subject of general medicine. In orthopaedic surgery, which is concerned chiefly with the phenomena of statics and of locomotion, the subject is obviously of particular interest and importance. Nicholas Andry's *L'Orthopédie,* written in 1741, from which the name of the specialty has been adopted, consists largely of a consideration of body mechanics. It is essential that the broad outlines of the subject of postural mechanics be understood, both as underlying all orthopaedic therapy and as applying to the prevention and treatment of the individual disease entities.

Body mechanics has been defined as "the mechanical correlation of the various systems of the body with special reference to the skeletal, muscular, and visceral systems, perhaps with the circulatory and nervous systems as well. Normal body mechanics may be said to obtain when the mechanical correlation is most favorable to the function of these systems." It is obvious that good body mechanics means a high degree of physiologic efficiency, and that this in turn means a greater resistance to the onset of disease as well as a greater capacity for recovery to the normal state.

Normal Posture.—The basic concept of body mechanics is an optimum standing posture. Familiarity with this correct standing posture is prerequisite to an understanding of the most efficient use of the body in any physical activity. In the theoretical *ideal standing posture* the center of gravity lies directly over the center of support. The line of weight-bearing which passes through the mastoid process falls across the greater trochanter and the tibial tuberosity and reaches the ground at the base of the fifth metatarsal bone. The feet are so placed that the line of the Achilles tendon is perpendicular to the ground and bisects the

367

posterior surface of the os calcis. The knees and hips are straight. The lumbar spine is practically flat against a string stretched from the seventh cervical vertebra to the gluteal fold, as is the dorsal spine, and the long axis of the neck is vertical. There is no lateral curvature. The shoulder joints lie in the midaxillary plane of the body. The chest is moderately elevated in a position midway between full inspiration and complete expiration, and the abdominal musculature is under sufficient tension to form a straight line between the xiphoid process and the pubis.

From this theoretically ideal posture, met with only in highly trained individuals, the average *normal posture,* as obtained by analysis of a large number of examinations, shows significant variations (Fig. 135,*A*). The feet may be very slightly pronated. The lumbar spine is slightly concave backward, the dorsal spine slightly convex backward, and the long axis of the neck inclined slightly forward. The chest is slightly depressed and the abdominal musculature is sufficiently relaxed to allow slight prominence of the abdomen.

It must be kept in mind that this description of normal posture applies to a composite or average individual with bodily proportions and relationships of given magnitude. Since different individuals are not uniform but present varying bodily proportions, it is evident that there will be significant minor differences between the group normal posture and the individual normal. Postural details will obviously vary with the physical build peculiar to the individual.

Body Types.—By studies of the physical characteristics of large groups of individuals it has been shown that in addition to the average body type, which indeed forms numerically a minority, there are two general structural types with anatomic characteristics sufficiently distinct to permit of easy recognition and with specific susceptibilities to certain disease processes.

The slender individual of *hyperontomorphic, asthenic,* or *carnivorous type* is lean and lanky, of rather delicate build, and of high-strung temperament (Fig. 134,*A*). The vertebrae are small, and the mobility of the spine is increased. The torso is long and narrow with most of the increased length in the thorax rather than in the abdomen. The ribs are lengthened and their downward inclination increased. The chest expansion is poor. Because of the narrow thoracic outlet the liver occupies a low position. The stomach is similarly low, and its loose attachments permit an increased drop on standing. The small intestine is definitely shortened, which may interfere with the absorption of nutriment. The mesentery is long, with the result that when the individual stands the small intestine lies largely in the upper pelvis. The large intestine is relatively long and its transverse portion redundant and low. Retroperitoneal fat is diminished; ptosis of the kidneys and drag upon the sympathetic plexuses are facilitated. The hands are long and slender, and the feet are highly arched. Statistics have shown that individuals of this type have a relatively high susceptibility to tuberculosis, to mental diseases, and to rheumatoid arthritis.

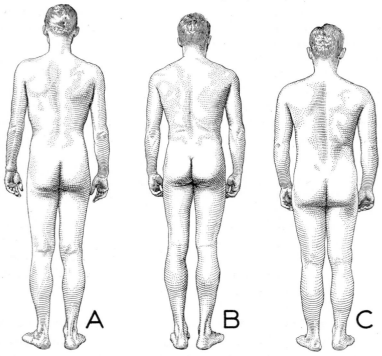

Fig. 134.—Body types. *A*, Slender (hyperontomorphic). *B*, Intermediate. *C*, Stocky (hypo-ontomorphic).

The contrasting stocky body type is known as *hypo-ontomorphic, sthenic,* or *herbivorous.* These individuals, characteristically of placid temperament, are sturdy and heavy, with bones which are relatively large and dense (Fig. 134,*C*). The neck is short and thick, the shoulders massive, and the back broad. The chest is wide, short and deep; its volume of expansion is large. The ribs are nearly horizontal and the subcostal angle wide. The lumbar region is short and strongly built. Four instead of five lumbar vertebrae occur not uncommonly. The abdomen is long in relation to the thorax. The stomach is situated transversely and empties well. The small intestine is definitly lengthened, facilitating increased absorption. The large intestine is short, and the mesenteric attachments are short and strong, lessening the likelihood of visceroptosis. Extraperitoneal fat is abundant. Flexibility of the spine is decreased, and the lumbar curve and the forward inclination of the pelvis are diminished. The extremities are short, thick and heavy; the arches of the feet low. Arteriosclerosis, chronic renal disease, and osteoarthritis are especially likely to occur in this type of individual.

From the foregoing it will be apparent that there is a close relationship between individual body type and individual optimum posture. In general it is the individuals of hyperontomorphic type who experience most difficulty in acquiring or maintaining correct postural habits; yet these same asthenic individuals derive relatively greater physiologic benefit from proper body mechanics than do persons of intermediate or sthenic body type.

Faulty Posture.—The typical attitude of poor posture of severe degree is too familiar to require an extended description (Fig. 135,*B*). The head protrudes, the shoulders are rounded and drooped, the chest is flat, and the thoracic spine has an increased posterior convexity. The lumbar lordosis is exaggerated and the abdomen is protuberant, particularly in its lower half. The pelvic inclination is increased. The knees are slightly flexed, and the feet are pronated. All degrees of these postural aberrations are encountered.

The term *round shoulders* has been used to designate faulty posture in which drooping of the shoulders and increased convexity of the dorsal spine are conspicuous. In such cases the postural abnormalities are never limited to the shoulder girdle and chest, however, but are present throughout the body. Well-marked cases exhibit changes in the anteroposterior curves of the entire spine. The head is carried forward, and the lumbar lordosis is either exaggerated or flattened. The chest is narrow and flat. The vertebral borders of the scapulae are likely to be prominent. The abdomen sags forward, particularly in its lower part. Flattening and pronation of the feet are frequently associated.

That clinical symptoms may be caused by defective posture is not surprising in view of the abnormal stresses to which the viscera and their supporting structures are subjected. Forward drooping of the head puts a strain upon the ligamentum nuchae and may cause an aching in the neck. Diminished thoracic expansion results in lowered pulmonary and circulatory efficiency. Ptosis of the abdominal viscera exerts an unfavorable effect on the processes of digestion by increasing directly the

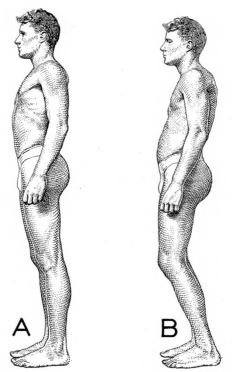

Fig. 135.—Posture in intermediate body type. *A,* Excellent. *B,* Poor.

burden of mechanical work performed by peristalsis and probably also by interfering indirectly with intestinal tonus as the result of pull on the nerves in the mesentery. Clinically these changes result in disorders of digestion and often lead to chronic constipation. The distorted lines of weight-bearing, together with the weak muscular support, place upon the hips, the knees, and particularly the complex arches of the feet an abnormal strain which may well exceed the physiologic reserve and cause troublesome aches. In other cases the relationship between faulty posture and symptoms, while equally significant, is less direct. The constant muscular and ligamentous strain associated with poor posture and ptosis may cause a very definite susceptibility to fatigue and may lead gradually to considerable loss of weight.

Corrective Measures.—It is obviously necessary, before ascribing a patient's complaint to posture alone, to rule out by a very careful clinical and laboratory study any other possible cause for the symptoms. Every such case should be thoroughly considered from the general medical and general surgical viewpoints. When, however, exhaustive diagnostic studies have been completed, many cases will still remain in which the major pathologic processes can be ascribed to defective posture alone. In this group of patients very gratifying results may be obtained by conscientious application of the principles of correct body mechanics.

The first step in the treatment of faulty posture is to secure the patient's cooperation in the program of rehabilitation. He should then be given a clear idea of the postural defects which are present and of the proper mechanical relationships which are to be gained. He must be taught that the influence of any system of corrective exercises will depend upon their being executed while the parts of the body are in proper mechanical relationship, and that exercises may even be harmful when these conditions are not fulfilled. A system of muscle training exercises for daily use is then to be adopted, suited to the characteristics of the individual case and so graduated as to lead by easy stages to the desired endurance level. Light corrective braces may be worn between exercises, but it must be emphasized that such apparatus is only a temporary expedient and is to be discarded as soon as possible. As muscular vigor begins to return, the relief and gratitude exhibited by many of these patients, whose chronic distress has been the result simply of careless and defective posture, is striking. With the physical improvement there develops often an increased mental independence and vigor which make the weeks or the months of muscle training a distinctly worthwhile investment. Proper postural habits once acquired will usually be retained with a minimum of effort.

Biophysics of the Locomotor System.—No discussion of the postural relationships of the body at rest can be complete without calling attention to the vastly more complex subject of the physiology, normal and pathologic, of the body in motion. This subject, called by Howorth "dynamic posture," is so intricate that its investigation has hardly been begun, and few data capable of practical application have as yet been accumulated. However, a start has been made, most notably in the field of the biomechanics of gait. The development by Schwartz and by Saunders and Inman of an accurate method of recording and analyzing the mechanical elements of gait is of fundamental value. Steindler has published an exhaustive study of the mechanics of normal and pathologic locomotion. It seems not unlikely that great advances in orthopaedic surgery will be made possible in the future by adding to the present morphologic concepts of the locomotor system an increased understanding of its detailed physiology.

PART II. PHYSICAL THERAPY

Introduction.—Physical medicine comprises the evaluation and treatment of disease and injury by physical agents and includes physical therapy, occupational therapy, physical rehabilitation, and convalescent training. Physical therapy is the oldest of these divisions of physical medicine. Despite the long and honorable history of physical therapy, it is only in recent decades that its methods have been widely accepted and systematized as an essential part of scientific therapeutics. During the First World War physical therapy was extensively used in the late treatment of wounds of various kinds, and its methods became highly popularized. This resulted in the development, fostered by commercial interests, of many new machines for supplying appropriate thermal or electrical energy. In some quarters the very number and mechanical complexity of these devices have served to obscure the underlying therapeutic principles and to bring discredit upon physical therapy as a whole. It cannot be emphasized too much that the selection of treatment must be based on physiologic principles. For successful results sound judgment and good technic are essential. When physical therapy is prescribed and practiced with these principles in mind, it forms an extremely valuable and in fact indispensable part of orthopaedic treatment.

During the Second World War the value of physical medicine and particularly physical therapy received greatly increased recognition. Large departments of physical therapy functioned actively in all military hospitals. Increased numbers of personnel were trained in the principles of physical therapy, and new procedures for their application were developed. For any program of physical therapy to be effective in treatment of the individual case, it is essential that two preliminary and fundamental requirements be satisfied. These are (1) that an adequate amount of rest be assured and (2) that the principles of good body mechanics be followed. The importance of rest as a supplement to the more vigorous methods of treatment can scarcely be overemphasized. Adequate rest should be assured both for the diseased member itself and for the body as a whole. An example of local rest is the use of a removable splint for the immobilization of an arthritic joint between diathermy treatments. For rest of the entire body, which is indicated after any severe systemic disease, a definite program of short daily periods of recumbency is often employed. During any period of rest or of activity the maximum physiologic benefit will be derived only if the requirements of good body mechanics are constantly fulfilled.

Exclusive of rest, the major agencies of physical therapy are four: *heat, massage, exercise,* and *light.* There are innumerable special procedures by which these fundamental agencies may be applied: thus diathermy is a specialized technic for the use of heat; and electrical stimulation is a specialized and artificial form of exercise. *Hydrotherapy* adds no independent therapeutic principle but in many instances makes possible a more convenient and effective application of heat, massage, or exercise.

Heat.—In physical therapy, heat is used chiefly because it has a local analgesic action, the exact mechanism of which has not been fully explained, and because by dilating the capillaries it tends to increase the local circulation. The accompanying psychic effect is also of value. The increased circulation is extremely beneficial in improving the nutrition of the tissues and in accelerating local processes of absorption and repair. Dry heat is commonly applied by means of a hot water bottle, an electric pad, an infrared lamp, or electric lamps arranged in a hood or "baker." Diathermy has the advantage of warming the deeper tissues in addition to the surface structures. Short-wave diathermy utilizes a current of very high frequency; this has not been proved to be more effective than diathermy of longer wave length but is usually more conveniently applied. Moist heat, usually applied by means of whirlpool baths, tub baths, or compresses is preferable to dry heat in most cases because the layer of water tends to soften the skin and is also an excellent conductor of heat. The warm *paraffin bath* provides an excellent means of applying heat intensively to hand or foot. More heat (an additional ten degrees Centigrade) can be applied to a part of the body with a paraffin bath than with a water bath without danger of causing a burn. *Contrast baths,* or soaks involving immersion alternately in hot and in cold water, are of value in restoring circulatory tone by inducing alternate dilation and contraction of the small blood vessels.

Heat is commonly used as a preliminary to massage or exercise or both, although it may be used alone when more vigorous physical therapy is contraindicated. When local heat is used, the danger of burns must be kept constantly in mind and precautions taken accordingly. Although the possibility of damage from an excess of heat is an obvious one, burns from hot water bottles are still common, and too much diathermy, especially of the short wave type, may injure deep structures such as synovial membrane or hyaline cartilage.

Massage.—Like heat, massage induces a local vascular dilation and an increased circulation. It is said that the red cell count and hemoglobin are raised if the area of massage is at all extensive. The technical varieties of massage are numerous. Essentials are that it be begun slowly and gently, with stroking chiefly in a centripetal direction, and that it be increased in vigor gradually and never to the extent of causing pain. Massage is of chief value in improving the nutrition and tone of tissues after immobilization or paralysis and in accelerating the absorption of edema or hemorrhage following trauma. It is usually preceded by the application of heat and is itself often used advantageously as a preliminary to exercise.

Exercise.—Two forms of exercise, *active* and *passive,* are often considered together but have contrasting therapeutic uses.

Active exercise is movement performed by the patient himself. Such movement may be either assisted or resisted by the physical therapist. Active exercise involves autonomous use of all local parts of the locomotor system. It brings about a marked increase of local circulation and acceleration of local metabolism and prevents the development of adhesions and contractures. With regulated active exercise, as, for instance, following the prolonged immobilization of a fracture, the muscles can be expected to show a gratifying increase of power. The resistive exercises of DeLorme, which are a form of graded active exercises against resistance, are of great value in restoring muscle strength in conditions such as quadriceps atrophy after injury of the knee. This was well demonstrated in many military hospitals during World War II. Such exercises are now being extensively employed in the development of weak muscles after infantile paralysis. In disabilities of the upper extremity and particularly of the hand, active exercise is often best prescribed in the form of *occupational therapy* or *work therapy*. The construction of simple objects and other activities in the workshop may serve to stimulate the patient's interest as well as to improve the local disorder. Occupational therapy for the injured worker should include physical activity as nearly as possible identical with that of his former job. Such therapy frequently accomplishes rehabilitation from both physical and psychic standpoints, restoring strength and confidence and minimizing disability.

In *passive exercise* the affected joint is carried through its range of painless movement by the physical therapist. It is useful in preserving joint mobility and thereby preventing contractures. As relaxation of the patient is essential, considerable care must be taken not to cause pain or fear. Forced movement may lead to tissue damage and loss of mobility.

The *electrical stimulation* of muscles, contractions being induced by the application of electrodes to the overlying skin, is a form of artificial exercise which is useful in maintaining the nutrition and mobility of muscles and tendons during the early stages of nerve recovery after paralysis. It should never be used in preference to ordinary active exercise.

Exercise, particularly of the active type, is important in the after-treatment of fractures. Each case must be considered individually, and the time for beginning motion must be varied with the site and nature of the injury and with the age and general condition of the patient. In all cases sufficient time for early union must be allowed before motion is started, and such motion must be begun gently and increased gradually.

It is often advantageous to combine exercise with hydrotherapy. This may be accomplished by the use of the small arm or leg tank or on a larger scale by means of a Hubbard tank or therapeutic pool. Warm water exerts a direct sedative effect tending to decrease muscle spasm and apprehension, removes by its buoyancy the strain which weight-bearing imposes upon weakened structures, and opposes to active exercise a gentle equalized resistance. Hydrogymnastics may be of most striking value in the convalescent stage of poliomyelitis but are of benefit also in the treatment of other types of paralysis, arthritis, postoperative disabilities, and a wide variety of other osteoarticular disorders.

Light.—Although the therapeutic power of light and particularly of its ultraviolet components has at times been greatly overrated, it possesses a very definite and very important place in physical therapy. Ultraviolet irradiation causes a chemical reaction in the body, the exact characteristics of which are not well known. It is of specific benefit in rickets and osteomalacia. It has long been known to be of value in bone and joint tuberculosis. In the treatment of a wide variety of conditions with which a state of chronic malnutrition is associated, ultraviolet light is a useful adjunct. Sunlight is still the best source of therapeutic irradiation, although most of the ultraviolet lamps now on the market are effective and convenient. It cannot be too much emphasized that light therapy, unless intelligently prescribed and carefully administered, possesses the potentiality of causing serious tissue injury.

CHAPTER XVIII

AFFECTIONS OF THE SPINE AND THORAX

In this chapter abnormal curvatures of the spine and deformities of the chest are discussed. Affections of the lower part of the lumbar spine and of the sacrum and coccyx are so common and important that they have been placed in a separate chapter under the heading, "Affections of the Low Back."

PART I. AFFECTIONS OF THE SPINE

Scoliosis

Definition.—Scoliosis or lateral curvature of the spine is a condition in which a series of vertebrae remain persistently deviated from the normal spinal axis; the lateral deviation is invariably accompanied by some degree of rotation of the vertebrae. Scoliosis is a deformity rather than a disease and is most often secondary to pathologic changes outside of the spine itself.

Incidence.—Lateral curvature is one of the most common deformities of the spine. Its onset occurs usually during the years of growth. The factors which result in scoliosis are often established long before the child reaches school age, and definite deformity is usually recognizable before the age of fourteen years. In the early school ages scoliosis is slightly more common in boys, but during adolescence it occurs three to five times as often in girls.

Classification and Etiology.—For purposes of description, cases of scoliosis can be conveniently classified in two ways: (1) according to the causative agent and (2) according to the shape and level of the curvature.

The etiologic classification is necessarily imperfect since our knowledge of the causes of scoliosis is incomplete. One large group of cases is made up of patients whose spinal curvature is a result of temporary postural influences; such postural scoliosis is not accompanied by asymmetrical changes in the individual structures of the spine and is relatively

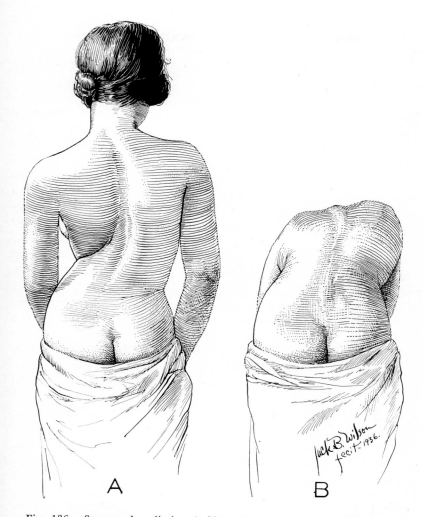

Fig. 136.—Structural scoliosis. *A,* Note right dorsal, left lumbar curvature with high right shoulder and prominent left iliac crest. *B,* Posterior prominence of the right side of the back associated with the rotation of the vertebrae is accentuated when the spine is flexed.

easy to correct. This type of case is termed *functional* or *nonrigid scoliosis. Structural, rigid,* or *fixed scoliosis* (Fig. 136), on the other hand, is characterized by definite morphologic abnormalities, and it is with this group of cases that therapeutic effort is most concerned. In children, cases of functional scoliosis sometimes progress, develop morphologic changes, and so undergo transition into the structural type.

The causes of structural scoliosis are numerous. A small group of the cases is definitely congenital in origin; a clear example is lateral curvature due to the presence of a hemivertebra. Pathologic changes in the bones, such as those of rickets and osteomalacia, may so impair the strength of the spinal column that postural and gravitational stresses cause the development of scoliosis. Asymmetrical paralyses, as found in poliomyelitis, amyotonia congenita, or muscular dystrophy, frequently lead to scoliosis by destroying the normal balance of the supporting musculature. The collapse of the lung and the contraction of the thoracic wall in chronic empyema often lead to curvature of the spine. A similar type of scoliosis follows the rib resections of thoracoplasty in the treatment of pulmonary tuberculosis. In many instances of scoliosis, however, the pathogenesis is unknown. In these cases of so-called *idiopathic scoliosis* the underlying factor has generally been assumed to be a functional weakness or insufficiency of the spine, and by some observers such weakness has been thought to be of hormonal or congenital origin. It is possible that in some cases the curvature results from asymmetrical growth at the epiphyseal plates of the vertebrae.

In the regional classification of scoliosis three types of curvature are outstanding. These are (1) the C-shaped, left total curve, with its apex usually at the lower dorsal level, which is usually postural, paralytic, or congenital in origin; (2) the S-shaped compound curve, consisting usually of a primary right dorsal curve and secondary left cervical and left lumbar curves, which is often idiopathic in type; and (3) primary left or right lumbar curvature. Other varieties of lateral curvature occur but are less common.

Pathology.—The extent of the pathologic changes varies with the degree of lateral curvature. All the structures of the concave side are compressed, while those of the convex side may remain normal or even appear stretched (Fig. 137). The vertebra at the middle of the curve shows the greatest change, being wedge-shaped. Those above and below it are usually lozenge-shaped. The intervertebral disks are com-

pressed on the side of the concavity and may project on the opposite side
as a result of the pressure. The anterior longitudinal ligament is thickened
on the concave side and thinned on the convex side. As the deformity
increases, a proliferation of bone takes place, and later ossification of the
ligaments may occur; these changes may progress until there is ankylosis

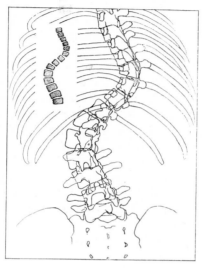

Fig. 137.—Structural scoliosis. Note rotation of vertebrae and wedging of
vertebral bodies at apices of curvature. The wedging is clearer in the inset.
(Tracing from roentgenogram.)

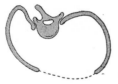

Fig. 138.—Cross-section of thorax in scoliosis, showing distortion of ribs
associated with rotation of the vertebra. (After Hoffa.)

of the spine at the level of greatest distortion. Two or three vertebrae
may be fused. The muscles become atrophic and on section may
exhibit fatty and fibrous degeneration. Due to rotation of the vertebrae,
which is invariably present, the ribs on the side of the convexity are thrust
backward with an increase in their angularity; this produces the so-called
"razor back" deformity. When the curve affects the lower part of

the spine, the pelvis may be distorted. Changes in the anterior chest wall include a flattening and diminution of thoracic capacity on the convex side of the curve and a prominence and increased capacity on the concave side (Fig. 138). All of the organs of chest and abdomen may be distorted by the abnormal pressure and strain put upon them by changes in the shape of the thorax.

Clinical Picture.—As a rule there is no complaint until deformity of the back is noticed, and, since the deformity is of very gradual development, it may reach considerable proportions before its presence is observed. The patient may be brought to the doctor because of a high shoulder, a prominent hip, or a projecting shoulder blade. When the patient is a young girl, the deformity is often first noticed by her dressmaker. Occasionally the child may complain of fatigue and backache before a deformity is noted. As the deformity progresses, the discomfort may become more marked. Pain developing in the lumbar region may be due to pressure of the ribs upon the crest of the ilium. There may be shortness of breath, due to diminished respiratory capacity, and gastrointestinal disturbances from crowding of the abdominal organs. In patients with only slight deformity, symptoms may not appear until later in life.

The physical examination should include careful note of the following points: (1) inspection of the natural, relaxed standing position; (2) estimation of the shape and degree of spinal curvature, the number of vertebrae involved, and the level and extent of the maximum deviation; (3) estimation of the degree of rotation or twisting of the vertebrae; and (4) estimation of the amount of spinal flexibility. Each of these factors is important in determining the treatment.

In left total scoliosis the deformity is a long single curvature with its convexity to the left. In the majority of cases of structural scoliosis the backward rotation is on the side of the convexity, the slight prominence of the ribs posteriorly causing a corresponding asymmetry of the thorax. The shoulder on the side of the convexity is held elevated and anterior with respect to the other shoulder. In cases of purely postural character the curvature can be straightened voluntarily and undergoes complete spontaneous correction during recumbency. Right total scoliosis is much less common than left and presents converse deformities.

The compound or S-shaped type of curve is found in the majority of the cases of so-called idiopathic scoliosis and in 30 per cent of the entire group of scoliosis patients. The deformity consists most often of a primary dorsal curve convex to the right and of secondary cervical and lumbar curves convex to the left. The curvature cannot be corrected voluntarily and does not disappear in recumbency although in recumbency it may be less pronounced. The asymmetry and rotation in this type of scoliosis may be very marked. The rotation deformity is best observed when the patient is made to bend sharply forward.

Simple lumbar scoliosis is most commonly convex to the left with the apex of the curvature at the level of the second lumbar vertebra. The iliac crest is more prominent on the side of the concavity, while there is fullness of the back on the side of the convexity. Single dorsal curves tend to develop accentuation of the normal dorsal kyphosis, a rotation deformity, and secondary curves in the cervical and lumbar regions.

Diagnosis.—In making the diagnosis of scoliosis, the examiner must attempt to determine the basic etiologic factor. It should be remembered that scoliosis is not a primary disease of the spine but is a resultant of the action of certain mechanical forces upon the spine. When the diagnosis is being made, the posture, the rotation, the lateral deviation, and the limitation of normal mobility should be carefully noted. The roentgenograms may show the character of the curve, the presence of bony defects, and the degree of distortion of the individual vertebrae. This information is helpful in determining the etiology, and the roentgenograms provide also a valuable graphic record of the degree of curvature.

Prognosis.—Structural scoliosis is essentially a self-limited condition; in most cases progression of the curvature ceases spontaneously at or before the age of fifteen years. In many instances, however, the deformity tends to progress rapidly during the growing period of childhood and therefore constitutes a serious therapeutic problem until arrest of any advancing curvature can be assured. Every case demands careful attention and supervision over a long period of time.

Without treatment the postural curvatures may remain stationary, as may the deformities of structural scoliosis in adults, but the structural curvatures in growing children often increase to cause marked deformity and disability.

With treatment scoliosis of the postural type may be completely cured. The structural type in young children may be prevented from becoming worse and often may be greatly improved; rarely, however, is complete correction of the curvature obtained.

The earlier the treatment is started, the better the prognosis. The C-shaped curvatures are more amenable to treatment than are the compound or S-shaped curves. Rachitic scoliosis often responds poorly to treatment. In children scoliosis due to chronic empyema tends to progress to severe deformity despite any form of treatment.

Treatment.—The basic principles of treatment are (1) to prevent the increase of scoliosis, when the tendency toward curvature is recognized at an early stage; (2) to overcome the rigidity of the spine, when the deformity has become established, by means of mobilizing exercises; (3) to secure as much correction of the deformity as possible; (4) to develop sufficient muscle strength to maintain the correction; (5) to supply artificial support of the spine when the muscle strength is inadequate to maintain the correction; and (6) to prevent overfatigue and other deleterious influences which might lead to an increase of the curvature.

Prophylactic Treatment.—Recognition of the earliest stage of scoliosis is essential. Prophylactic treatment in the majority of instances is concerned with the preschool child rather than the older boy or girl. Improper postural influences in school, such as the poorly designed school desk, are to be regarded not as causing scoliosis but simply as aggravating an already existing disorder. Unilateral defects of sight or hearing may play an etiologic rôle and should be corrected. Exercises to maintain the mobility of the spine and to strengthen the weaker groups of muscles are important. When rickets is suspected, medical antirachitic measures, massage and exercise, and prevention of improper posture are essential. When an increase of the curvature is considered likely, the patient should be examined at frequent intervals.

Treatment of Established Scoliosis.—The treatment of most cases of scoliotic deformity falls into three mutually complementary stages: (1) *mobilization* of contracted structures by means of exercises, (2) *correction* of the curvature by application of straightening forces, and (3) *maintenance* of the correction by brace or spinal fusion. The technical procedures by which these objects are best attained vary with the characteristics of the individual case. The following methods are in common use:

1. *Corrective Exercises Alone.*—Properly directed exercises may mobilize the curved portions of the spine in selected cases and

strengthen certain muscle groups to aid in maintaining the corrected position. As muscular weakness always accompanies the deformity and as maintenance of the improved position of the spine always requires greater muscle strength than was present before correction, it is essential that an attempt be made to increase the power of the supporting musculature. Corrective exercises should be performed for from one to three hours daily; they are best carried out under careful supervision in a gymnasium and should be continued for many months. Progressive diminution of the curvature is an indication that sufficient gymnastic work and exercise are being carried out. Any increase of the deformity necessitates change to a different method of treatment. After an adequate period of supervision the exercises may be carried on at home. Little improvement is to be expected unless the patient is willing to work faithfully with the exercises. Elaborate gymnastic apparatus is often used, especially in Europe, to help in the process of muscle development but is in no way indispensable for proper strengthening of the musculature. Good general hygiene, including a nutritious diet and plenty of fresh air, is important. Excess weight should be eliminated. Any complicating factor, such as unequal leg length or a flatfoot deformity, must be treated.

2. *Corrective Exercises, Passive Stretching, and Supports.*—It is sometimes desirable to stretch the spine, either in suspension with the use of the *Sayre head halter* or in recumbency on the *Lovett stretching board.* This treatment should be carried out before the corrective exercises are begun. In order that the improvement secured by stretching and exercise may be retained, a corset brace or removable plaster jacket should be worn at all times when the patient is not engaged in special exercises.

The *compensation method of Steindler,* when properly carried out, is a useful treatment for selected cases; however, in a few clinics it is thought to be of little value. In this method no attempt is made to mobilize or to correct the primary rigid curve, since such attempts are often ineffectual and frequently cause an increased flexibility and collapsibility of the entire spine. Carefully selected exercises are employed, however, to develop upper and lower compensatory curves which will so realign the body that the head and shoulders will be held squarely over the pelvis and the pelvis squarely over the ankles. This treatment is followed by a period of fixation in a brace which maintains the compensatory curves. When the brace is later removed, systematic exercises are instituted to provide muscle strength adequate to insure maintenance of the compensation. If it is apparent that muscular support sufficient to preserve the alignment cannot be secured, operative stabilization of the spine is indicated.

3. *Corrective Plaster Jackets.*—By means of plaster jackets much of the abnormal curvature may often be corrected. The jackets should be preceded by corrective exercises to effect mobilization. Plaster is then applied with the patient either in suspension or in recumbency; the recumbent position facilitates the application of side pulls to correct the lateral deviation and of twisting forces to counteract the rotation. After as much improvement as possible has been obtained by a series of plaster jackets, a laced plaster jacket, a corset with multiple parallel flexible stays (Hoke type), or a brace with axillary crutches should be worn for many months in order to maintain the correction. Corrective gymnastic exercises should then be taken for a long period of time.

Many modifications of the simple plaster body jacket have been devised; only a few of the more important adaptations can be mentioned here. The *Cook* or *Sayre fenestrated jacket* is fitted with large pads which exert corrective pressure through appropriately placed windows. In the *Abbott method* a jacket is applied while the patient lies with the spine flexed upon a special frame fitted with ratchets and bandages to exert corrective forces, and pressure is later applied by means of windows and pads. The *Galeazzi corrective jacket* is applied with the patient standing, the spine in anterior flexion, and its curvature and torsion corrected by mechanical apparatus acting upon pelvis and shoulders. In many clinics these jackets are no longer used.

In other methods the principle of a hinged jacket is utilized, facilitating continuous gradual correction of the curvature. The *Brewster turnbuckle jacket,* composed of two girdlelike sections, is fitted with a hinge on the side of the convexity and a turnbuckle on that of the concavity. The *Milwaukee brace* combines the hinge principle, pressure pad on the convex side of the curve, and longitudinal stretching between head and pelvis. The *Risser plaster jacket* is much used; it consists of a body cast which incorporates one or both thighs and the head and neck and is provided with anterior and posterior hinges and a turnbuckle on the side of the concavity; after correction has gradually been effected, stabilization is secured by means of operative fusion performed through a window in the posterior aspect of the cast.

4. *Operative Treatment.*—The operation of spinal fusion is the most effective means of treating severe and increasing scoliosis. Stabilizing operations are indicated when rapid increase of the curvature cannot be prevented by the use of corrective exercises, corsets, braces, and plaster jackets. In certain clinics operation is advocated for all forms of paralytic scoliosis, of increasing idiopathic scoliosis, and of any other type which is accompanied by marked deformity in adolescence. Of 425 cases of idiopathic scoliosis reviewed in 1941 by a committee of the American Orthopaedic Association, approximately 50 per cent required stabilizing operations. In this series of cases treated in 16 American clinics, spinal fusion after correction by means of a turnbuckle cast yielded results which were imperfect and in some cases unsatisfactory, but which were better than those obtained by any other form of treatment. In some clinics the spinal fusion is done in two stages preceded by a period of recumbency upon the hyperextension Whitman frame with the application of head and pelvic traction (Fig. 69), while in others the two-stage operation is performed before recumbency and correction of the curvature. Operative fusion of a long segment of the spine, the level depending upon the details of the individual curvature, may be carried out according to the Hibbs technic (Fig. 74), or according to a modification of this method. Kleinberg inserts on the concave side of the spine an autogenous bone graft or a beef bone graft in order to stimulate new bone production on the side of greater stress. A portion of a rib is sometimes used for the same purpose. All stabilizing operations upon the spine should be followed by rest in bed, preferably in a plaster cast, for a period of from ten to fourteen weeks, after which an ambulatory plaster jacket or strong spinal brace or corset must be worn for an additional period of at least nine months. During this time the new bone will become firm and the fused area will grow sufficiently strong to prevent progression of the scoliosis. Some surgeons, believing that a certain amount of early activity stimulates the production of new bone, recommend shorter periods of recumbency and immobilization, while others advise six months of recumbency.

In paralytic scoliosis associated with asymmetrical weakness of the muscles of the abdomen, considerable improvement of the deformity

may result from surgical reinforcement of the weakened abdomina
muscles by the use of long strips of fascia lata (Lowman operation).

In congenital scoliosis caused by a lumbar hemivertebra, operativ
removal of the extra bone segment, followed by stretching and turnbuckl
casts, may result in considerable correction of the deformity.   Thi
operative treatment is extremely formidable and accompanied by som
risk.   In some hands equally good results have been obtained by con
servative methods alone.

Kyphosis (Round Back)

Anteroposterior curvature of the spine in which the convexity i
directed posteriorly is called *kyphosis*. The thoracic and sacral level
of the normal spine exhibit this type of curvature. Posterior convexity o
abnormal degree results from pathologic changes located primarily in th
vertebral bodies, the intervertebral disks, or the supporting musculature

Kyphotic deformity occurs not uncommonly in children and young
adults.   Types resulting from faulty posture and from diseases such a
tuberculosis or chronic arthritis have been described in preceding chapters
Other entities which may cause kyphosis in youth include *vertebra*
epiphysitis and *vertebral osteochondritis*.

Kyphotic deformity seen in the middle or late age groups is ofter
termed *adult round back*. Its causes include postural influences anc
common bone and joint diseases as well as degenerative spinal lesion
peculiar to adult years.

Vertebral Epiphysitis

(Osteochondritis Deformans Juvenilis, Scheuermann's Disease
Adolescent Kyphosis)

The term *vertebral epiphysitis* has been applied to a chronic affection of the epiphyses of the vertebral bodies which is evidenced clinically
by fatigue, backache, and kyphosis of gradual development (Fig. 139)
The process always involves a number of contiguous vertebrae and usually is most marked in the lower or middle portion of the dorsal spine
Vertebral epiphysitis makes its appearance at puberty and is self-limited,
its active course lasting usually for two or three years.

Etiology.—Roentgenographic evidence suggests that the process is
a disturbance of the ossification of the epiphyses.   The etiologic agent
has not been established.   Hypotheses of the causation include (1)

mpaired circulation associated with rapid growth, similar to that some-
imes believed to occur in coxa plana; (2) disturbances of the calcium-
ohosphorus metabolism causing bone changes similar to those of
ate rickets or osteomalacia; (3) disturbance of epiphyseal growth by
orotrusion of the intervertebral disks through deficient cartilage plates.

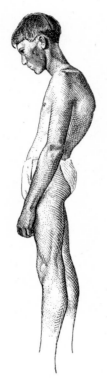

Fig. 139.—Vertebral epiphysitis, showing pronounced dorsal kyphosis and
sociated poor posture.

Roentgenographic Picture.—In early cases the bone edges above
nd below the intervertebral spaces appear cloudy and mottled. The
oiphyses are irregular in outline, particularly at their anterior edges,
1d may appear fragmented. The intervertebral spaces may be narrowed.
s healing takes place, the fragmentation disappears, and the bone out-
nes become relatively more distinct but remain irregular. There is
ften a visible horizontal cleft in the middle portion of the vertebral

body, extending from the anterior margin posteriorly for about two-thirds of the depth of the body. The vertebral bodies appear wedge-shaped and atrophied, and in severe cases there may be evidence of bone absorption (Fig. 140).

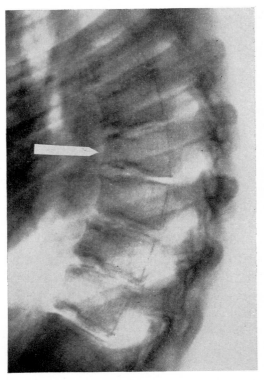

Fig. 140.—Lateral roentgenogram showing vertebral epiphysitis in boy fourteen years of age. Note the narrowing or wedging of the anterior portion of some of the vertebral bodies and the irregularity of their superior and inferior surfaces.

Clinical Picture.—The symptoms usually begin between the ages of twelve and sixteen years. The first subjective evidence may be fatigue and pain in the back and lower extremities. Undue prominence of the spinous processes of the vertebrae may be noticed, especially at the lower dorsal and upper lumbar levels, and gradual development of kyphosis takes place. The deformity persists in recumbency. Stiffness and tenderness may be present throughout the spine. Expansion of the chest is abnormally restricted. The affection sometimes progresses to the point of severe disability, while in other cases it causes very few symptoms.

Diagnosis.—Vertebral epiphysitis is to be distinguished from tuberculosis of the spine. In tuberculosis there is marked spinal rigidity, which is never striking in epiphysitis, and the roentgenograms show localized bone destruction and an angular rather than a rounded kyphosis. Vertebral epiphysitis is also to be differentiated from osteochondritis, which develops at an earlier age and is localized to a single vertebral body.

Treatment.—The therapy depends upon the severity of the symptoms. In the milder cases it may be advisable to institute only stretching and postural exercises. It is sometimes necessary to support the spine by means of a brace or plaster jacket. Occasionally, recumbency for a period of three months upon a Bradford or a Whitman frame may be indicated and should be followed by the use of a plaster jacket or brace.

Vertebral Osteochondritis (Calve's Disease)

Vertebral osteochondritis is a rare, obscure affection of unknown etiology. Unlike vertebral epiphysitis, vertebral osteochondritis develops usually in children between five and ten years of age and is characterized by pathologic changes localized in a single vertebral body. The lesion is found most often in the lower dorsal or lumbodorsal level of the spine.

Roentgenographic Picture.—In osteochondritis the vertebral body shows evidence of fragmentation while the adjacent intervertebral spaces appear normal or thickened. The affected vertebral body may be wedge-shaped or uniformly flattened. As healing takes place, there is a marked increase of bone density, similar to that found during the healing stage of tuberculosis of the spine.

Clinical Picture.—Vertebral osteochondritis is characterized by pain, fatigue, and an evident angular kyphosis. Sometimes night cries, muscle spasm, and tenderness are present.

Diagnosis.—Vertebral osteochondritis must be carefully differentiated from tuberculosis of the spine and tumor. It is to be distinguished also from vertebral epiphysitis, in which the changes always involve more than one vertebra.

Treatment.—The patient should be placed upon a frame in hyperextension with head and pelvic traction (Fig. 69) for a period of at least three months. This treatment should be followed by a plaster jacket or a brace for from three to six months, or longer. Usually the treatment has little apparent influence in shortening the course of the disease. Rarely it may be advisable to stabilize the spine by operative fusion (Fig. 74).

ADULT ROUND BACK

Etiology.—Adult round back may be due to faulty posture alone or to an occupation which requires constant flexion of the spine; to old age with its constant atrophy of the intervertebral disks *(senile kyphosis)*; to atrophy of the vertebral bodies *(senile osteoporosis)*; or to a pathologic entity such as rickets, scoliosis, fracture, osteitis deformans, arthritis, muscular dystrophy, infantile paralysis, acromegaly, osteomalacia, hyperparathyroidism, tuberculosis, or other diseases which affect the spine. Atrophy of the intervertebral disks sometimes takes place in middle life; it may progress to cause a single long kyphosis with flattening of the lumbar and cervical portions of the spine and forward projection of the head.

Pathology.—In adult round back due to lesions of the intervertebral fibrocartilages, the pathologic changes which occur in the disks are characteristic. The normal disk, as demonstrated by Schmorl, comprises a central portion, the *nucleus pulposus*, consisting of a semifluid medium under pressure, and a peripheral portion, the *annulus fibrosus,* which forms a fibrocartilaginous capsule. Two thin plates of hyaline cartilage separate the disk from the bones above and below. These cartilage plates are in contact with the superior and inferior surfaces of the vertebral bodies. In 30 per cent of all adult spines protrusion of the disk tissue into the spongy bone of the vertebral bodies has been found. This lesion may occur in any case of abnormal anteroposterior spinal curvature, whether in a child or in an adult.

Gradual collapse of the intervertebral disks allows adjacent vertebral bodies to become approximated. As a result of the irritative changes, new bone formation occurs about the edges of the vertebral bodies. If in addition the anterior portion of the cartilaginous plates is destroyed, bridges of new bone may develop across the intervertebral spaces and create an ankylosis.

In adult round back from senile osteoporosis the disks remain relatively normal, but the spongy bone within the vertebral body becomes atrophic and the cortex becomes thinned. This osteoporosis is presumably a manifestation of disuse atrophy. In the thoracic spine the vertebral bodies may become wedge-shaped, while in the lumbar region they may assume a biconcave or hourglass contour as seen in lateral roentgenograms. The osteoporosis may lead to pathologic compression fractures of the vertebral bodies.

Clinical Picture.—The deformity of kyphosis is of characteristic appearance and may be associated with considerable pain, weakness of the back, and general fatigue. The aching and tiring of the back usually occur below the level of the kyphosis. Seldom is there any localized tenderness; it may be present, however, in senile osteoporosis with recent compression fracture.

Treatment.—Attempt should be made to maintain correct posture; exercises to strengthen the muscles of the back and abdomen and to expand the chest will sometimes aid in accomplishing this. In more advanced cases it may be necessary to apply a light spinal brace or corset. If the symptoms are located in the cervical spine, a Thomas collar may be used to support the head and so relieve the constant dragging sensation. In some cases a period of immobilization on a Whitman frame is advisable, and, rarely, operative fusion of the spine may be indicated for the relief of intractable backache. For senile osteoporosis, the administration of calcium and vitamins with particular attention to increase in vitamin D intake may be helpful, and in many cases symptomatic improvement has followed treatment with the sex hormones.

Posttraumatic Kyphosis (Kümmell's Disease)

Posttraumatic kyphosis is a chronic affection of the adult spine characterized clinically by the delayed development of deformity following trauma and pathologically by rarefaction and collapse of the affected vertebral body. Either a single severe injury or repeated slight injuries may be the causative agent. A trophic disturbance of the vertebral body, due presumably to circulatory changes following trauma, has been suggested as a factor in the pathogenesis. It is not unlikely that posttraumatic kyphosis is a result of an unrecognized fracture of a vertebral body.

Pathology.—Following the injury, gradual absorption of bone is believed to take place, leading to roentgenographic changes suggesting a rarefying osteitis and culminating in collapse of the body of the vertebra.

Clinical Picture.—The clinical course can be divided into three stages. The first of these begins with the injury and ends after a day or two when the immediate symptoms subside. The second stage is one of quiescence; the patient has no symptoms and is able to resume his ordinary occupation. After weeks, months, or even years of latency, the third stage, marked by deformity and discomfort, begins. Its outstanding feature is the development of kyphosis, which is most often located in the dorsal spine. Occasionally, especially in untreated cases, there may be weakness and considerable pain in the muscles of the back and lower extremities. Severe cases may be attended by extreme pain localized in the back; it may radiate down the legs when the lesion is in the lumbar area.

Diagnosis.—In the differential diagnosis tuberculosis, vertebral osteochondritis, osteoarthritis, tumor, metastatic malignancy, and senile osteoporosis must be considered.

Prognosis.—When no neurologic symptoms have developed, the patient usually improves greatly within a few months of the beginning of treatment and is able to resume his former occupation.

Treatment.—When pain is a prominent symptom, recumbency, preferably in hyperextension in a plaster shell, is the most desirable form of treatment. Hyperextension exercises should be carried out daily. A brace should then be worn for a period of a year. If the symptoms persist, operative stabilization of the spine is indicated (Fig. 74).

Lordosis (Hollow Back)

Anteroposterior curvature of the spine in which the concavity is directed posteriorly is termed *lordosis*. Pathologic lordosis is less common than pathologic kyphosis. It is usually secondary to other deformity of the spine or to deformities of the lower limbs. It is often found in association with flexion contracture of the hip, congenital dislocation of the hip, coxa vara, progressive muscular dystrophy, paralysis from poliomyelitis, obesity of the abdomen, dorsal kyphosis, congenital abnormality of the spine, spondylolisthesis, and shortening of the Achilles tendons.

Clinical Picture.—Constant aching throughout the lower part of the back, protrusion of the abdomen, and generalized fatigue are often present. A waddling gait suggestive of congenital dislocation of the hip may be noted. The patient tires easily and does not have the average amount of bodily vigor; these symptoms are often found in young children and may be very disturbing to the parents.

Treatment and Prognosis.—Therapy should include general postural exercises with particular effort to strengthen the abdominal and the gluteal muscles. A strong support for the back with a lower abdominal pad is usually helpful. The result of treatment is often complete relief of the backache, but frequently the improvement will not be permanent unless the pathologic factor underlying the deformity can be remedied.

Traumatic Neurosis of the Spine

There can be no doubt that injuries of the back are sometimes followed by pains and aches generalized over the whole body. These symptoms may undermine the patient's psychic stability and lead to the development of a frank neurosis or abnormal psychosomatic state.

Clinical Picture.—Dull pain and aching are present throughout the back and neck. If the pain is radiating, it most often runs up the back from the coccyx to the occiput. Much of the discomfort may be localized about a prominent spinous process. There may be hypersensitiveness of this region and of other areas over the spine. The posture is often poor. General hyperirritability, twitching, and aching of the whole body may be present. There may at first be evidence of slight injury of ligaments and muscles with accompanying pain and muscle spasm. Most of the symptoms are entirely subjective and inconstant, changing from day to day and producing no muscle spasm or limitation of motion. When there is an element of compensation or litigation, the symptoms are nearly always more marked, are likely to be exaggerated, and usually persist until settlement of the claim is made. Settlement is often followed immediately by recovery.

Diagnosis.—In the diagnosis of traumatic neurosis great care must be taken in an effort to exclude all possibility of an organic lesion. The diagnosis is necessarily influenced by the psychic state of the patient and by his past history.

Treatment.—The back should be treated with local physical therapy. It may be wise to insist on the patient's wearing a back support in the form of a corset or brace for a limited period. Postural exercises form an important part of the treatment. Static abnormalities of the feet or knees, if present, should be corrected. It is most important for the physician to gain the confidence of the patient and to employ adequate and well-planned psychotherapy.

PART II. DEFORMITIES OF THE THORAX

Deformities of the thorax are observed not uncommonly. In many of the cases the disability is slight and little can be accomplished by treatment.

1. Flat Chest

This deformity often accompanies round shoulders or round back. In some cases it is apparently the cause of round shoulders.

Treatment.—Selected exercises are indicated in an effort to increase the chest expansion and to strengthen the back muscles as a means of improving the posture.

2. Pigeon Breast (Pectus Carinatum)

In this type of chest deformity the sternum projects forward and downward like the keel of a boat. There is a definite increase of the anteroposterior diameter of the thorax. The prominence may be more marked on one side than the other. The deformity is almost always of acquired type and often accompanies rickets. Occasionally pigeon breast is secondary to extreme tuberculous involvement of the dorsal spine (Fig. 67).

Treatment.—Deep breathing and postural exercises to strengthen the muscles of the back are indicated. Occasionally pressure upon the sternum with deep inspiration may tend to reduce the deformity. Braces similar to hernial trusses have been applied in an effort to exert constant corrective pressure upon the sternum. Such braces are not indicated except in cases of extreme deformity, since they are most uncomfortable and since the resulting correction often proves to be of only slight degree. In a few cases pigeon breast has been observed to improve spontaneously.

3. Funnel Chest (Pectus Excavatum)

In funnel chest the body of the sternum is depressed, the costal cartilages are angulated posteriorly, and the lower rib surfaces show an outward flare. The lateral diameter of the thorax is increased. It is believed that shortening of the central tendon of the diaphragm causes the sternal depression, while shortening of the lateral tendon pulls inward the ribs to which it is attached and produces the flared appearance of the lower ribs. The deformity is often progressive. Severe forms of funnel chest are usually of congenital origin. They cause considerable disfigurement, especially in girls, and may be associated with serious cardiorespiratory embarrassment.

Treatment.—Any obstruction of the upper respiratory passages should be eradicated. Postural gymnastics may be tried but are usually ineffective. Severe cases should be treated by the thoracic surgeon. In patients under one year of age, only mobilization of the sternum by division of the xyphosternal junction and separation of the sternum from the diaphragmatic attachments are done. In older patients an extensive operation consisting of division and resection of the deformed costal cartilages, wedge osteotomy and elevation of the sternum, and division of all the sternal and anterior costal attachments of the diaphragm may be necessary.

CHAPTER XIX

AFFECTIONS OF THE LOW BACK

The term "affections of the low back" is used in this chapter to include the common lumbosacral and sacroiliac joint syndromes, spondylolisthesis, injuries of the lumbar intervertebral disks, coccygodynia, and herniation of fascial fat.

The frequency with which affections of the low back are encountered brings them constantly to the attention of every practitioner of medicine. Patients whose low back pain is caused by visceral rather than musculoskeletal lesions or is an hysterical conversion symptom associated with tension, nervousness, and chronic fatigue are problems for the internist and psychiatrist respectively rather than the orthopaedist. However, low back pain, with or without sciatic pain, is the commonest complaint with which orthopaedic surgeons are confronted in adults. The variety of bone, joint, muscle, ligament, and nerve lesions which may cause low back pain and the difficulties encountered in their treatment make these affections formidable orthopaedic problems. In each case the diagnosis and treatment must be based upon a careful evaluation of the clinical and roentgenographic findings in the light of available information on the various recognized types of low back lesions.

Classification.—For clarity of description, cases characterized by low back pain may be discussed according to the following outline:

1. Lesions peculiar to the low back.
   A. Ligamentous and muscular injuries of the normal low back. Of these, the syndrome of lumbosacral instability resulting from acute or chronic traumatic influences is the most important.
   B. Abnormalities of the bony structures of the low back. Among these are congenital anomalies, spondylolisthesis, and prespondylolisthesis.
   C. Injuries of the lumbar intervertebral disks.
   D. Herniation of fascial fat.
2. Common osteoarticular lesions of infectious, neoplastic, or traumatic nature affecting the low back.
3. Visceral lesions with pain referred to the low back.

1. A. Ligamentous and Muscular Injuries of the Normal Low Back

The majority of cases of low back pain of orthopaedic nature fall into this group. The mechanism of injury is either an episode of violent trauma or continued mechanical strain of postural or occupational type. In most cases the lesion itself is presumably a tear or stretching of ligaments which support and limit the mobility of a joint. There is considerable evidence for the belief that in many cases the lesion may be a tear of the posterior longitudinal ligament, a tear of the annulus fibrosus, or traumatic changes within the disk substance. Muscle injury may be associated. The hemorrhage and organization which follow an injury may cause the ligaments to lose their normal tone and strength and so lead to a state of chronic relaxation which predisposes the joint to further injury. During pregnancy temporary relaxation of the ligaments of the sacroiliac joints occurs normally.

Most of the cases of this type can be classified into two groups: (1) lumbosacral sprain and (2) sacroiliac sprain. The lumbosacral joint, situated at the critical level between movable and immovable portions of the spine, is particularly liable to injury from forces applied in an obliquely anteroposterior direction, as in violent flexion or hyperextension of the spine, falls upon the buttocks, and gravitational stresses associated with excessive lordosis. Lumbosacral sprains are therefore very frequently encountered. The sacroiliac joints, on the other hand, are large in area and protected by strong ligamentous structures; they may nevertheless be injured occasionally by violence applied to the low back in a rotary or obliquely lateral manner, although in recent years many observers have denied the existence of true sacroiliac sprain.

Clinical Picture.—The symptoms and physical signs are very similar to those of other affections of the low back and warrant detailed analysis. Many of these symptoms and signs are identical with those of rupture of an intervertebral disk, which are described on pp. 414-415.

Localized Pain.—Pain in the low back is the outstanding symptom. The discomfort is often localized to a single area. At times it may be generalized across the whole back, however, and the area of maximum intensity may shift from one side to the other. If pain in the low back is precipitated or aggravated by motion, it will in most instances be relieved by recumbency.

Radiating Pain.—Radiation of pain into the legs is a frequent symptom in low back affections; it is thought to be due either to an irritation of the nerve roots of the lumbosacral plexus which are adjacent to the lumbosacral and sacroiliac joints or to a protrusion of a ruptured intervertebral disk, which will be discussed later. Long fourth or fifth lumbar transverse processes also may cause irritation of the nerve roots. The lower intervertebral foramina may be narrowed and irregular, causing nerve irritation. The sciatic nerve may be affected by spasm or sustained contraction of the pyriformis muscle, over which the nerve passes after it emerges from the pelvis. In partial or complete sacralization of the fifth lumbar vertebra there may be irritation of the nerve fibers of the lumbosacral plexus, causing radiation of pain into the leg and spastic scoliosis *(Bertolotti's syndrome)*. Localized numbness or hyperesthesia of the leg is frequently observed.

Radiation of pain into the legs usually follows the distribution of the sciatic nerve. In other instances the pain follows the course of the superior gluteal nerve into the buttock or exhibits lumbar radiation into the groin and lateral side of the thigh.

Tenderness.—There is usually localized pain on firm pressure over the affected area. When the lumbosacral joint is involved, the tenderness is usually most acute over the lumbosacral supraspinal ligament though it may be present over the iliolumbar ligament of either side or may be generalized across the whole low back. When the sacroiliac structures are affected, tenderness may be present about the inferior sacroiliac ligaments and the greater sciatic notch.

Muscle Spasm.—In patients who are having low back pain there is often marked spasm of the lumbar muscles. The spasm may be equal on the two sides; it is often asymmetrical, however, causing curvature of the spinal column, the so-called "sciatic scoliosis." Spasm may be present also in the hamstring muscles, making it impossible to flex the hip while the knee is extended. There also may be spasm of the tensor fasciae latae muscle and a contracture of the fascia lata.

Abnormal Limitation of Mobility.—There is usually marked limitation of motion from muscle spasm, especially in the acute cases. Tests of mobility dependent upon the localization of the muscle spasm are of value in differential diagnosis and should be carried out in the standing, sitting, and lying positions. In the standing position, flexion and hyperextension may be sharply limited. Rotation of the lower portion of the spine is often restricted, the patient being able to turn slightly more toward the normal side than toward the affected side. Flexion in the sitting position may be definitely restricted.

Posture.—In acute low back affections the lumbar spine is often flattened and deviated away from the affected side (sciatic scoliosis) (Fig. 141). In chronic conditions, however, the spine may be deviated toward the affected side. It is believed that the position of scoliosis is adopted because it relaxes the tension upon the plexus from which the sciatic nerve is formed. The lateral curvature is rarely associated, however, with true sciatic neuritis. When the scoliosis persists for a long time, it may cause the development of a compensatory curvature.

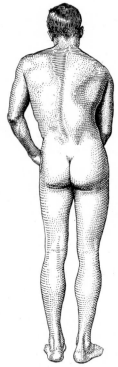

Fig. 141.—Lateral curvature of the lumbar spine in acute affection of the low back (sciatic scoliosis).

Special Tests of Passive Mobility.—A number of passive mobility tests have been devised or popularized by various observers and are of value in the clinical analysis of low back affections. The following tests are in common use:

1. Extreme flexion of both thighs upon the abdomen, with the knees flexed, places the lumbosacral joint under flexion stress while causing no unilateral rotary stress of the sacroiliac joints or stretching of the sciatic nerves. Lumbosacral pain produced by this maneuver is therefore an indication of a disorder of the lumbosacral joint.

2. Straight-leg-raising, i.e., flexion of the hip while the knee is held in extension (Fig. 142), stretches the sciatic nerve and places a rotary and flexion stress upon the low back structures. It causes pain when sciatic irritation is present (Lasègue's sign).

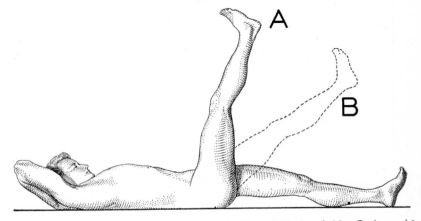

Fig. 142.—Straight-leg-raising test. *A*, Normal limit of hip flexion with knee extended. *B*, Limitation of hip flexion due to pain in the presence of sciatic irritation.

3. When the hip of the affected side is flexed, extension of the knee will cause pain in the affected side of the low back (Goldthwait sign). The mechanism is similar to that of the preceding test.

4. Forcing the hip of the affected side into flexion, abduction, and external rotation with the knee flexed places a stress upon, and causes pain in, the affected side of the low back (Faber sign).

5. When the hip and knee of the affected side are flexed and the hip of the opposite side is then hyperextended, the affected side undergoes a rotary stress which results in pain (Gaenslen sign).

6. Pain in the low back and lower extremity on passive flexion of the knee while the patient lies prone on a firm table indicates the presence of an orthopaedic lesion in the low back region (Nachlas sign).

7. Contracture of the iliotibial band may be demonstrated by the following test: The patient lies on his sound side with the thighs flexed enough to obliterate the lumbar lordosis. Grasping the ankle lightly with one hand and steadying the hip with the other, the examiner flexes the knee to a right angle, abducts the hip widely, and extends the hip. If the iliotibial band is shortened, the hip tends to remain passively abducted (Ober sign).

8. Forceful and prolonged lateral compression of the iliac crests, while placing no stress upon the lumbosacral joint, sometimes produces pain in the affected sacroiliac structures.

Roentgenographic Examination.—Roentgenograms are often of little help toward making a positive diagnosis. They are of great assistance, however, in ruling out conditions such as neoplasms or tuberculosis. The presence of bony anomalies, such as sacralization of the fifth lumbar vertebra (Figs. 144 and 145), should be looked for. Occasionally calcification is seen within the iliolumbar ligaments. In lumbosacral affections the plane and smoothness of the articular facets, the width of the intervertebral disk spaces, and the degree of the lumbosacral angle are to be noted. Arthritic spurring and bridging may be seen. The roentgenograms should include anteroposterior, lateral, and oblique views. A search for defects of the isthmus or pars interarticularis should be made, and any forward displacement of a vertebral body should be noted. The examiner should also look for destructive changes and increased bone density about the sacroiliac joints.

Differential Diagnosis.—Ligamentous and muscular injuries of the low back must frequently be differentiated from (1) arthritis of the lumbar spine or sacroiliac joints, (2) fracture of the body or processes of the last lumbar vertebra, (3) spondylolisthesis and prespondylolisthesis, (4) rupture of an intervertebral disk, (5) tuberculosis, (6) malignancy, (7) fatty and fibrous nodules overlying ligaments and muscles, (8) traumatic neurosis, and (9) malingering. When the diagnosis is being made, the visceral diseases which may cause low back pain must be considered. A history of aggravation of the pain by exercise and of relief during recumbency suggests that the symptoms are of osteoarticular rather than visceral origin.

Treatment.—Brief presentation of the more important therapeutic principles and their clinical application will be made. In the majority of cases nonoperative treatment of ambulatory or recumbent type is indicated. In certain selected cases, however, operative treatment is to be preferred.

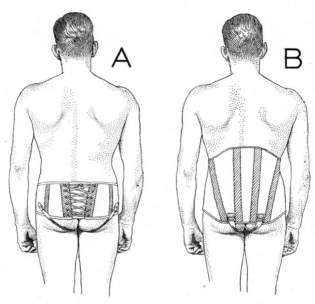

Fig. 143.—*A*, Sacroiliac belt; *B*, lumbosacral support. These are constructed of heavy canvas with stays of spring steel.

1. *Conservative Treatment.*—The principles of the treatment of ligament and of muscle injuries of the normal low back are essentially the same. The primary requisite is rest and support. In the acute phase absolute recumbency is a necessity; the patient should lie supine in bed upon a firm, hard mattress or on a mattress which is separated from the bedsprings by a fracture board. Occasionally it is advisable to apply traction to one or both legs in order to relieve muscle spasm and pain. Recumbency may sometimes be made more effective by placing a pillow under the knees or under the painful portion of the back. Recumbency should continue until all pain and muscle spasm subside. It is always advisable to accompany the rest in bed with local heat and massage, maintaining constant warmth over the painful area by means of an electric pad or a hot water bottle. Daily diathermy treatment of the low back often helps to relieve the pain. Aspirin may be helpful. Acute

cases attended by muscle spasm may be relieved by Tolserol or Myanesin or by dilute procaine solution given intravenously. In moderately acute cases in which the symptoms improve rapidly with recumbency, it is usually possible to allow gradual return to walking in one or two weeks, provided that the back be firmly strapped with adhesive plaster or supported with a snugly fitting low back brace or corset. In sacroiliac affections the strapping should exert lateral compression upon the ilia but need not extend above their crests, while in lumbosacral affections it should reach up above the rib margins. If sufficiently prolonged support cannot be derived from strapping, a belt or brace should be worn (Fig. 143). Occasionally it is necessary to obtain still stronger support by the application of a light plaster cast. Such a cast should be well moulded to the patient's torso and should extend well down over the iliac crests.

When walking is allowed, it is sometimes desirable to have the patient begin with crutches. Often an acute case will become chronic if weight-bearing without proper support of the back is allowed too soon. When the patient is permitted to be up, it is advisable to begin posture exercises to increase the strength of the back muscles. Too much emphasis cannot be placed upon the necessity of warning the patient to be careful about lifting and bending. He should not be allowed to return to strenuous work until the prescribed exercises can be performed without causing pain. If an exciting cause such as faulty posture or a focus of infection is present, especial attention should be given to its eradication. Intestinal stasis should be corrected by appropriate catharsis.

Cases of only moderate severity may be treated without the initial period of recumbency.

2. *Manipulative Treatment.*—When the response to conservative therapy is unsatisfactory, manipulation of the low back may break up painful adhesions, decrease muscle spasm, and thus lead to relief of the symptoms. Manipulation is frequently indicated in persistent cases associated with local and radiating pain and deformity of the low back. Although manipulation without anesthesia will lead in many instances to relief, it is the author's belief that the best results are obtained with the use of general or spinal anesthesia. In the presence of muscle spasm, the manipulation may be more effective if preliminary doses of curare are administered intramuscularly.

For cases characterized by persistent lumbosacral pain, the manipulation consists of forced hyperextension and forced flexion of the lumbar spine. It may be followed by a plaster body cast for from two to eight weeks and then by a back brace for several weeks. If a cast is not used, hot applications and deep massage should be started immediately after manipulation and continued until the symptoms subside.

For sacroiliac affections the manipulation should consist of gradually forced flexion of the hip with the knee extended, followed by forced adduction of the flexed hip. It should be continued until spasm of the hamstring and tensor fasciae latae muscles has been completely overcome. Occasionally a distinct clicking sound will be noted during manipulation, and, if the patient is not under anesthesia, he may experience sudden relief of pain. The manipulation is best followed by recumbency, physical therapy with emphasis on gradually increasing exercises, and a sacroiliac belt to support the low back when the patient returns to walking.

3. *Operative Treatment.*—Operative measures include injections, myotomy, fasciotomy, removal of abnormal bone formations, and joint stabilization or arthrodesis. These procedures may be used also in the treatment of abnormalities of the bony structures of the low back, described in the following section.

The injection of acutely tender, sharply localized areas of the low back with procaine or Xylocaine is often very helpful.

Injections of the sciatic nerve with procaine, normal salt solution, or quinine urea sometimes lead to relief of persistent sciatic pain. Epidural injection of from 100 to 200 cc. of weak procaine solution or normal saline into the sacral canal will often cause partial or complete relief of persistent sciatic pain when it is caused by a ruptured intervertebral disk.

Operations for the relief of sciatic pain have been described in which either the tensor fasciae latae or the pyriformis muscle is sectioned, or the ligaments and muscle attachments are stripped from the posterior superior iliac spine and the adjacent iliac crest. Complete recovery from persistent pain has in some instances followed these procedures.

For chronic cases in which careful therapy as outlined above has been unsuccessful, operative stabilization of one or more joints of the low back is indicated for the relief of pain and the prevention of recurrences. For instability of the lumbosacral joint, arthrodesis may be performed according to the Hibbs technic (Fig. 74). For pain of sacroiliac origin the joint may be fused according to one of the methods described on page 179.

As a rule, lumbosacral fusion should be followed by from six to twelve weeks in bed and then by use of a back brace for a period of from six to twelve months. After all arthrodesis operations sufficient recumbency must be allowed for the grafts to become firmly attached and the formation of new bone to take place. A great many failures are undoubtedly due to over-enthusiasm on the part of the surgeon in allowing the patient to sit, stand, and walk too soon after operation.

When a large last lumbar transverse or spinous process or an abnormal lumbosacral articular facet is associated with severe pain either localized or radiating, removal of the abnormal process or facet will sometimes afford permanent relief.

1. B. Abnormalities of the Bony Structures of the Low Back

A great many of the cases of low back pain present roentgenographic evidence of anomalous bony development. In interpreting the relationship of these abnormalities to the clinical symptoms, the examiner must remember that similar anomalies are often present in individuals who are symptom-free. Nevertheless, most statistical studies support the natural inference that anomaly of the bony structure of the low back renders it less stable than the normal back and more inclined through faulty mechanics to development of the ligamentous and muscular affections which have been described.

The most important bony anomalies of the low back are the following (Fig. 144):

1. *Sacralization of the Last Lumbar Vertebra.*—This term is applied to a bony conformation in which one or both of the transverse processes of the last lumbar vertebra is long and wing-shaped, and either articulates with, or is fused to, the sacrum or ilium or both (Fig. 145). The condition is found in 3.5 per cent of all individuals, and in over half of this number low back pain is a common experience. A lumbosacral fusion may be indicated if conservative measures fail to relieve the pain.

2. *Elongation of the Transverse Process of the Last Lumbar Vertebra.*—Abnormally long fifth lumbar transverse processes are found in 25 per cent of the cases of low back pain. Such processes may occasionally impinge upon the ilium, and the resulting friction may give rise to the formation of a painful bursa. In such cases excision of the elongated process may be indicated.

3. *Defect of the Neural Arch (Spina Bifida Occulta).*—Clefts are frequently found in the vertebral laminae (Fig. 146) and may be associated with underdevelopment of the supporting ligaments. Partial or complete lack of fusion between the laminae of the last lumbar vertebra or of the first sacral segment is common; this imperfection has been found

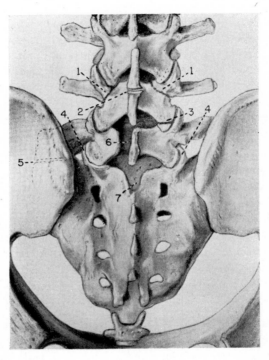

Fig. 144.—Congenital anomalies of the lumbar spine. (1) Bilateral isthmus defect, (2) impingement of third and fourth lumbar spinous processes, (3) fissure defect of lamina at the articular facet, (4) tropism or change of normal angle of articular facet, (5) sacralization of fifth lumbar transverse process with pseudarthrosis, (6) spina bifida occulta, fifth lumbar vertebra, and (7) spina bifida occulta, first sacral segment. (In section by Freiberg, edited by Bancroft and Marble: Surgical Treatment of the Motor-Skeletal System, J. B. Lippincott Company, 1951.)

in 5 per cent of all spines examined by roentgenograms. At the affected level the spine is weakened and prone to injury. If there are pain and weakness at the lumbosacral joint and conservative therapy is ineffective, a fusion operation is indicated.

4. *Variation of the Spinous Processes.*—When the neural arch has failed to fuse, the spinous process may be attached to only one lamina. In other instances the spinous process associated with normal laminae may be large and elongated so that it touches the spinous process of the vertebra

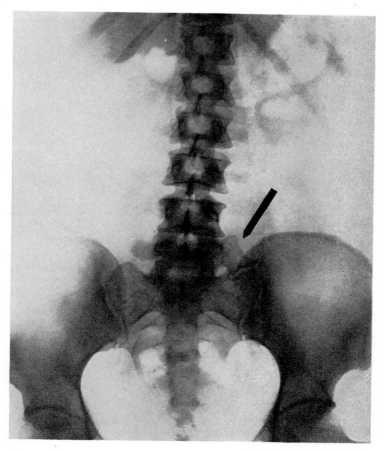

Fig. 145.—Roentgenogram showing congenital anomalies of the lumbar spine. The left transverse process of the lowest of six lumbar vertebrae is sacralized.

above or below (Baastrup's disease). Constant irritation caused by this friction may give rise to the formation of a painful bursa. In such cases the large spinous process should be excised.

5. *Variation of the Lumbosacral Angle.*—Wide variations of the angle between the upper surface of the sacrum and the horizontal plane when the patient is standing are not uncommon, and in many instances an abnormally horizontal sacrum is associated. In this type of case the lumbosacral joint is prone to injury from strain with the subsequent formation of small bony spurs about the margins of the vertebral bodies. The treatment is the same as that of lumbosacral sprain.

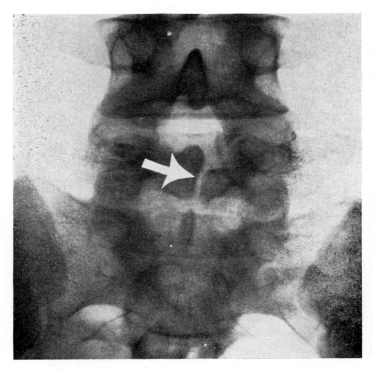

Fig. 146.—Roentgenogram showing spina bifida occulta of the fifth lumbar vertebra. Note cleft in the laminal arch.

6. *Variation of the Articular Facets.*—Variations in the size and plane of these small but important joint surfaces are common. This variation is spoken of as *tropism* (Fig. 144). The facets between the last lumbar vertebra and the sacrum are particularly important in this respect. When abnormally disposed, they form a source of mechanical weakness which

under the influence of postural stresses may lead to irritation of the lumbosacral plexus and result in pain radiating to the lower extremities. If the articular surfaces of the lumbosacral facets occupy an anteroposterior rather than their normal transverse plane, there is a tendency for gravitational stresses to cause sprain of the lumbosacral joint. Asymmetry in the planes of the two articulations is particularly likely to form the mechanical basis for sprain. Occasionally a facetectomy or a spinal fusion operation may be indicated to relieve the symptoms.

7. *Constitutional Variations.*—The entire structure of the spine varies with the development of the body as a whole, and individuals of certain body types are particularly susceptible to low back strain. Individuals with long, narrow backs or with flat backs are especially liable to pain in the low back region. In the tall, thin type the presence of a sixth lumbar vertebra is not uncommon, while short, stocky individuals sometimes have only four lumbar vertebrae. The treatment is the same as that of lumbosacral sprain.

8. *Isthmus Defects.*—Absence of bony continuity at the pars interarticularis, or isthmus, of the fifth lumbar vertebra is found in about 5 per cent of adult skeletons. It is called spondylolysis; when bilateral it is sometimes termed prespondylolisthesis. The defect is more often bilateral than unilateral. It may lead to low back pain and spondylolisthesis. Its treatment is the same as that of spondylolisthesis.

Spondylolisthesis

Spondylolisthesis is a forward displacement of the fifth lumbar vertebra and spinal column upon the sacrum or, less commonly, of the fourth lumbar vertebra and spinal column upon the fifth lumbar vertebra (Fig. 147*A*). Rarely either the fourth or the fifth lumbar vertebra may be displaced forward while the vertebrae above and below remain in their normal position. Posterior displacement of the last lumbar vertebra upon the sacrum, constituting the reverse of the usual spondylolisthesis, has been described, but evidence for its existence as a pathologic entity is not convincing.

Etiology.—The underlying cause of spondylolisthesis is an absence of bony continuity at each isthmus, the narrowest part of the neural arch. The pathogenesis of isthmus defects has not been established; they are believed to result from fracture, possibly at birth, or from anomalous development of the vertebra. Bilateral isthmus defects divide the vertebra into two separate pieces of bone. The anterior portion is made up of the body, pedicles, transverse processes, and superior articular processes. The posterior portion, often referred to as a separate neural arch, consists of the laminae, the inferior articular processes, and the spinous process. When a bilateral isthmus defect is present, the bony anchorage of the vertebral column to its base on the sacrum is lost and its stability is altogether dependent upon the ligaments. The presence of a bilateral isthmus defect without forward displacement of the vertebral body, called *prespondylolisthesis* or *spondylolysis* is thought to be a frequent cause of low back pain.

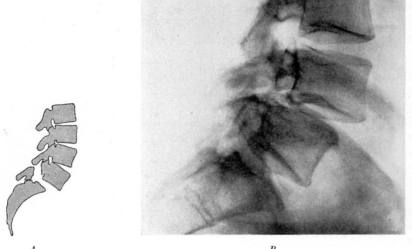

A. *B.*

Fig. 147*A.*—Spondylolisthesis. Note the defect in the pedicles of the last lumbar vertebra, which allows the vertebral body to slip forward upon the sacrum.

Fig. 147*B.*—Lateral roentgenogram showing spondylolisthesis. Note marked slipping forward of fourth lumbar vertebra upon the fifth.

The immediate or exciting cause of spondylolisthesis is believed to be trauma. Although the slipping or listhesis may be caused by a single severe injury, chronic postural strains are more often responsible. Contributing factors in the etiology of spondylolisthesis are (1) the normal mobility of the lumbosacral joint, (2) the normal laxity of the lumbosacral ligaments, and (3) the normal inclination of the upper sacral surface. Progressive increase of slipping in adults is uncommon. The symptoms are probably caused by narrowing of the intervertebral disk with degenerative changes in the disk and proliferative bone changes about the intervertebral foramina. Rarely the body of a vertebra together with its intact neural arch may become displaced forward when articular facet lesions are present; this condition has been termed *pseudospondylolisthesis*. The diplacement may produce symptoms of pressure upon the roots of the cauda equina.

Clinical Picture.—Pain may be severe, slight, or entirely absent. It is often well localized in the lumbosacral joint region but may radiate down one or both legs along the course of the sciatic nerve and especially into the distribution of the peroneal nerves. There is often complaint of stiffness of the back, and all of the symptoms become worse with exercise and strain. Prior to the onset of frank symptoms there may have been recurrent episodes of fatigue and weakness. Upon examination the low back appears lordotic. The spinous process of the detached neural arch is prominent on palpation and often is evident on inspection. There is a tender depression just above it. The sacrum is much nearer vertical than normally. The torso is shortened, the ribs may rest upon the iliac crests, and the abdomen may protrude. In severe cases the pelvic inclination is decreased and the body is swayed backward. There may be marked limitation of anteroposterior motion in the affected area and considerable spasm of the erector spinae muscles. There may also be spasm of the hamstring muscles. When the condition is severe, the gait is sometimes awkward and waddling. In some cases the projecting vertebra is palpable on rectal examination.

Spondylolisthesis is frequently found in women and is an important complication of pregnancy.

Diagnosis.—Because of similarities in the clinical appearance of the back, spondylolisthesis of severe degree is occasionally confused with congenital dislocation of the hips, tuberculosis of the lumbar spine, and rickets. It may be impossible to differentiate clinically between spondylolisthesis with slight displacement and lumbosacral sprain or ruptured intervertebral disk. In spondylolisthesis the roentgenograms show the pathognomonic findings, however, of isthmus defects and the unmistakable forward slipping of the body of one vertebra on another.

Treatment.—For cases in which the symptoms are trivial, no treatment is indicated other than posture exercises, physical therapy, and precaution against overexercise or injury. Immobilization of the spine in a flexed position, by means of a plaster cast extending from the lower part of the thighs to above the costal margins, will relieve most of the acute pain. The cast should be followed by a back brace. In the milder cases an ambulatory plaster jacket or brace, together with posture exercises to strengthen the muscles of the back, may be adequate treatment.

When there is progressive increase of pain or recurrence of acute episodes of trauma which the patient cannot well avoid, operative fusion of the last two or three lumbar vertebrae to the sacrum is indicated. This should be followed by from six to twelve weeks of recumbency and then by a brace for a period of from six months to a year following the date of operation. The functional results are very satisfactory. In the rare cases in which there is evidence of pressure upon the cauda equina, laminectomy should be carried out.

1. C. Injuries of the Lumbar Intervertebral Disks

In the lower lumbar region, injury of an intervertebral disk with herniation of its nucleus pulposus into the spinal canal is a frequent cause of low back and sciatic pain. The same type of herniation of the nucleus pulposus may occur in the cervical spine with radiating pain into the shoulders and arms, and in the dorsal spine with radiating pain around the thorax. These herniations are observed much less frequently than those in the lumbar spine.

Etiology and Pathology.—Degenerative changes in the posterior longitudinal ligament and annulus fibrosus may weaken the periphery of the disk and predispose it to injury. In the most important type of disk lesion, the nucleus pulposus ruptures through a weak area of the annulus fibrosus, bulging into the anterolateral aspect of the spinal canal and compressing the nerve root at that level as it enters the intervertebral foramen. The disks between the fourth and fifth lumbar vertebrae and the fifth lumbar and sacrum are the most common sites of rupture. In many cases more than one disk is involved. Ruptures of the disks in the upper lumbar spine constitute only about 2 per cent of the cases. Early protrusions are not irreversible but may undergo spontaneous reduction. Considerable evidence suggests that traumatic and degenerative changes in the disks, without actual rupture, are an important cause of back pain.

Clinical Picture.—The greatest incidence is in healthy adults between the ages of thirty and forty. Men are affected twice as often as women. A majority of the patients recall an episode of trauma such as a lifting or pushing strain associated with the onset of symptoms. However, many give no history of injury. In many instances low back pain precedes the onset of lower extremity pain by months or years, sciatica coming on when the posterior protrusion of the disk becomes great enough to compress the nerve root. Usually the lower extremity pain is temporarily aggravated when intraspinal pressure is increased by coughing or sneezing. The symptoms are usually intermittent, recurrent attacks of severe pain being precipitated by episodes of minor trauma. The lower extremity pain may be accompanied by numbness and tingling.

The physical signs of spasm of the lumbar muscles, decrease of lumbosacral flexibility, and limitation of straight leg raising by pain are usually obvious. The lumbar lordosis may be decreased, and sciatic scoliosis due to muscle spasm may be present. Firm pressure over or beside the fifth or fourth spinous process will usually cause pain. Every patient who shows these low back signs should have a neurologic examination of the lower extremities. Common signs of nerve root pressure which suggest the diagnosis are diminution or loss of the ankle or knee jerk, a localized hypesthesia to pin prick, and slight weakness in dorsiflexing the ankle against resistance. In late cases atrophy of the muscles of the lower extremity may be obvious.

Diagnosis.—Presumptive diagnosis of intervertebral disk rupture is made on the history and physical findings. It must be remembered, however, that bony lesions about the intervertebral foramina or within the spinal canal or a thickened ligamentum flavum can cause an identical clinical picture. The most important entities requiring differentiation are ligamentous and muscular injuries of the low back, chronic arthritis, prespondylolisthesis and spondylolisthesis, and spinal cord tumors. The possibility that both a bony lesion and a disk lesion may be present must be kept in mind. According to some reported series, the roentgenogram shows a narrowing of the intervertebral space in a high percentage of the cases of ruptured disk. Roentgenographic visualization of the spinal canal with contrast media should be reserved for atypical cases. Only about two-thirds of the positive myelographic studies have been confirmed at operation.

Treatment.—In almost all cases treatment should begin with conservative measures designed to support the back and to relieve irritation of the nerve root. A plaster body jacket or a wide lumbosacral support or corset reinforced with a snug-fitting lumbar pad or shingle will often provide adequate relief and promote gradual recovery in several weeks' time. A firm mattress and fracture board often help by splinting the back at night. Heat and massage hasten symptomatic relief, and as the pain subsides special exercises should be started. The patient should be cautioned against sudden stooping, twisting, or lifting strains, and sometimes it is wise to have the patient change to a more sedentary occupation.

Patients who are not satisfactorily relieved after a thorough trial of conservative treatment should have excision of the protruding nucleus pulposus. The indications for surgical treatment are stronger (1) if the symptoms are severe, (2) if the extremity shows increasing atrophy of the muscles or other evidence of a progressive nerve lesion, (3) if the patient is young and vigorous and must return to strenuous physical activity, and (4) if the patient is not affected by psychoneurosis or medicolegal influences. The advisability of combining spinal fusion with excision of the disk must always be considered. The age and occupation of the patient and the strength of his low back structures as indicated by the clinical, roentgenographic, and operative findings are factors strongly influencing the decision. Some observers believe it is always advisable to fuse the spine if there is roentgenographic evidence of a congenital lumbosacral anomaly. Recent statistics show that excision of the disk accompanied by fusion is more often followed by complete and lasting relief of symptoms than is excision of the disk without fusion. However, only a very small percentage of the backs now operated upon for intervertebral disk rupture alone are being fused.

Prognosis.—Doubtless many cases of minor disk injury recover with little treatment. The majority of cases treated conservatively also improve satisfactorily, but in some instances the symptoms recur on subsequent trauma. In intractable cases the severe lower extremity pain can usually be cured or greatly reduced by excision of the disk. The combined operation of disk removal and spinal fusion may improve the prognosis for permanent relief of both the low back and the sciatic pain.

1. D. Herniation of Fascial Fat

Following a systematic survey of fibrositis in the lumbar and gluteal regions in 1944, a new concept of the cause of low back pain in some individuals was advanced by Copeman and Ackerman. Careful plotting of localized "trigger points" in a series of patients produced a definite "pain pattern". A thorough anatomic study revealed that this pattern was the same as the "basic fat pattern" which was constantly present, even in the most cachectic individuals in whom other fat was absent. It was noted that the "trigger points" with subjective pain might arise during any pyrexial illness or trauma, and that although the subjective pain disappeared, the trigger point, which could be detected by tenderness on palpation, remained.

Careful physical examination to localize the trigger point is essential. Palpation of, or pressure on, this area may reproduce complaints which have been severe enough to incapacitate the patient.

Surgical exploration of these trigger points has disclosed herniation of fat lobules through the neighboring fascial structures. The herniation has been of three types: (1) non-pedunculated, as, for instance, in the angle of the deep fascia where it splits to invest the sacrospinalis muscle, or along the crest of the ilium; (2) pedunculated, which is believed to be the late result of strangulation of a hernia originally of the non-pedunculated type; and (3) foraminal, found only along the edge of the sacrospinalis muscle where the posterior primary rami of the first, second, and third lumbar nerves pierce the deep fascia. Examination of the foraminal type has shown herniation where the nerve passes out together with a small artery and vein. Normally at these foramina are narrow folds of fascia which occlude the openings on flexion of the back. Herniation is thought to take place when the folds fail to function.

Pathologic study of the material excised at operation has shown lobulated masses of adipose tissue, and sometimes tough fibrous connective tissue showing evidence of edema and hemorrhage. Nerve tissue has been seen in some sections but is not a consistent finding.

Treatment.—Infiltration of the trigger point with procaine may bring complete relief of varying duration. A technique of "teasing" the lobule with the infiltrating needle, which results in releasing the constricting fascial bands or lobular capsule, has been described as effective in some cases. Excision of the herniated lobule, or of the fatty and fibrous tissue underlying the trigger point when a definite herniation cannot be found, is usually productive of lasting relief.

2. Common Osteoarticular Lesions of Infectious, Neoplastic, or Traumatic Nature

Specific pathologic conditions of the bones and joints, not limited necessarily to the lumbosacral or sacroiliac joints, often cause low back pain directly or lead to an impaired mechanical resistance which augments the incidence of sprain. Low-grade infections, neoplastic processes, and old fractures are examples. The commonest disease of this nature, however, is chronic osteoarthritis. In young adults, Strümpell-Marie arthritis is a frequent cause of low back pain. In stout individuals over forty years of age with proliferative bone changes about the joint margins, susceptibility to low back pain following acute or chronic strain is greatly increased, and the symptoms are likely to persist for long periods. Arthritic changes in the lower lumbar and lumbosacral articular facets constitute a common and important cause of low back pain and may be associated with pain which radiates to the legs. In women, low back pain is sometimes associated with a localized increase of density in the ilia adjacent to the sacroiliac joints; this condition has been called *osteitis condensans ilii*. In adolescents sacroiliac symptoms are sometimes associated with roentgenographic changes in the sacroiliac joint surfaces resembling bone destruction and suggestive of osteochondritis. The postural stresses associated with conditions such as flat feet or inequality of leg length may also predispose the individual to low back sprain.

3. Visceral Lesions With Pain Referred to the Low Back

Low back pain unassociated with local osteoarticular changes may be caused by any of a wide variety of visceral diseases. This pain, although located definitely over a bone or joint by the patient, is entirely of referred type. Pain referred to the low back is particularly common in the course of the following diseases:

1. *Gastrointestinal Diseases.*—Because of overloading of the colon with fecal matter, pain may be referred to the low back by irritation of the lumbar nerves. A spastic colon is occasionally the cause of pain in the low back. A wide variety of other gastrointestinal diseases,

including disorders of the duodenum, appendix and rectum, produce low back pain at times. Intra-abdominal adhesions and hernias also form a frequent source of discomfort referred to the low back.

2. *Urologic Diseases.*—Most of the diseases of the genitourinary tract may at times cause disabling low back pain. This is particularly true of the infections and tumors of the prostate gland.

3. *Gynecologic Diseases.*—That lesions of the female pelvic organs can cause low back pain has been established by studies of large series of cases. The exact frequency with which this occurs, however, is uncertain. Retroversion and retroflexion of the uterus appear to be frequent causes of pain in the sacral and lower lumbar regions.

4. *Lesions of the Central Nervous System.*—Tabes, meningitis, syringomyelia, lateral sclerosis, and similar conditions occasionally give rise to pain in the low back. Tumors of the spinal cord are often accompanied by low back pain. Tumors of the cauda equina are likely to be evidenced by pain radiating into one or both legs and by spasm of the hamstring muscles.

5. *Sciatic Neuritis.*—Primary sciatic neuritis, a rare affection, is usually accompanied by pain referred to the low back.

6. *Lesions of the Retroperitoneal Structures.*—Infections and tumors in the retroperitoneal area may cause pain in the low back.

7. *Generalized Infectious Diseases.*—Diseases such as influenza, undulant fever, and septicemia are often accompanied by pain in the low back.

Coccygodynia (Painful Coccyx)

Pain about the coccyx and lower part of the sacrum, or coccygodynia, is in most cases a result of sprain of the sacrococcygeal ligaments and often follows a direct blow or fall, such as may be occasioned by sitting down suddenly or sliding down a flight of stairs. It is sometimes caused by sitting for a long period on a hard surface. The pain is not always experienced immediately after the injury but may develop gradually later. Coccygodynia sometimes begins insidiously without evident trauma and may be a result simply of faulty posture. In some cases an inflammatory reaction within the pelvis may be the etiologic factor.

Clinical Picture.—There is usually an aching, nagging pain located near the sacrococcygeal junction. At times there may be shooting pains in the buttocks or even down into the legs. These pains are especially severe when the patient is sitting on a hard surface or when arising after sitting for any length of time. There may be considerable pain on defecation. The patient often complains of being nervous and irritable and may develop a psychoneurosis on account of the pain, with exaggeration of all symptoms. Examination shows a tender coccyx which on rectal examination is sometimes rough and angulated. It may be abnormally mobile or fixed.

Diagnosis.—The diagnosis, while not difficult, should be made with caution since pain in the coccygeal region is often associated with arthritis of the low back or with psychoneurosis. Roentgenograms occasionally show deviation of the coccyx forward or to one side as a result of either injury or developmental variation.

Treatment.—In acute traumatic cases showing displacement of the coccyx, the deformity may be reduced by gentle manipulation, especially if the coccyx has been angulated forward and its motion appears to be restricted. Hot baths, strapping of the low back, and massage may afford considerable relief. The patient should be instructed to sit on cushions or soft chairs. Occasionally, however, sitting upon cushions which are very soft may cause the buttocks to spread and may thus increase the pain. The use of a large rubber ring is sometimes indicated to relieve the pressure occasioned by sitting. An alternative method is to have the patient sit on a firm cushion which is placed forward in the chair. The application of a thick piece of felt, with an opening cut out over the coccyx to prevent pressure, is another method of treatment. All exercise which increases the pain should be avoided.

If the pain cannot be relieved by nonoperative measures, excision of the coccyx, which can be carried out very simply, will often relieve the patient of all symptoms. Before resort is made to operation, however, great care should be taken to remove all contributing causes of the discomfort, since in occasional cases the diagnosis is somewhat uncertain and the relief of pain following operation is incomplete. If a psychoneurosis is present, it should be treated before surgery is contemplated.

Comment.—There can be no doubt that the present treatment of low back pain is not uniformly satisfactory. In many cases the symptoms are unnecessarily prolonged because of poor judgment on the part of the physician in not insisting upon rest of the back in the acute stage, with efficient support and gradual resumption of activity. Many unnecessary operative fusions for low back pain are performed because of the urgeon's unwillingness to carry out efficient conservative therapy. On he other hand, fusion is frequently done for economic reasons, since the patient cannot afford a long period of conservative care and must be protected against the possibility of recurrence when he resumes his occupation. In such instances operation is unquestionably indicated. One cannot be too cautious, however, in operating upon the back of a patient who has a compensation or insurance claim pending, who shows any evidence of an abnormal psychosomatic state, or who is in the military service.

There is no doubt also that many unorthodox practitioners of medicine and members of the medical cults thrive on the common failure of physicians to appreciate the proper treatment of low back pain. Most of the work of this group involves manipulation to break up adhesions and so relieve pain. The patient is told that a dislocated joint or bone has been put back into place, a statement which makes a profound impression on the layman's mind. Much misunderstanding on the part of the patient will be avoided if the physician can recognize and explain carefully to the patient the true nature of the problems involved in the treatment of low back pain.

CHAPTER XX

AFFECTIONS OF THE HIP

Introduction.—The ball-and-socket structure of the hip joint permits of a wide range of motion which is exceeded by no other joint the body except the shoulder. At the same time a remarkable degree of stability is provided by the close fit of the femoral head into the acetabulum and its deepening lip, the cotyloid cartilage and by the support of the strongest capsular ligaments and the thickest musculature of the body. Of all the joints the hip is most deeply situated. This relative inaccessibility increases the difficulty of diagnosing hip lesions, render thorough operative exposure of the joint arduous, and so plays a large part in making affections of the hip a major part of orthopaedic surgery.

The especial affections of the hip which are discussed in this chapter can be grouped conveniently according to the location of the lesion. *Coxa plana* and *slipping of the upper femoral epiphysis* are common and important entities characterized by pathologic changes in the epiphysis or at the epiphyseal line. *Congenital coxa vara* and *coxa valga* marked by alterations in the angle of femoral neck to femoral shaft, a less common. *Pathologic dislocation of the hip* and *intrapelvic protrusion of the acetabulum* are characterized by a changed relationship between femur and pelvis. To be remembered also in the diagnosis of hip affections are lesions of the soft tissues, which include *synovitis, bursitis, and snapping hip.*

Coxa Plana (Legg-Perthes' Disease, Avascular Necrosis of the Capital Femoral Epiphysis, Flat-Headed Femur)

Coxa plana is a flattening of the epiphysis of the head of the femur due to osseous changes without primary involvement of the articular cartilage. It was described in 1909 by Legg of Boston and by Waldenstrom in Sweden, and in 1910 by Calvé in France and Perthes Germany. Before the affection was recognized as an independent entity these cases were believed to represent a mild form of tuberculosis of the hip.

Coxa plana occurs in children between the ages of three and twelve years and is found much more commonly in boys than in girls. It is seen most frequently in children who are of stocky, heavy type but who are otherwise normal. It is sometimes bilateral.

Etiology.—The cause of the pathologic changes occurring in coxa plana has not been definitely established. Because of the predominance in boys, it is the author's opinion that a sex hormone is the most likely underlying cause. Most observers believe that trauma or strain is a primary factor. Slight injury of the femoral head, resulting in a disturbance of the circulation between epiphysis and femoral neck, may be responsible. Chronic infection of low grade has been cited as an etiologic factor because occasionally a staphylococcus has been cultured from the joint or the epiphysis. Sometimes children exhibit a partial subluxation of the hip as a result of an unusual shallowness of the acetabulum and an increase in the anteversion of the neck of the femur; it has been supposed that weight-bearing on abnormal joint structures of this kind may result in a flattening of the head of the femur.

Pathology.—Massive subchondral necrosis of the bone and marrow of the entire epiphysis of the femoral head takes place. This is followed by disintegration and absorption of the dead bone and its replacement by granulation tissue. Finally collapse of the head occurs, producing a characteristic flattening deformity. As new bone is formed, healing takes place and the fragmented areas become reorganized into a smooth regular mass of bone, which never, however, regains the shape and appearance of a completely normal epiphysis. The articular cartilage usually remains smooth. The synovial membrane and capsule become thickened. The ligamentum teres may undergo either atrophy or hypertrophy; its blood vessels usually show obliterative changes as healing takes place.

Clinical Picture.—The most constant early sign is a limp, which is associated with muscular spasm and may or may not be accompanied by pain. The pain is often referred to the inner side of the thigh or knee. As the disease progresses, the limp persists and may become more severe. The hip suffers slight limitation of all motions, and particularly of internal rotation and abduction. In rare instances all of the symptoms may be exaggerated and the disability may be severe. A moderate flexion and adduction deformity with prominence of the greater trochanter may develop. There is atrophy of the muscles of the hip, thigh, and leg. Thickening of the joint capsule is sometimes palpable, giving a boggy

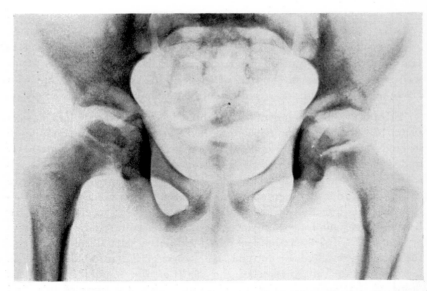

Fig. 148A.—Roentgenogram showing coxa plana (Legg-Perthes disease) of the right hip in a boy five years of age. Note irregularity and increased density of capital femoral epiphysis.

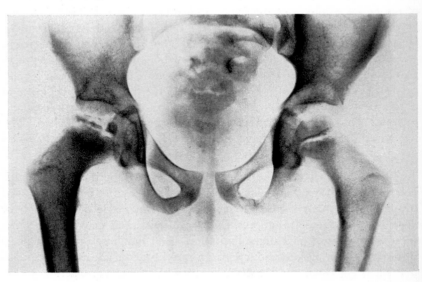

Fig. 148B.—Roentgenogram showing coxa plana of the right hip (same case as Fig. 148A), nine months later. Note fragmentation of epiphysis with areas of absorption and widening of the neck of the femur. Treatment was rest in bed and traction.

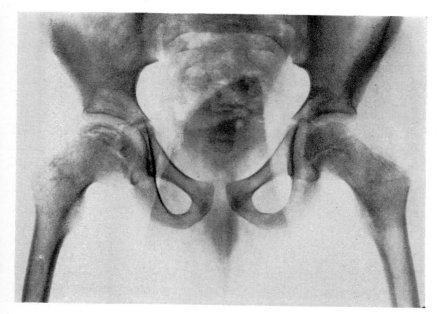

Fig. 148C.—Roentgenogram showing coxa plana of the right hip (same case as Fig. 148A), four years later. Note regeneration of capital epiphysis with rounding of head and recalcification which is not yet complete. Widening of neck and recalcified epiphysis is quite marked.

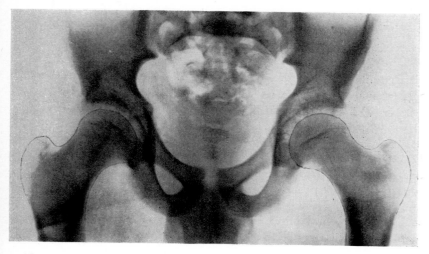

Fig. 148D.—Roentgenogram showing coxa plana of the right hip (same case as Fig. 148A), seven and one-half years later. Note well-formed, smooth, rounded head of femur with almost normal-appearing epiphysis and neck as compared with left hip. (Outlines of heads and necks have been retouched.)

feel, and usually slight shortening of the leg is demonstrable. During the stage of repair the signs and symptoms become less severe and the hip may appear almost normal. Later in life, however, the hip may show evidence of a degenerative process which has the appearance of an osteoarthritis (*malum coxae senilis,* page 228).

Roentgenographic Picture.—The stages of degeneration and repair can be visualized by roentgenographic examinations (Figs. 148*A* to 148*D*). Small areas of resorption appear in the femoral neck adjacent to the epiphyseal plate. In early cases the epiphysis shows thinning or flattening and in some instances definite fragmentation. Within the head appear dense areas which become less conspicuous as healing takes place. The neck becomes very broad and short and may present a coxa vara. The acetabulum changes in shape to correspond with the deformity of the femoral head. Two distinct types of deformity of the head are observed: (1) the *cap type,* in which the head of the femur has the appearance of a jockey cap, and (2) the *mushroom type,* in which the entire head is flattened. During the stage of fragmentation the epiphysis may appear to break into several parts, and later, during the stage of repair, these can be seen to coalesce into a single mass of healing bone. Flattening and broadening of the head may cause it to protrude laterally from the acetabulum.

Diagnosis.—Coxa plana is to be differentiated from early tuberculosis, rheumatoid arthritis, synovitis, slipping of the upper femoral epiphysis, congenital dysplasia of the hip, and congenital coxa vara.

Prognosis.—Coxa plana is a self-limited disease with a constant tendency toward spontaneous recovery. The prognosis in the mushroom type of head is better than that in the cap type. It is more favorable in younger children than in older. It has been repeatedly demonstrated that relieving the strain of weight-bearing by means of traction, recumbency in plaster or splints, or crutches during the stages of degeneration and repair minimizes the progressive distortion of the head. The symptoms may disappear but further flattening of the head is likely to develop and persist. The functional end result when weight-bearing is prevented may be almost normal, but, on the other hand, there may be a permanent limp and restriction of hip motion.

Treatment.—The primary consideration is rest, particularly from the strain of weight-bearing. When pain, muscle spasm, or deformity is present, skin traction is indicated. Rest in bed should be continued until there is no pain or muscle spasm on motion and until there is definite roentgenographic evidence of repair. The hip should then be protected either by the use of a Thomas walking caliper splint which allows no weight-bearing through the hip joint, by the use of crutches accompanied by a high-sole shoe on the sound leg, or by the use of a sling from the lower leg of the affected side to the shoulder of the same side, allowing weight-bearing on the sound leg with crutches. In some clinics skin traction in bed is continued until roentgenographic evidence of nearly complete repair is present, which may be as long as twelve to twenty-four months. Following this treatment, strenuous activity involving weight-bearing should be avoided until the roentgenograms indicate that an end stage of repair has been reached. It is probable that healing is to some extent delayed by the use of plaster spica casts and traction braces because of the resultant bone atrophy. Drilling of the femoral head in order to effect revascularization has been recommended as leading to an earlier and more complete repair, but the end results have not proved this procedure to be of value. Operative measures which can be expected to afford most relief from pain in the adult with severe disability are (1) a reconstruction operation, (2) a subtrochanteric osteotomy, or (3) an arthrodesis.

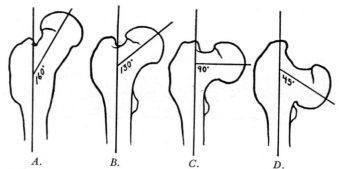

A.   B.   C.   D.

Fig. 149.—Angles of femoral neck to shaft. A, coxa valga; B, normal; C, moderate coxa vara; D, severe coxa vara.

Coxa Vara

Coxa vara is an abnormality of the upper end of the femur, consisting of a decrease in the angle of the shaft to the neck (angle of inclination) and hence resulting in a shortening of the extremity (Fig.

149). All cases of coxa vara can be classified according to whether the primary anatomic change is in the neck (*cervical*), in the head (*epiphyseal*), or in both neck and head (*cervico-epiphyseal*).

Etiology.—Coxa vara may be congenital or acquired. The acquired form is by far the more common. It may develop as a result of one of the following affections of growing or adult bone: rickets, osteomalacia, and osteitis deformans; or as a result of one of the following diseases: osteomyelitis, pyogenic epiphysitis, arthritis, and tuberculosis. It may occur also in the end stages of coxa plana or of congenital dislocation of the hip with or without reduction. Acquired coxa vara may also follow a slipping of the capital femoral epiphysis, an intertrochanteric fracture of the femur which has not been properly reduced, or a greenstick fracture of the neck of the femur in childhood.

Congenital coxa vara is of especial interest and importance and will be discussed as a separate entity.

Congenital Coxa Vara

Congenital coxa vara is usually first observed in early childhood but may not be recognized until later in life. It is usually bilateral and of the cervical type. It is sometimes associated with other congenital defects, especially in the femur.

Etiology.—Congenital coxa vara may be a primary developmental anomaly or may be secondary to some intrauterine affection of bone, such as achondroplasia.

Clinical Picture.—Often the first evidences of the affection appear after an episode of slight trauma. The complaint may be that of weakness and stiffness in the leg together with an awkward gait or a definite limp. The range of abduction and internal rotation is usually restricted, while that of external rotation and adduction may be increased. A deformity characterized by prominence of the greater trochanter and external rotation of the leg may develop. The amount of actual shortening depends upon the extent of the depression of head and neck of the femur on the shaft; it is usually from 2 to 4 cm. Atrophy of the muscles is always marked. There is usually little or no associated pain. At times all of the discomfort is referred to the thigh or knee.

In bilateral coxa vara there may be a characteristic gait, the so-called "duck waddle," in which the body sways from side to side.

Roentgenographic Picture.—In the young child, in addition to the decrease of the angle of the head and neck to the shaft of the femur, a most characteristic roentgenographic change is the demarcation of a triangular area of bone in the lower side of the neck close to the head. The epiphyseal line lies on one side of this area, and across the neck on the other side is an abnormal band of decreased density. The head of the femur is situated low in an acetabulum which is often shallow and sloping and which may appear abnormally wide (Fig. 150A).

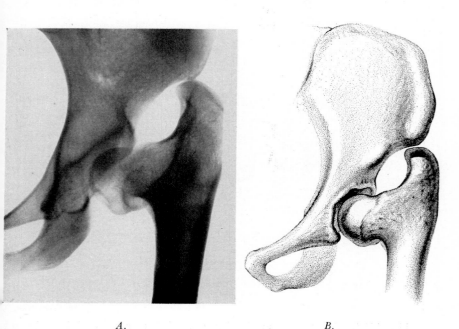

A.   *B.*

Fig. 150.—Congenital coxa vara in adult. Note acute angle between femoral neck and shaft, extreme elongation of the greater trochanter, and shallowness of the acetabulum. *A*, Roentgenogram; *B*, Drawing from roentgenogram.

In older cases the depression of the head and neck on the shaft becomes more marked, and the triangular area of bone fuses to the neck to assume the appearance of a dependent lip. There is usually a marked upward prominence of the greater trochanter and upper part of the shaft (Figs. 150A and 150B).

Diagnosis.—The diagnosis is made from the clinical picture together with the roentgenographic evidence of decrease in the angle of the neck of the femur to its shaft.

Differential Diagnosis.—Tuberculosis, slipping of the capital femoral epiphysis, congenital dislocation or subluxation of the hip, and coxa plana must be carefully differentiated from congenital coxa vara.

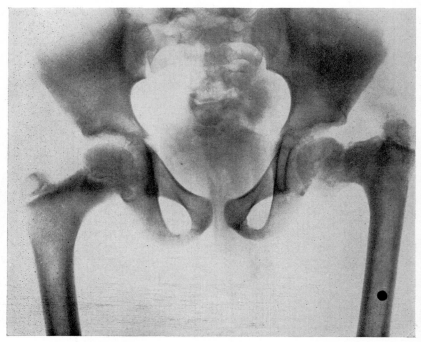

Fig. 151*A*.—Roentgenogram showing congenital coxa vara of left hip in boy eleven years of age. The neck-shaft angle of the left femur is 75 degrees as compared with 120 degrees on the right. Note distortion of the epiphysis and neck with prominence of greater trochanter. Left leg is one inch shorter than right leg.

Treatment.—When there is little deformity, protection of the hip against the strain of weight-bearing constitutes adequate treatment and active motion may be allowed. Drilling of the femoral neck and epiphysis in congenital coxa vara has been reported to retard progression of the deformity. If practicable, the hip should be kept in an abducted position. When the deformity is severe, it may be advisable to manipulate the hip under anesthesia and to immobilize it in plaster in full abduction, internal rotation, and extension. After three weeks the immobilization should be followed for a period of from three to six months by the use of a caliper brace to protect the hip from strain during walking. Fixed adduction deformity should be corrected by a cuneiform osteotomy through the neck or subtrochanteric area (Figs. 151*A* and 151*B*). The author prefers a subtrochanteric osteotomy. In advanced cases with disability late in life, a reconstruction operation or arthrodesis is indicated for the relief of pain.

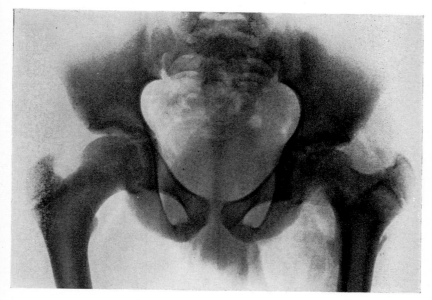

Fig. 151*B*.—Roentgenogram showing congenital coxa vara of the left hip (same case as Fig. 151*A*), three years following subtrochanteric osteotomy. Neck-shaft angle is now 120 degrees on the left and 125 degrees on the right. Note continued prominence of the left greater trochanter. Leg length is equal.

Slipping of the Capital Femoral Epiphysis (Epiphyseal or Adolescent Coxa Vara, Epiphyseolysis)

Slipping of the upper femoral epiphysis is most often observed in children between ten and sixteen years of age, is more common in boys than in girls, and may be unilateral or bilateral. In most cases a history of trauma or strain can be elicited, but the traumatic episode is often trivial and the possibility of a low-grade infection at the epiphyseal line cannot be excluded. Slipping of the upper femoral epiphysis occurs in two types of children: (1) fat children with undeveloped sexual characteristics (*Fröhlich's syndrome* or *endocrine type*) and (2) very tall,

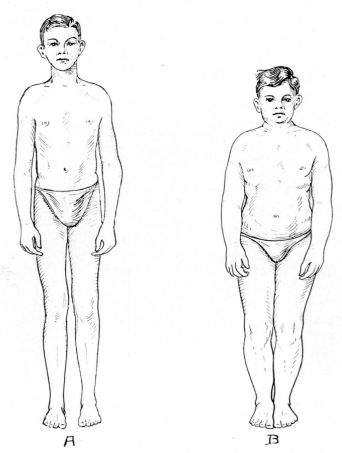

Fig. 152.—Types of children in whom slipping of the upper femoral epiphysis is most often observed: *A*, tall and slender; *B*, obese (Fröhlich's syndrome).

thin children (Fig. 152). A great many of these patients give a history of rapid skeletal growth immediately preceding displacement of the epiphysis.

In all cases a vascular disturbance at the epiphyseal line presumably precedes the epiphyseal displacement, but an endocrine disturbance is probably the main causative factor. Some observers are of the opinion that the cause is an imbalance between the pituitary growth hormone and the sex hormones. Slipping of the epiphysis may follow increased strain without obvious trauma, as occurs in the extremely obese child. As a result of trauma, which may be of any degree from slight to violent, the epiphysis may be completely loosened and displaced. The head of the femur becomes displaced downward and backward on the neck (Fig. 153), which retains its normal angle but which later may show evidence of torsion. When trauma is the exciting cause, the deformity is usually unilateral; cases not precipitated by an episode of trauma are often bilateral. Forty per cent of the cases are bilateral. Some observers believe that trauma alone never can cause the slipping, but that there first must be a disturbance of bone formation at the epiphyseal line.

Clinical Picture.—When there is no history of trauma, the onset is usually very gradual, the early symptoms being fatigue after walking or standing and later a slight amount of pain, stiffness, and a limp. The diagnosis should be suspected in any adolescent who has these symptoms and shows a slight restriction of internal rotation of the hip. After trauma the symptoms may either develop immediately or come on gradually. The degree of trauma apparently has little effect on the extent of the disability. The affected extremity gradually becomes shorter and smaller, and the range of motion, especially of internal rotation and abduction, becomes restricted. Hyperextension may be more easily carried out on the affected side than on the normal. When the affected hip is flexed, it tends to abduct and rotate externally. When the displacement of the epiphysis is marked, the leg assumes a position of flexion, abduction, and external rotation. At first the discomfort may consist of referred pain in the knee, but later the pain is located in the hip. There is usually pain about the anterior aspect of the hip when the limits of its range of motion are reached. Tenderness may be present about the anterior and lateral aspects of the hip.

Roentgenographic Picture.—Four roentgenographic stages of the affection have been described: viz., preslipped, slipped, quiescent, and residual. In the early stages the epiphyseal line is abnormally wide and irregular. Slipping can sometimes be recognized in the lateral roentgenogram before it becomes apparent in the anteroposterior view. When slipping has taken place, there is noted a displacement of the neck upward and forward on the head of the femur so that the lowest point of the proximal end of the neck projects as a beaklike process (Fig. 153). There is evidence of slight torsion in the neck. The upper part of the neck is lengthened, the lower part is shortened, and the whole neck becomes bowed and exhibits coxa vara. New bone may form between the lower border of the neck and the overhanging head. In advanced stages the femoral head appears quite atrophic, especially in its lower half, and the neck is very thick and short. When the trauma has been severe, the roentgenogram may demonstrate complete separation of the head from the neck of the femur.

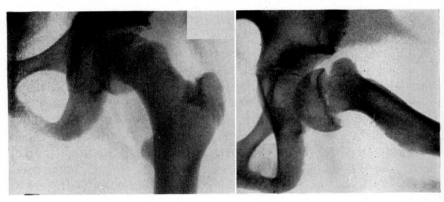

A.   *B.*

Fig. 153.—Anteroposterior (*A*) and lateral (*B*) roentgenograms showing slipping of upper femoral epiphysis in girl eleven years of age. Note upward slipping of the neck of the femur. The head has become displaced downward and also backward.

Diagnosis.—Slipping of the upper femoral epiphysis is to be differentiated from early tuberculosis of the hip, coxa plana, congenital coxa vara, subacute infectious processes, and fracture. Roentgenograms are necessary to establish the diagnosis; a lateral view is essential in addition to the usual anteroposterior film.

Treatment.—The object of treatment is to correct the displacement with a minimum of trauma and to maintain the correction until bony union between neck and epiphysis has taken place. In some early

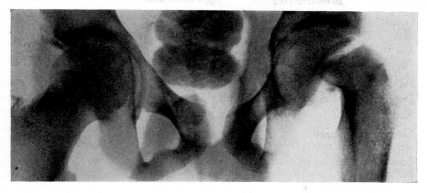

Fig. 154*A*.—Anteroposterior roentgenogram showing slipped capital femoral epiphysis of the left hip in a boy fourteen years of age. Note upward displacement of neck of femur.

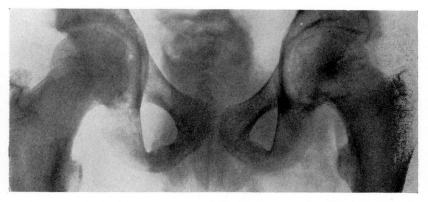

Fig. 154*B*.—Roentgenogram showing slipped capital femoral epiphysis of the left hip (same case as Fig. 154*A*), two months after reduction by skeletal traction and closed manipulation. Note almost normal relationship between capital epiphysis and neck of the femur.

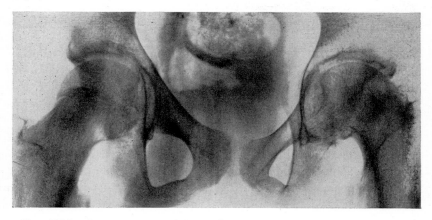

Fig. 154*C*.—Roentgenogram showing slipped capital femoral epiphysis of the left hip, eighteen months following reduction. Note that the epiphyseal line has completely disappeared on the left, but there is some deformity present. The motion in the left hip was approximately 50 per cent normal.

cases traction, preferably skeletal, in a position of slight abduction and internal rotation for approximately two weeks will reduce the displacement. In the early case with moderate or severe displacement of the epiphysis, reduction may sometimes be accomplished by the same maneuver which is used for the reduction of a fracture of the neck of the femur, viz., upward traction with the hip and knee flexed, followed by gradual extension, full abduction, and internal rotation (Figs. 154A, 154B, and 154C). Forceful manipulation is contraindicated by the danger of causing serious intra-articular damage. The corrected alignment can be maintained by means of prolonged traction, by a hip spica cast with the hip extended, abducted, and internally rotated, or by the insertion of the three-flanged nail of Smith-Petersen or the multiple pins of Moore or Knowles. Drilling across the epiphyseal line is sometimes carried out in an effort to hasten consolidation.

In the preslipping stage, which can be recognized roentgenographically by a widening and irregularity of the epiphyseal line, internal fixation by wires or pins, or immobilization in plaster for a twelve-week period is indicated. When weight-bearing is allowed, a Thomas walking caliper splint may be used for protection of the hip. At times it may be preferable to use a high-sole shoe on the normal leg and crutches for several months.

Cases with only slight displacement (less than 1 cm. in both anteroposterior and lateral roentgenograms) which is not corrected by a trial period of traction should be treated in the same way as those in the preslipping stage, no attempt being made to correct slight degrees of deformity by manipulation or operation.

Forceful manipulation of the hip in the late case is usually inadvisable because of the danger of causing further interference with the blood supply of the epiphysis. For the same reason open reduction should be avoided when possible. In late cases with severe deformity the function of the hip can often be improved by a transcervical or a subtrochanteric osteotomy. In still later cases in adult years, a reconstruction operation or an arthrodesis is sometimes indicated.

If the patient is obese, his weight should be reduced. A well-balanced, multi-vitamin diet is always indicated. In all degrees of slipping, rest of the hip and protection from weight-bearing are important. The opposite hip should be watched for any clinical or roentgenographic sign of early slipping since bilateral involvement is common.

Prognosis.—Cases with slight slipping treated early have a favorable prognosis. Late cases with severe displacement often have a permanent disability after any form of treatment.

Coxa Valga

Coxa valga is an increase in the angle of the neck of the femur to its shaft, in contrast to coxa vara which is a decrease of this angle (Fig. 149). Coxa valga tends to produce an increase in the length of the extremity.

Etiology.—Coxa valga is most often of congenital origin. The condition is always present in infants before weight-bearing is begun. It is sometimes found in association with rickets, infantile paralysis, cerebral palsy, pseudohypertrophic muscular dystrophy, congenital dislocation of the hip (Fig. 28), and any affection of infancy and childhood which has prevented normal weight-bearing. In occasional cases coxa valga is thought to be a result of injury.

Clinical Picture.—In extreme cases there is an awkward gait and the thigh is outwardly rotated and abducted. When roentgenograms are being made, the extremity should be held in a neutral position as regards rotation.

Treatment.—Therapy should be directed toward lessening the limitation of adduction. In most cases, however, no treatment is required. The hip may be manipulated under anesthesia, forced into an attitude of adduction, and immobilized in plaster. In rare instances an osteotomy to decrease the angle of the neck of the femur to its shaft may be indicated. If the patient has not borne weight on the leg and there is no reason for his not bearing weight, he should be encouraged to stand and to walk.

Pathologic Dislocation of the Hip

Pathologic dislocation of the hip is not a specific disease entity but is a complication of many affections of the hip. It develops as a result of (1) erosion of bone about the acetabulum, the femoral head, or both, or (2) paralysis of the muscles and relaxation of the other soft tissues around the hip joint. In most cases the head of the femur becomes displaced upward and posteriorly.

Etiology.—Tuberculosis of the hip, in which gradual erosion of the acetabulum and destruction of the head of the femur may take place, results often in pathologic dislocation of the hip (Fig. 76*B*). Dislocation often follows pyogenic arthritis or osteomyelitis of the upper end of the femur. In these conditions the dislocation is in large part due to relaxation of the ligamentous supports following distension of the joint capsule by fluid; the relaxed ligaments allow displacement of the head of the femur to the dorsum of the ilium. Pathologic dislocation is occasionally seen in infantile paralysis and cerebral palsy. It may follow the general muscular atrophy of prolonged febrile illness. Occasionally it may accompany rheumatoid arthritis or neuropathic arthropathy. Flexion and adduction of the hip, accompanied by pain, are important factors leading to dislocation.

Treatment.—Preventive therapy is imperative. The possibility of dislocation should be anticipated and should be guarded against by preventing flexion and adduction. If there is likelihood of displacement, the leg should be kept in traction. As soon as a dislocation is recognized, it should be corrected. Occasionally before reduction can be accomplished, it may be necessary to remove by open operation the fibrous material which has filled the acetabulum. In some cases in which the dislocation cannot be reduced, it is advisable to displace the femoral head anteriorly, since this increases the stability of the joint. In selected cases a subtrochanteric osteotomy, a Lorenz bifurcation operation, or a reconstruction operation may be desirable. A shelf operation (Fig. 29) often provides satisfactory stability and is sometimes indicated in dislocation following paralysis. In many cases arthrodesis is the procedure of choice.

Intrapelvic Protrusion of the Acetabulum (Arthrokatadysis, Otto Pelvis, Protrusio Acetabuli)

Intrapelvic protrusion of the acetabulum is an uncommon affection of undetermined etiology. In some cases it is of congenital or familial origin. In other instances it is probably secondary to common affections such as rheumatoid or low-grade pyogenic arthritis. It is characterized by a deepening or inward protrusion of the acetabulum which allows the head of the femur to project farther into the pelvis than normally (Fig. 155). The roentgenograms usually show thinning and eburnation of the walls of the acetabulum, but occasionally there is evidence of increased bone formation. There may be narrowing of the joint space and absorption of cartilage. Usually little change occurs in the head of the femur, but occasionally it is irregular or enlarged. Some observers believe that the thinning of the acetabular wall is a late result of osteochondritis of the acetabulum in youth. The affection is found more often in females than in males and may be either bilateral or unilateral. The youngest reported patient was eight years old. This affection is frequently observed in the Negro race.

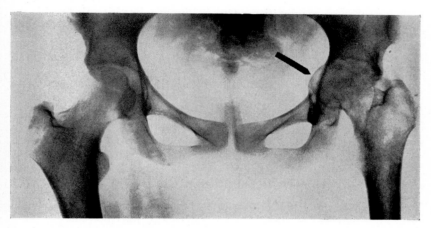

Fig. 155.—Roentgenogram showing intrapelvic protrusion of the acetabulum (protrusio acetabuli) in the left hip in a girl fourteen years of age. (Courtesy Childrens Seashore House, Atlantic City, N. J.)

Clinical Picture.—Limitation of motion develops gradually over a period of years. Abduction and rotation are especially restricted. There may be little or no pain except when osteoarthritic changes are superimposed. In the end stage, ankylosis of the hip usually results.

Treatment.—Little treatment is indicated unless the deformity is accompanied by pain, in which event rest and traction for several weeks, followed by the use of a Thomas walking caliper splint, may result in symptomatic improvement. Night traction may be used for a long period. If disabling pain persists, arthrodesis or arthroplasty may be indicated.

Synovitis of the Hip

Etiology.—Synovitis of the hip is usually caused by an injury or strain of the joint. It may be associated with structural changes, such as those found in coxa plana, or may possibly be the result of a low-grade infectious process with superimposed strain. It occurs most often in children.

Clinical Picture.—There is usually pain upon pressure anteriorly or over the greater trochanter. Muscle spasm is a constant finding. A limp is usually associated. The hip is often held in a flexed and abducted position although it may be adducted.

Diagnosis.—Synovitis of the hip joint is to be distinguished from acute or subacute epiphysitis and from iliopsoas bursitis. In bursitis the characteristic localization of the pain and tenderness is helpful in making the differentiation. Osteomyelitis, pyogenic arthritis, tuberculosis, coxa plana, and slipping of the upper femoral epiphysis must also be ruled out before the diagnosis can be made.

Treatment.—For both acute and chronic cases rest and hot applications are indicated. When the pain is severe, fixation in traction, followed by a plaster cast, may be advisable. Synovitis is not in itself serious and usually clears up rapidly. If there is a more serious underlying lesion of the hip, however, the synovitis may recur.

Bursitis in the Region of the Hip

Eighteen or more bursae about the hip have been described, but of these only four are of clinical importance (Fig. 156).

1. **The iliopectineal or iliopsoas bursa** is located between the iliopsoas muscle and the iliopectineal eminence, on the anterior surface of the hip joint capsule, and frequently communicates with the joint cavity.

Clinical Picture.—Tenderness is usually present over the anterior aspect of the hip at about the middle of the inguinal ligament. Pain caused by pressure upon the femoral nerve in this area may radiate down the front of the leg. The hip is usually held in flexion, abduction, and external rotation. Pain is elicited upon attempting to extend, adduct, or internally rotate the hip.

Diagnosis.—Femoral hernia, psoas abscess pointing in the groin, synovitis, and infections of the hip joint are to be considered in the differential diagnosis.

Treatment.—The patient should be placed at rest in bed with traction applied to the lower extremity. Hot applications should be placed over the area of tenderness on the anterior aspect of the hip. If the bursa is acutely inflamed, antibiotic therapy should be used. The bursitis usually subsides completely within several weeks.

2. **The deep trochanteric bursa** is located behind the greater trochanter and in front of the insertion of the gluteus maximus muscle.

When the deep trochanteric bursa is enlarged, the normal depression behind the greater trochanter is completely obliterated. At this point there may be marked tenderness. The leg is usually held in an abducted and externally rotated position, which relaxes the tension upon the gluteus maximus muscle. Pain may radiate down the back of the thigh, and any motion of the hip joint may cause discomfort.

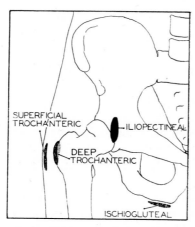

Fig. 156.—Most commonly affected bursae about the hip.

Deep trochanteric bursitis is to be differentiated from infection of the hip joint and from osteomyelitis of the upper end of the femur.

When a pyogenic infection is present, treatment with an antibiotic is indicated. When suppuration has not occurred, rest and heat constitute adequate treatment. For tuberculous infection complete excision of the bursa is advisable.

3. **The superficial trochanteric bursa** is located between the greater trochanter and the skin.

Tenderness and swelling may be present over the bursa, but there is no pain on motion of the leg.

The therapy is the same as that outlined for deep trochanteric bursitis.

4. **The ischiogluteal bursa** is located superficial to the tuberosity of the ischium. Chronic ischiogluteal bursitis is sometimes spoken of as "weaver's bottom." It develops in tailors, boatmen, and other individuals whose occupation necessitates prolonged sitting upon hard surfaces.

Tenderness over the tuberosity of the ischium is constant, and there may be pain radiating down the back of the thigh along the course of the hamstring muscles.

If the inflammation is not severe, heat and rest will usually cause the symptoms to subside. Procaine injections may be helpful. Persistence of pain, however, indicates complete excision of the bursa.

Snapping Hip

Snapping hip is an uncommon affection. With the knee flexed, active internal rotation of the hip will sometimes give rise to a snapping noise. It may be present with every step. It is caused by the slipping to and fro over the greater trochanter of a fibrous band on the deep surface of the gluteus maximus muscle. The snapping can seldom be heard with passive motion. It is not always associated with pain but may, at times, be very annoying to neurotic patients who have a tendency to overemphasize all symptoms.

Treatment.—Sometimes immobilization of the hip in plaster will lead to complete subsidence of the symptoms. In order to obtain permanent relief, however, it is often necessary to divide the tendinous band; it may then be sutured to the underlying structures or behind the greater trochanter. The symptomatic results are not always satisfactory, especially if the condition has been present for a long time.

CHAPTER XXI

AFFECTIONS OF THE KNEE

Introduction.—The knee is the largest joint in the body. In general it is hingelike in character, and its stability is dependent upon (1) an intricate group of strong ligaments and (2) the supporting muscles and tendons. The motions of the knee joint are an extensive anteroposterior, rotatory gliding movement and a very limited rotation of the flexed tibia upon the femur. Flexion of the knee takes place actually between the semilunar cartilages and the femur. Rotation has been shown to take place between the semilunar cartilages and the tibia.

The knee joint is formed by the articulation of the two rounded condyles of the femur with two shallow depressions in the tibia which are also called condyles. Between the condyles of the tibia is the tibial spine, which divides to form medial and lateral tubercles. Immediately anterior to the tibial spine is a flattened triangular area on the antero-superior aspect of the tibia, at the base of which lies the tibial tuberosity. On either side of the joint are strong collateral ligaments which prevent lateral displacement, and behind the knee is the posterior ligament which forms the floor of the popliteal space. Between the corresponding condyles of femur and tibia are semilunar cartilages or menisci, each of which acts as a wedge-shaped cushion between the tibia and femur and helps to maintain tension in the two cruciate ligaments. The cruciate ligaments extend from the intercondylar notch of the femur to the upper surface of the tibia. The anterior cruciate ligament prevents forward displacement of the tibia, and the posterior cruciate ligament prevents backward displacement. The synovial membrane constitutes the lining of the joint and is continued above into a large anterior pocket called the suprapatellar bursa or quadriceps pouch. Behind the patellar ligament and projecting into the anterior portion of the joint is the infrapatellar fat pad, which is extrasynovial and changes shape with every movement of the joint. This pad is connected with the inter-condylar notch of the femur by the ligamentum mucosum. About the joint, in addition to the tendons and muscles, are bursae, blood vessels, and nerves.

Internal Derangements of the Knee Joint

This term is commonly applied to those intra- and extra-articular affections of the knee, most often of traumatic origin, which are the result of lesions of the semilunar cartilages, the joint surfaces, the ligaments, the fat pads, or the synovial membrane. The more common derangements include (1) lesions of the semilunar cartilages, (2) rupture of the internal and external lateral ligaments, (3) rupture of the cruciate ligaments, (4) injury of the tibial spine, (5) loose bodies, osteochondritis dissecans, and synovial chondromas, (6) hypertrophy and pinching of the infrapatellar fat pad and synovial membrane, and (7) exostoses.

1. Lesions of the Semilunar Cartilages

Displacements and tears of the semilunar cartilages constitute by far the most frequent type of internal derangement of the knee joint. The internal cartilage is injured from five to fifteen times as frequently as the external; the reasons for this are two: (1) a difference in structure, the inner cartilage being longer, less securely attached, and bifurcated at its anterior pole; and (2) a difference in etiology, the mechanism of injury which causes damage of the internal cartilage being more common than that which affects the external. It is convenient to consider the etiology and symptomatology of injuries of each cartilage separately.

A. Injuries of the Internal Semilunar Cartilage

Etiology.—Derangement of the internal semilunar cartilage is usually caused by a sudden internal rotation of the femur upon the fixed tibia while the knee is abducted and flexed. The damage occurs most frequently about the anterior portion of the cartilage. A greater degree of knee flexion at the instant of injury causes the tear to be situated nearer the posterior end of the cartilage. If the anterior portion of the cartilage is torn and slips into the joint, it may lodge between the joint surfaces, prevent complete extension, and give rise to so-called "locking." If the rotary strain is severe, the connection between the cartilage and the internal lateral ligament may be torn, allowing the cartilage to slip into the joint. With extension of the knee the free border of the cartilage may be caught between the condyles and be split longitudinally. This produces the so-called "bucket-handle" type of cartilage, in which the inner portion may be easily displaced centrally between the joint surfaces and cause locking. When the joint is "unlocked," the cartilage becomes dislodged from between the articular surfaces.

Pathology.—The lesion (Fig. 157) may consist of (1) a tearing of the anterior or posterior part of the cartilage with or without displacement; (2) a transverse tear through the central portion or through any other portion of the cartilage; (3) a longitudinal splitting with or without the displacement characteristic of the "bucket-handle" cartilage; or (4) a simple loosening of the cartilage at its peripheral attachment, allowing it to slip into and out of the joint. Any one of these lesions may

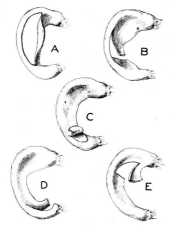

Fig. 157.—Types of semilunar cartilage injury: *A,* Longitudinal splitting (bucket-handle type); *B,* tear of middle third; *C,* tear of anterior tip; *D,* longitudinal splitting of anterior third; *E,* tear of posterior third. (After Henderson.)

give rise to the symptoms of a joint derangement. When the cartilage is partially torn from its peripheral attachment, it may heal without difficulty if further displacement is prevented. Tears limited to the central rim of the cartilage probably never heal. At operation, the "bucket-handle" lesions are as common as all the other lesions combined.

Clinical Picture.—An accurate history is most important, since often the diagnosis is based more upon the history than upon the physical findings. A typical history is that of a ball player whose knee is suddenly twisted inward (Fig. 158). Acute pain on the inner side of the knee accompanies the injury, and the player is likely to fall to the ground. His knee cannot be straightened, and the joint may swell rapidly. If the leg be pulled when it is found that he cannot straighten the knee, the player may feel something in the knee snap back into place. Instantly he is relieved of the sharp pain and is able to get up and walk. In other instances the history may be that of a coal miner who is working on his knees and who feels something give way in his knee when he turns to shovel coal. Symptoms and signs identical with those of the former case then follow.

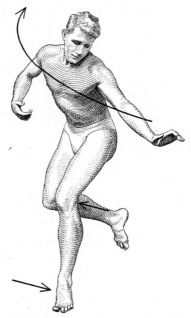

Fig. 158.—A mechanism of injury commonly resulting in tear of the internal semilunar cartilage. Note abduction and flexion of left knee and external rotation of left foot as the trunk twists to the right.

If the condition remains untreated, the disability persists for a variable length of time. Following the initial accident the feeling of a slipping within the knee, with pain referred to the inner side of the joint, may recur frequently. Such episodes may be precipitated by external rotation of the foot or abduction of the ankle.

Examination of the affected knee brings to light a number of signs. In acute cases there may be lateral instability and extensive effusion of blood in the joint. In the presence of this effusion it is difficult to diagnose the exact type of injury. As the swelling subsides, the originally unstable knee may gradually regain its stability as the torn capsule heals. Localized tenderness is present at this stage, either about the anterior tip of the internal semilunar cartilage or about the medial or posterior margins of the joint surfaces. Forced adduction often elicits pain on the medial aspect of the knee. If the cartilage remains displaced, full extension will be impossible. Partial locking is present in approximately 70 per cent of the cases in which the diagnosis can be made definitely. Hamstring muscle spasm often prevents complete extension of the knee and must be differentiated from true locking. When a posterior tear has caused displacement, it may be impossible to flex the joint fully; this locking will persist until the dislocation of the cartilage is reduced. Tears of the posterior half of the cartilage may be demonstrated by the McMurray or "click" test. Holding the tibia in extreme external rotation and abduction, the examiner slowly extends the knee from the fully flexed position; an appreciable clicking and transient pain indicate the presence of a posterior tear.

When the displacement recurs frequently, the patient always feels insecure. Often a little twist or misstep will again throw the cartilage out of its normal position. The patient may learn to reduce the displacement without assistance. Recurrent displacement is usually accompanied by a moderate increase of joint fluid. The swelling will persist as long as any part of the torn cartilage is irritating the synovial membrane. Occasionally in recurrent cases the cartilage is displaced toward the medial side, and a mass can be felt along the medial border of the joint. In such cases the cartilage can usually be pushed in with the fingers. Atrophy of the muscles of the thigh and leg is always present in chronic cases.

B. Injuries of the External Semilunar Cartilage

The mechanism of injury is the converse of that causing damage of the internal semilunar cartilage. The foot is usually fixed firmly upon the ground, and the femur rotates outward upon the tibia while the knee is adducted and flexed. The pathologic changes are similar to those in injuries of the internal cartilage.

Clinical Picture.—The symptoms and signs are essentially the same as those of injury of the internal cartilage with the exception that they are referred to the lateral side of the knee and are often less severe. After injury of the external cartilage, straightening or fully flexing the knee will at times produce a loud crack or snap which can be felt on the lateral side of the joint as the knee jerks into place. This has occasioned the term "trigger knee." For a posterior tear of the external cartilage the McMurray test is the same as that described for the internal cartilage except that the tibia is placed in extreme internal rotation and adduction instead of external rotation and abduction.

Diagnosis.—The diagnosis of a derangement of either cartilage is based upon the characteristic history and physical signs. Locking is typical but may occur also in other types of internal derangement. Roentgenograms yield little relevant information but should be taken in order to exclude fracture, loose bodies, exostoses, arthritis, and aberrant calcification. In addition to the usual anteroposterior and lateral roentgenograms, a posteroanterior picture should be taken with the knee flexed to 90 degrees; this shows the intercondylar space and is sometimes called the tunnel view. In some clinics the diagnosis is based chiefly on the results of pneumoarthrography, or roentgen examination after the injection of air or oxygen into the joint. The author feels that this should be used only as an aid in diagnosis and never should full dependence be placed upon these roentgenographic findings, which to some observers are very difficult of interpretation.

Treatment.—For derangement of either cartilage the treatment is essentially the same.

If the joint capsule is distended after a recent injury, the fluid should be aspirated as it is usually bloody and will predispose to the formation of adhesions. Application of ice is always helpful in acute knee injuries. If, following an initial injury, the knee is locked, an attempt should be made to reduce the displacement of the cartilage; this may be done by the application of traction or by resort to manipulation. In the case of the internal cartilage the knee should be flexed, abducted, externally rotated, and then quickly internally rotated and extended. For displacement of the external cartilage, the knee should be flexed, adducted, internally rotated, and then quickly externally rotated and extended. If the cartilage dislocation can be reduced, the joint should be immobilized for three weeks or more. A dressing of soft glazed cotton rolls, broad splints, and elastic cloth bandages, or a light plaster cast, is a most comfortable and efficient means of immobilization. Following treatment by splinting, the shoe should be built up ¼ inch on the medial side for cases of displacement of the internal cartilage, or on the lateral side for displacement of the external cartilage. Such a shoe minimizes strain in walking. The patient should be cautioned against weight-bearing with the foot turned to one side or the other. Massage of the thigh and exercise of the quadriceps muscle should always be employed to aid in maintaining muscle tone and strength. Active resistive exercises are most effective in building up both strength and size of the quadriceps muscle; they are excellent for the acutely injured knee before weight-bearing is allowed and will result in a more rapid absorption of the effusion.

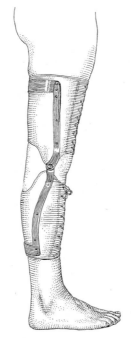

Fig. 159.—Modified Jones knee cage for protection and support of injured knee. (After Bennett.)

If the knee remains weak and stiff after the original displacement, continued physical therapy is indicated in order to strengthen the muscles and to restore normal mobility. It may be desirable to manipulate the knee gently under anesthesia. A brace, such as the Jones knee cage or one of its modifications (Fig. 159), is often indicated to prevent strain upon the knee. If pain and limitation of extension persist, the cartilage should be removed.

If the displaced cartilage is unquestionably palpable, if displacement has occurred more than once, or if the symptoms persist after immobilization, an exploratory operation is indicated. It is often impossible to make a specific diagnosis before operation. If it is clinically definite that displacement or laceration of the cartilage has occurred, the operation should not be delayed, for arthritic changes may develop in the joint when the torn semilunar cartilage is allowed to remain as an irritant to the synovial membrane and hyaline cartilage. When, in exploring the joint, the cartilage is found to be loosened or torn in any part it should be removed as completely as possible. Some surgeons advise long exploratory incisions for all knee operations, while others reserve the long incisions for cases in which the diagnosis is obscure. Usually a short oblique or curved incision is made directly over the front portion of the affected cartilage; through this the joint is examined and the torn cartilage removed. If removal of the entire cartilage through an anterior skin incision is found to be impossible, the skin incision may be extended posteriorly and a second capsular incision may be made posterior to the collateral ligament.

Instruction and practice in forceful voluntary contraction of the quadriceps muscle should be begun before operation and resumed on the first postoperative day. On the fourth or fifth postoperative day, walking with crutches may be started if the knee is not supported, and without crutches if an elastic bandage or a thin cylinder cast has been applied to protect the knee. At the end of a week, massage and more strenuous quadriceps exercises are begun; they are continued until normal mobility and strength have been regained. As the patient resumes normal active use of the knee in from ten days to three weeks, it is sometimes advisable to protect the joint with a brace (Fig. 159). Unrestricted exercise should not be allowed for about twelve weeks after operation. After the removal of a cartilage it may be advisable to build up the heel of the shoe ¼ inch on the affected side in order to lessen the strain on the knee. Removal of the cartilage does not in itself impair the muscle strength or function of the joint to any appreciable exent.

C. CYSTS OF THE SEMILUNAR CARTILAGES

Semilunar cartilage cysts are six to twelve times as common in the external cartilage as in the internal cartilage.

Etiology.—The cyst of the semilunar cartilage is thought to represent (1) the end-result of a localized degenerative process within the cartilage, (2) a congenital defect in the development of the cartilage, or (3) a ganglion-like structure resulting from trauma between the peripheral surface of the cartilage and the synovial membrane.

Pathology.—The cysts are more often multiple than single. They contain a soft, gelatinous material and are sometimes lined by cells resembling endothelium.

Clinical Picture.—The symptoms and signs are similar to those of semilunar cartilage injuries; there is, however, no locking or sudden effusion. Cysts may appear following injury of the knee. Sometimes many years elapse, however, between the injury and the appearance of the cysts. There is sometimes a continuous, dull ache in the affected joint. The discomfort is always worse after activity and relieved by rest. The typical cyst is found on the lateral side of the joint as a tense, slightly tender swelling which may become as large as a walnut.

Treatment.—Complete excision of the cyst and the affected cartilage is indicated.

D. Discoid Cartilages

As a result of an uncommon developmental anomaly, the external semilunar cartilage is sometimes discoid rather than semilunar in form. A discoid cartilage may be present in each knee. It is often associated with a high fibular head.

Clinical Picture.—The most characteristic clinical feature is a loud click which is felt and heard when the knee joint is flexed or extended; this occurs usually near the limits of knee motion. The joint does not lock. The typical patient is in his teens, has noticed a painless clicking for a variable length of time, and with or without minor trauma of the knee begins to have an aching pain on the lateral aspect of the knee and a feeling of weakness in it. Examination confirms the clicking on motion and may disclose tenderness over the lateral cartilage. As the discoid cartilage is thicker than normal, roentgenograms may show a widening of the space between the lateral condyles of femur and tibia.

Treatment.—In the presence of symptoms the treatment is excision of the entire discoid cartilage.

2. Rupture of the Internal and External Lateral Ligaments

Etiology.—The internal or medial collateral ligament is ruptured by stresses resulting from forceful eversion of the foot and abduction of the knee, usually when the knee is slightly flexed and the extensor mechanism relaxed. The external ligament, less frequently injured, may be ruptured by forceful adduction of the internally rotated knee. Rarely does rupture of a lateral ligament occur without injury of the adjacent semilunar cartilage.

Clinical Picture.—There is an increase in the lateral mobility of the knee with tenderness over the injured ligament. When the internal lateral ligament is ruptured, the tenderness is usually greatest over its inferior attachment. There may be an associated increase of joint fluid, swelling, and ecchymosis. Rarely is an unmistakable defect in the region of the affected ligament palpable. Tenderness may be very persistent. On motion of the knee there are definite weakness, instability, and occasionally a sensation of slight catching within the joint.

Treatment.—After recent rupture of the internal or external lateral ligament the knee should be maintained in complete extension for a period of from three to four weeks. During this time the splints may be removed for daily physical therapy. If the injury is severe, active and passive movement of the joint should not be permitted, but if it is slight they may be allowed. Often the attachment of the internal semilunar cartilage is torn when rupture of the internal lateral ligament occurs, and in cases of this type it is most important that the knee be put completely at rest. Exercise of the quadriceps muscle should be started immediately after the injury in order to forestall muscle atrophy. These exercises must be carried out frequently and forcefully if a strong knee is to be obtained. Full weight-bearing should not be permitted until there is no tenderness over the torn ligament and no pain on abduction or adduction of the knee. When the patient begins to walk, it is best that a knee brace be applied to prevent excessive lateral motion and hyperextension. The heel of the shoe on the affected side should be raised ¼ inch in order to prevent strain of the ligaments. When injuries of the collateral ligaments are carefully treated from the beginning, a complete restoration of function may be expected.

If the acute rupture is complete as indicated by extreme lateral instability of the knee, or if, despite a vigorous and prolonged course of quadriceps exercises, the ligaments remain relaxed, an operative reconstruction is to be considered. For reinforcement or reconstruction of the external ligament a flap of fascia lata and a portion of the biceps tendon may be used. Where the collateral ligament is relaxed but not completely ruptured, Mauck's operation of transplanting the distal end of the ligament with its bony attachment downward on the tibia is often successful in improving the stability of the joint. The internal lateral ligament may be reinforced or reconstructed with the tendons of the gracilis and semitendinosus muscles. The intact semitendinosus tendon may be transplanted into the medial condyle of the femur, as described recently by Bosworth. The results of these reconstructive operations are often very satisfactory.

3. Rupture of the Cruciate Ligaments

Etiology.—The cruciate ligaments are ruptured only by severe trauma. The anterior cruciate ligament may be damaged by the same type of trauma which causes injury of the internal semilunar cartilage, and the posterior cruciate ligament by the same trauma which injures the external semilunar cartilage. Forced hyperextension of the knee and internal rotation of the tibia on the femur, with rupture of the internal lateral ligament, may at the same time produce a rupture of the anterior cruciate ligament. If the ligament itself does not break with this type of violence, avulsion of the medial tubercle of the tibial spine may occur. Any force which displaces the tibia backward on the femur while the knee is flexed may cause rupture of the posterior cruciate ligament. Falling on the flexed knee in such a manner that the force of the impact is received on the upper end of the tibia, instead of on the patella, may cause rupture of the posterior cruciate ligament. Rupture of either cruciate ligament is always attended by injury of the joint capsule.

Clinical Picture.—Rupture of a cruciate ligament is followed by extreme swelling and marked instability of the knee joint. When the anterior cruciate ligament is torn or stretched, the tibia can be displaced forward on the femur. When the posterior cruciate ligament is torn or stretched, the tibia can be displaced backward on the femur when the knee is flexed. Lateral as well as anteroposterior instability may be present. Occasionally both ligaments are torn; this results in extreme instability and is likely to be associated with complete dislocation of the knee.

Treatment.—Following recent injury of a cruciate ligament, the knee should be immobilized in slight flexion, preferably by means of a plaster cast, for a period of at least two months. Immobilization should be followed by a snugly fitting knee cage (Fig. 159) which allows only limited motion. For old patients with little or no disability, treatment is not indicated.

Operative reconstructions of the cruciate ligament are not always functionally successful, although in skilled hands the results are sometimes excellent. The anterior cruciate ligament is best reconstructed by the use of fascia lata. The posterior cruciate ligament is sometimes reconstructed by utilizing the semitendinosus tendon. Often a reefing of the capsule on the medial aspect of the knee, fascia lata being used for reinforcement, will improve the stability of the joint. After these operations the knee should be fixed in plaster for one month or more, following which a knee cage allowing limited motion is worn for several additional months. After all cruciate ligament injuries and reconstructive operations physical therapy is indicated and must include a strenuous program of resistive exercises to build up the strength of the quadriceps muscle.

4. Fracture of the Tibial Spine

Etiology.—Fracture of the tibial spine is usually caused by a mechanism of injury similar to that which results in rupture of the cruciate ligaments. Avulsion of the whole tibial spine or of either intercondylar tubercle may occur. With the severe trauma of violent abduction or adduction the whole spine may be broken and one of the intercondylar tubercles depressed. Fracture of the medial tubercle of the spine results from the same type of violence as that which causes injury of the anterior cruciate ligament. The medial tubercle, when detached, usually becomes displaced anteriorly. Fracture of the lateral tubercle of the spine is caused by forcible abduction of the tibia and direct contact with the lateral condyle of the femur.

Clinical Picture.—Fracture of the tibial spine occurs usually in adolescents. The injury is followed quickly by severe swelling of the joint, tenderness, pain, and inability to extend the knee completely. There is usually a bony block causing locking, which is the outstanding symptom. There may also be considerable anteroposterior instability of the joint.

Treatment.—If little or no displacement of the fragment has occurred, immobilization for four weeks, followed by the use of a knee cage, may be sufficient. Aspiration should be done before immobilization is effected. Quadriceps exercises should be started early and gradually increased. If the fragment is displaced, it may be possible by means of manipulation to force it back into position; immobilization should then be used for eight weeks. In most cases, however, open operation is indicated. Small fragments which do not weaken the attachment of the cruciate ligaments may be excised. The after-care is the same as that of arthrotomy for the removal of a semilunar cartilage. If the fragment is large and includes the attachment of one or both cruciate ligaments, it should be replaced in the upper surface of the tibia and fixed by a single screw or by a suture passed through two drill holes from the anterior tibial cortex to the intercondylar area. This procedure should be followed by immobilization for a period of from eight to twelve weeks.

5. Loose Bodies

Loose bodies are often found in the knee, elbow, and shoulder joints and are frequently referred to as "joint mice." In one series of such cases 90 per cent of the involvement occurred in the knee. The presence of intra-articular loose bodies is more frequently observed in men than in women.

Etiology.—Loose bodies may form in the joint as the result of disease or of trauma. They often consist of a structureless fibrinous material; the so-called "rice" or "melon seed" bodies found in association with the chronic synovial reaction of tuberculosis, syphilis, and osteoarthritis are of this type. Occasionally loose bodies arise by the formation and proliferation of cartilage within the synovial villi, forming the so-called synovial chondromas.

Timbrell Fisher has classified loose bodies as (1) those associated with an underlying pathologic process of recognized nature, such as chronic arthritis, tabes, tuberculosis, or purulent arthritis; (2) those which arise from the cartilage or bone of normal joints, such as the loose bodies of osteochondritis dissecans, detached articular ecchondroses, or detached intra-articular epiphyses; and (3) those bodies, such as the synovial chondromas, which form following an obscure pathologic change within the synovial membrane.

Clinical Picture.—Loose bodies usually cause a chronic intra-articular inflammation which is attended by an increase of joint fluid. There may be an associated weakness and instability of the joint. Following motion there is sometimes a sudden, intense pain, occurring when the loose body becomes wedged between the articular surfaces and causes a locking of the joint. In successive episodes of this kind the site of pain may vary widely. Loose bodies which are completely unattached may be found in any part of the joint, and their position may change between successive examinations. This variability of location, commonly determined by roentgenograms, is characteristic. Occasionally the body remains attached by a pedicle, occupies a more constant position in the joint, and can be palpated. Loose bodies can cause all degrees of joint symptoms and disability, from vague pain to extreme swelling and locking.

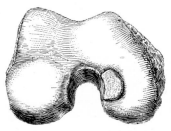

Fig. 160.—Osteochondritis dissecans of internal condyle of femur. Note partial detachment of fragment of cartilage and bone from lateral portion of internal condyle.

Osteochondritis dissecans is a joint affection characterized by ischemic necrosis and partial detachment of a fragment of cartilage and under-lying bone from the articular surface (Fig. 160). In more advanced cases the fragment is completely detached and its area of origin is recognizable as a shallow crater in one of the articular surfaces. The most common site of osteochondritis dissecans is the lateral portion of the articular surface of the internal condyle of the femur, in the neighborhood of the insertion of the posterior cruciate ligament. Osteochondritis dissecans has been demonstrated also, however, in the ankle, hip, elbow, and shoulder joints. It is seen most commonly in adolescence or early adult life but occurs also in children. Males are affected more frequently than females. The fragmentation is thought by some observers to be the result of trauma, the circulation being impaired and a subsequent disturbance of bone nutrition taking place. It is believed by others to be caused by embolism of minute blood vessels supplying the affected area of bone and cartilage. The symptoms and signs are in general the same as those occurring with other types of loose bodies and include discomfort, weakness, fatigue, and catching or locking of the joint. If the diagnosis is made before separation of the fragment has taken place, however, complete rest of the joint from weight-bearing for several months may bring about a reversal of the pathologic process, followed by complete disappearance of the roentgenographic changes and by clinical cure.

Synovial chondromas (osteochondromatosis) constitute a rare affection in which pedunculated and loose cartilaginous bodies arise within the synovial membrane. The knee joint is involved most commonly. Cartilage cells develop in the synovial villi, presumably as a result of metaplasia of the connective tissue cells. The cartilaginous bodies may occur singly but are usually numerous. Many of them remain attached to the synovial membrane; frequently it becomes thickly studded with them. The loose bodies sometimes show lamination from the deposition of calcium salts; they may possess either a loculated central cavity or a center of bony consistency.

Diagnosis.—The diagnosis of intra-articular loose bodies, or *joint mice,* can be made from the history. Roentgenograms demonstrate the presence of loose bodies if they contain calcium or bone.

Treatment.—If the loose bodies are producing symptoms of mechanical interference, they should be removed. It is often advisable to make a long incision, because of the difficulty of finding the loose bodies and the danger of leaving any within the joint. If the bodies contain calcium, roentgenograms made in the operating room may be helpful. The removal of attached bodies is not technically difficult. Joints in which the synovial changes are generalized are best treated by synovectomy. Loose bodies often occur in the posterior part of the knee joint and require a posteromedial incision into the popliteal space. Care must be taken not to injure the popliteal nerves, which should be retracted laterally. The after-care consists of a short period of immobilization, followed by physical therapy including vigorous active exercise of the weakened muscles.

6. Hypertrophy and Pinching of the Infrapatellar Fat Pad and the Synovial Membrane

A. The Infrapatellar Fat Pad

The large pad of fat behind the patellar ligament may at times be pinched and caught when the knee is extended. With repeated trauma, hemorrhage occurs into the fatty tissue, and a hard organized swelling appears which may later become calcified. A similar process may take place on either side of the patellar ligament.

Clinical Picture.—Pinching of the hypertrophic infrapatellar fat pad is associated with pain beneath the patellar ligament. The knee becomes stiff and weak and may show an effusion. Extension may cause a stabbing pain in the anterior aspect of the knee.

Treatment.—In early cases nonoperative therapy is indicated. Raising the heel of the shoe from ½ to 1 inch sometimes affords relief. It may be necessary to apply a hinged knee cage to prevent the last 20 or 30 degrees of extension. Massage and exercises should also be used. If the symptoms persist, operative removal of the entire fat pad is indicated. After operation exercises should be continued and the knee may require the protection of a brace for a period sufficiently long to allow the muscles to regain their normal strength.

Hoffa's disease is a term sometimes applied to marked hyperplasia of the fatty tissue of the knee. Obesity is presumably a predisposing cause since the affection is more common in fat people than in thin. The symptoms are essentially the same as those of hypertrophy of the fat pad; there may be especial discomfort on starting to walk, and creaking of the joint is sometimes marked. The treatment is the same as that described above, with the additional factor, when indicated, of medical measures designed to effect weight reduction.

B. The Synovial Membrane

Hypertrophy of the synovial villi is a frequent result of chronic intra-articular inflammation. The villous processes become enlarged and elongated and occasionally form lobulated masses which have been called *arborescent lipomas.* This affection is a localized form of villous arthritis.

Clinical Picture.—There is usually a feeling of instability in the joint, together with locking which may be only momentary and accompanied by sharp pain. The symptoms are most often referred to the medial side of the patella. There may be an effusion into the joint. Thickening of the capsule is usually palpable.

Treatment.—Nonoperative therapy consisting of a brace to limit full extension and of physical therapy may prove sufficient to relieve the symptoms. If satisfactory relief is not obtained quickly, however, a synovectomy is indicated.

7. Exostoses

Occasionally a joint may become locked or obstructed by the slipping of a tendon or muscle over a bony projection. This sometimes occurs, for example, at the posterior part of the knee. The commonest exostosis about the knee arises from the posteromedial surface of the lower end of the femur and is extra-articular. A sense of discomfort and slipping may accompany every movement. More often, however, the symptoms are trivial. The treatment consists of complete surgical removal of the exostosis.

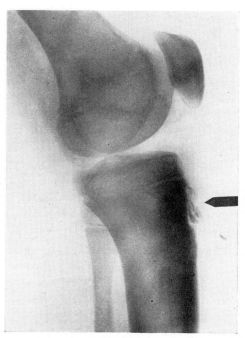

Fig. 161.—Lateral roentgenogram showing osteochondritis of the tibia tuberosity (Osgood-Schlatter's Disease) in a boy fourteen years of age. Note the fragmentation of the epiphysis of the tuberosity.

Osgood-Schlatter's Disease (Partial Separation of the Tibial Tuberosity, Apophysitis of the Tibial Tuberosity)

Osgood-Schlatter's disease is a partial separation of the tongue-like epiphysis of the tibial tuberosity apparently caused by the sudden or continued strain placed upon it by the patellar ligament during exercise

(Fig. 161). There is presumably a disturbance of the circulation of the epiphysis since it often becomes fragmented as does the epiphysis of the head of the femur in coxa plana. Osgood-Schlatter's disease occurs usually in active boys between ten and fifteen years of age and is especially common among those who ride bicycles. It is frequently bilateral.

Clinical Picture.—The disorder is associated with pain over the tibial tuberosity when the patellar ligament is tightened on strong extension or actively resisted flexion of the knee. The region of the tuberosity becomes enlarged and often is tender. The symptoms are sometimes acute and the tenderness extreme. Ecchymosis is occasionally observed. There is always aching in the area of the tuberosity on exercise, and particularly on climbing stairs and running.

Roentgenographic Picture.—The roentgenogram usually shows irregularity and slight separation of the epiphysis of the tibial tuberosity in the early stage and fragmentation of the epiphysis in the later stage. At times, however, little or no change may be visible. A film of the opposite knee should be taken for contrast, but often both knees are affected to the same extent and present an identical roentgenographic appearance.

Prognosis.—The outlook for cure is excellent as progression of the affection is self-limited and the symptoms nearly always respond favorably to treatment.

Treatment.—Immobilization in extension by means of splints or a plaster cast for a period of at least five weeks will usually cause the acute symptoms to subside completely, and no additional treatment may be needed. Weight-bearing is not prohibited. Following complete immobilization, however, it is often advisable not to allow full flexion for an additional period of several months. Complete avulsion of the tibial tuberosity sometimes necessitates operative reattachment. In rare cases extreme pain in the region of the tuberosity may suggest the presence of a low-grade osteomyelitis, in which event curettement of the affected area may be necessary before the symptoms will be relieved. In persistent cases it may be advisable to drill through the tuberosity to the upper end of the tibia in an effort to improve the local circulation. In untreated cases a fragment of the epiphysis may remain ununited and later require excision.

Recurrent or Habitual Dislocation of the Patella (Slipping Patella)

Recurrent dislocation of the patella occurs more often in females than in males and is usually unilateral. Inherited tendencies resulting in a low external condylar ridge are responsible for some of the cases. Recurrent dislocation of the patella is often associated with genu valgum and a general muscular hypotonia of the lower extremities. Direct trauma or strain is usually the precipitating factor.

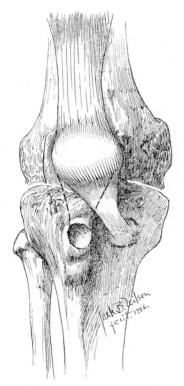

Fig. 162.—Operation for recurrent dislocation of patella. The patellar ligament with its bony tibial attachment has been transplanted medially.

Clinical Picture.—The dislocation is usually a lateral displacement which occurs on sudden contraction of the quadriceps muscle while the knee is extended or partially flexed and the extremity is externally rotated. It may occur with the knee in extreme flexion. Immediately following the dislocation, there is a sharp pain which may cause the patient to fall. The pain is particularly severe when the dislocation is infrequent; in some cases the displacement occurs very often and causes little discomfort. Dislocation of the patella may be followed by a slight or moderate amount of effusion into the joint, especially in the early stages of the disorder. The patient invariably complains of a constant feeling of weakness and insecurity and is very timid about taking strenuous exercise.

Treatment.—The patella may easily be replaced upon extension of the knee and flexion of the hip. In early cases the leg should be immobilized for a period of from five to six weeks. This should be followed by raising the inner side of the heel $\frac{1}{4}$ inch, walking with the toes turned in, and exercising the quadriceps muscle. In some cases the wearing of a knee cage (Fig. 159) is advisable.

In recurrent cases operation is indicated. Numerous surgical procedures involving the use of bone or soft tissue to hold the patella in place have been devised. One of the most successful operations is transplantation of the tibial tuberosity together with the patellar ligament from its normal position to the medial side of the anterior surface of the tibia (Fig. 162). After the tibial tuberosity and patellar ligament have been transplanted, it is usually advisable to reef the capsule on the inner aspect of the joint. Occasionally osteotomy is done to correct an associated genu valgum and in some instances patellectomy may be indicated.

Calcification of the Tibial Collateral Ligament (Pellegrini-Stieda's Disease)

Calcification of the tibial collateral ligament is a fairly common affection occurring usually in men between the ages of twenty-five and forty years. The deposits of calcium usually overlie the medial femoral condyle but have been observed also in the middle portion of the tibial collateral ligament just proximal to the level of the joint space. The calcification may be the result of involvement of the ligament by extension from inflammatory disease in adjacent structures such as bursae, tendons, ligaments, synovia, and bones. Trauma is most often the exciting cause, however, and may be of a single violent type or may consist of repeated minor injuries of the knee joint.

Clinical Picture.—Following traumatization, the medial aspect of the knee becomes sensitive to pressure. Complete extension of the knee is painful, and the joint is usually held in slight flexion. Slight swelling of the knee may be observed. Occasionally the calcified area can be palpated.

Diagnosis.—Dislocation of a semilunar cartilage and other internal derangements of the knee must be excluded before the clinical diagnosis can be made. The roentgenographic picture is pathognomonic.

Prognosis and Treatment.—In many cases the symptoms subside spontaneously without causing prolonged disability. Nonoperative treatment consists of rest and support during the acute stage. Physical therapy is helpful but should not be started until all of the acute signs have subsided. The operative treatment consists of excision of the calcification and plastic repair of the ligament. Occasionally the calcified mass recurs following resection.

Rupture of the Quadriceps Tendon and of the Patellar Ligament

The quadriceps tendon or the patellar ligament may be ruptured by the same type of violence as that which sometimes causes fracture of the patella, that is, sudden and violent contraction of the quadriceps muscle when the knee is flexed. Rupture of the tendon or the ligament is a much less common injury, however, than fracture of the patella.

Clinical Picture.—Rupture of the quadriceps tendon occurs more frequently than rupture of the patellar ligament and is seen most commonly in elderly persons. A definite tender depression can be seen and felt above the superior margin of the patella. The rupture may be associated with bloody effusion into the knee joint and resultant swelling.

Rupture of the patellar ligament results in upward displacement of the patella. A tender depression below the patella may be palpated but usually cannot be seen because of swelling of the infrapatellar fat pad.

Following rupture of either of these tendons, active extension of the knee is severely limited. In both conditions active flexion is of normal range but painful, while active extension is impossible in complete rupture and very painful in partial rupture.

Diagnosis.—The diagnosis is made from the history and the physical findings. Tendon rupture is to be differentiated from fracture of the patella by roentgenographic examination.

Treatment.—The treatment is surgical repair of the rupture. Suture should be followed by immobilization in extension for from six to eight weeks, after which a program of physical therapy including carefully graded exercise in flexion should be instituted.

Snapping Knee

In adults a snapping noise in the knee may be caused by a displacement of the external semilunar cartilage, especially if it is of discoid type, or by a sudden slipping of the biceps tendon or the iliotibial band. In early infancy sudden extension of the knee may cause the tibia to spring forward or rotate outward, producing an audible click; the mechanism is presumably a sudden and violent voluntary contraction of the muscular and tendinous structures about the joint. As a rule the symptoms of snapping knee are of trivial nature and there is no disability.

Treatment.—Supporting the knee with a brace or plaster splint, together with the use of massage, sometimes results in complete relief.

Intermittent Hydrarthrosis (Intermittent Hydrops or Synovitis, Quiet Effusion)

Intermittent hydrarthrosis is an insidious, painless synovitis which appears most often in young women and is characterized by the accumulation of synovial fluid at regular intervals of from five days to a month, each effusion persisting for several days and then regressing spontaneously. It appears most often in the knee but occurs also in the elbow and rarely in other joints. It is not accompanied by increase of local temperature nor by pain unless the swelling becomes extremely tense. There is, however, a feeling of stiffness and of slight discomfort about the joint. When the affection has become established, the swelling occurs in regular cycles, so that the patient can foretell exactly when the joint will become swollen. Between periods of swelling the joint appears in early cases to be normal, but in older cases it may be somewhat boggy and thickened.

Etiology.—Intermittent hydrarthrosis is thought by some authorities to be due to an endocrine disturbance. In young women it may be associated with the menstrual cycle. It has been known to disappear completely during pregnancy and to return following the termination of lactation. Other observers have offered the theory that intermittent hydrarthrosis may represent a trophic phase of a vasomotor neurosis, since in many respects it resembles a transient angioneurotic edema. The affection has been found to occur in association with the early stages of rheumatoid arthritis. In such cases many of the joints may be involved simultaneously.

Prognosis.—The periodic symptoms may continue for years. The outlook for cure is unfavorable except when a definitely controllable cause can be found.

Treatment.—In many cases the treatment is unsatisfactory. The administration of autogenous vaccines, gland preparations, or iodides by mouth has seemed helpful in some cases. Roentgen therapy is sometimes curative. Synovectomy offers an excellent chance for relief of the symptoms in a single joint. In some cases the symptoms have subsided following immobilization in plaster.

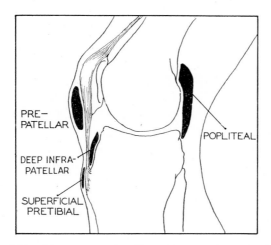

Fig. 163.—Most commonly affected bursae about the knee.

Bursitis

Eighteen or more bursal sacs about the knee have been described, but few of these are of clinical importance (Fig. 163).

The following bursae are most often affected:

1. *The prepatellar bursa* lies anterior to the lower half of the patella and the upper half of the patellar ligament; it occurs more constantly than any other bursa about the knee. It often becomes inflamed from the irritation of repeated or prolonged kneeling. Chronic prepatellar bursitis is spoken of as "housemaid's knee."

2. *The deep infrapatellar bursa* is situated between the lower portion of the patellar ligament and the tibia. When the bursa becomes swollen the normal depressions on either side of the patellar ligament disappear. Active flexion and extension of the knee are painful and limited.

3. *The superficial pretibial bursa* overlies the insertion of the patellar ligament into the tibia.

4. *The popliteal bursae* are found in the popliteal space and are numerous and inconstant. Of these, the *gastrocnemio-semimembranosus bursa* is of most clinical importance, as its distention by fluid is the usual cause of a *popliteal* or *Baker's cyst*. Bursae may develop also about the biceps tendon and between the semitendinosus and gracilis tendons and the tibia (the *anserina bursa*). Occasionally a tubelike extension of the synovial sac of the knee is present beneath the popliteus muscle. The popliteal bursae are often connected with the synovial cavity of the knee. When enlarged, they stand out as firm, hard swellings when the knee is extended but may disappear when it is flexed. Sudden trauma and strain are important factors in causing symptoms.

5. Variable bursae located beneath the tibial collateral ligament, described by V o s h e l l and B r a n t i g a n, may cause localized pain and tenderness, accompanied at times by a visible and palpable swelling.

Clinical Picture.—Any of these bursae may develop without pain or discomfort. Fatigue and weakness of the knee may gradually appear, especially in affections of the popliteal bursae and of those about the attachment of the patellar ligament. When the bursa becomes enlarged and tense, the swelling may be accompanied by extreme pain and by tenderness of varying degree. The prepatellar bursa is often the seat of an acute pyogenic infection.

Treatment.—In most cases the inflammatory symptoms subside with rest of the knee joint and hot applications. If a pyogenic infection is present, aspiration and antibiotic therapy are indicated. The greatly thickened prepatellar bursa resulting from longstanding chronic inflammation is treated by excision. Chronically distended popliteal bursae should also be excised. After the entire sac has been removed the bursa seldom recurs.

Involvement of the Knee in Hemophilia

Prolonged and repeated hemorrhage into the knee joint is a common manifestation of hemophilia, a hereditary disease of the blood which occurs in males and is transmitted by females. Involvement of ankle, elbow, hip, shoulder, or the joints of the fingers is also observed.

Pathology.—Repeated hemorrhage into a joint, precipitated by the trauma of motion, weight-bearing, or minor external violence, may be followed by incomplete absorption of the blood and later by organization. Degeneration of the articular cartilage, overgrowth of the synovium, and proliferation of bone at the articular edges may take place. In cases of recent hemorrhage a brown coloration of the joint structures is said to be characteristic. In late cases the pathologic changes may resemble those of rheumatoid arthritis, and the roentgenograms may show areas of cavitation in the atrophic bone.

Clinical Picture.—The patient is a male whose first episode of hemarthrosis has occurred, as a rule, during middle or early childhood. The involvement is usually monarticular. In cases of recent hemorrhage the joint capsule is distended, tender, and fluctuant, and motion of the joint causes discomfort. Discoloration of the skin is sometimes observed. Extensive hemorrhage is often accompanied by fever. Use of the joint intensifies the symptoms. Repeated hemorrhage may be followed by chronic swelling, discomfort on motion, muscle atrophy, and contracture.

Diagnosis.—Diagnosis of the acute case is made upon the history of trivial injury combined with the physical signs of hemarthrosis and is confirmed by the finding of a prolonged coagulation time. Late cases are less characteristic and must be differentiated with care from tuberculosis and chronic arthritis. In the differential diagnosis roentgenograms are of less value than an accurate history and physical examination.

Prognosis.—The initial hemorrhage is usually absorbed, and the prognosis for future joint function depends largely upon the patient's cooperation and good fortune in avoiding further episodes of trauma. Successive hemorrhages are likely to be followed by increasing disability, and the affected joint often presents finally a clinical and pathologic picture similar to that of rheumatoid arthritis.

Treatment.—In cases of acute hemarthrosis the extremity should be immobilized at once by means of a large cotton pressure dressing and splint. An ice pack should be applied about the affected area. In cases of extensive hemorrhage transfusion is the most valuable restorative measure. After subsidence of the hemarthrosis, physical therapy, consisting of heat, massage, and gentle motion, should be begun with extreme caution.   Protection from further traumatization is essential; when the knee joint is involved, this is often best accomplished by the use of a caliper brace to restrict knee motion and to relieve the stress of weight-bearing.   In late cases marked by deformity, gentle physical therapy should be supplemented by the cautious use of traction designed to effect gradual correction with a minimum of traumatization.

CHAPTER XXII

AFFECTIONS OF THE ANKLE AND FOOT

Disabilities of the foot are extremely common and form an important part of orthopaedic surgery. Commercial products for the relief of foot symptoms are widely advertised and are often used inadvisedly by the layman. Effective treatment is necessarily based upon an understanding of the mechanism of the normal and the pathologic foot.

The function of the foot is (1) to serve as a support for the weight of the body and (2) to act as a lever in raising and propelling the body forward in walking and running. The muscles of the leg supply the power, and the heads of the metatarsal bones serve as a fulcrum on which the weight is lifted.

The foot contains two main arches formed by bones and supported directly by ligaments and indirectly by tendons and muscles. A normal degree of motion and elasticity in these arches is necessary for proper function of the foot.

The longitudinal or long arch is made up of two components, the medial and the lateral. The medial component is the more important and comprises the os calcis, astragalus, scaphoid, three cuneiform bones, and first three metatarsal bones (Fig. 164,A) This arch rests on the head of the first metatarsal and on the os calcis. The lateral component of the longitudinal arch consists of the os calcis, the cuboid, and the fourth and fifth metatarsal bones, and is supported behind by the os calcis and in front by the heads of the fourth and fifth metatarsals. The anterior, transverse, or metatarsal arch is formed by the heads of the five metatarsal bones. Upon weight-bearing the anterior arch becomes flattened, but as soon as the weight is removed the metatarsal heads spring back into position and again form an arch.

The movements of the foot and ankle are most important in the diagnosis and treatment of disabilities of the foot. The ankle joint permits plantar flexion and dorsiflexion of the foot. The foot is inverted or in the varus position when it is so rotated that the plantar surface faces medially; the foot is everted or in the valgus position when the plantar surface is rotated outward (Fig. 165). These motions occur in the subastragalar joint between astragalus and os calcis and in the mediotarsal joints, between astragalus and scaphoid and between os calcis and cuboid. The primary motion of the mediotarsal joints, however, is adduction or inward swinging and abduction or outward swinging of the anterior portion of the foot. Pronation of the foot is a combination of eversion and abduction of the anterior portion of the foot; supination is a combination of inversion and adduction.

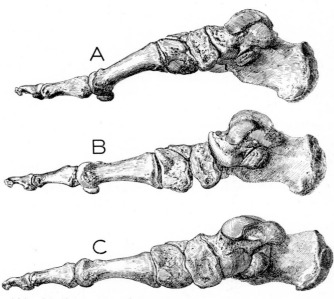

Fig. 164.—Medial aspect of bones of foot. *A*, Normal longitudinal arch; *B*, loss of arch in flexible flatfoot; *C*, absence of arch in rigid flatfoot, showing adaptive bone changes.

Static Disturbances of the Feet

This group of disorders includes all types of foot strain and disability which arise from relaxation of the arches and abnormal pressure upon the foot.

Predisposing Causes of Foot Strain.—Factors which may lead to strain of the foot are:

1. *Incorrect Shoes.*—Stiff leather shoes with pointed ends distort and compress the toes, making it impossible for the muscles to function normally. Muscle atrophy and loss of supporting power result. There can be little doubt that the modern shoe is the most important cause of many disabilities of the foot.

2. *Inadequate Muscular and Ligamentous Support.*—This may follow (a) rapid growth when muscle strength does not keep pace with the growth of the bony framework, and (b) prolonged illness or severe injury of the leg resulting in muscle atrophy and hypotonicity.

3. *Excessive Body Weight.*—Obesity often puts so much strain upon the foot on weight-bearing that the strength of the supporting ligaments and muscles is exceeded and the arches become abnormally depressed.

4. *Excessive Exercise.*—Too much standing, walking, or running, especially when the individual is not accustomed to such exercise or wears a flexible rubber-sole shoe, is a cause of foot strain.

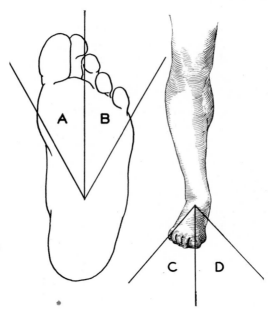

Fig. 165.—Terminology of motion in the tarsal joints. *A,* Forefoot adduction; *B,* forefoot abduction; *C,* eversion; *D,* inversion. (After Cave and Roberts.)

Flexible Flatfoot (Weak, Relaxed, or Flaccid Foot; Pes Planus)

A. In Adults

The principal characteristic of flexible flatfoot is the persistence of an attitude of eversion during periods of weight-bearing. Inversion of the foot is easily carried out, however, when the strain of weight-bearing is removed, and apparently restores the normal relationships among the bones of the longitudinal arch. Flexible flatfoot is more common in men than in women, and more common in the Negro race.

Etiology.—Various strains put upon the long arch during activity undoubtedly constitute a most important factor in the etiology. If the condition is allowed to continue, changes take place in the bones and joints and derange the mechanics of the arch. Occupations which require long periods of weight-bearing, minor congenital variations and relaxations of the joints, and abnormally long arches also may contribute to the development of flatfoot.

Pathology.—The ligaments of the longitudinal arch become weakened and relaxed. The architecture of the bones is changed to meet the new conditions of weight-bearing and pressure (Fig. 164,*B*). The plantar flexor and adductor muscles, which normally assist in maintaining the position of the arch, become weak and atrophic, and the lateral muscles are shortened.

Clinical Picture.—The earliest symptoms are discomfort in the feet and fatigue of the whole body following weight-bearing and activity. The patient tires easily and complains of a feeling of strain on the medial side of the ankle. This may be followed by dull aching in the leg and occasionally in the knee, hip, and back. There is a distinct loss of elasticity and spring in the step. The shoes feel tight and uncomfortable. There is considerable stiffness in the foot and pain upon starting to walk after resting. Cramps may occur in the legs at night and occasionally during the day; they are often associated with swelling of the feet. There may be uncomfortable burning sensations in the feet after activity, and often there are pain and tenderness beneath the scaphoid bone and internal malleolus and along the plantar surface of the medial portion of the foot. The leg seems to be displaced medially, and the weight falls upon the medial side of the foot. The weight-bearing axis, instead of passing between the first and second toes, falls medial to the great toe. Abnormal laxity of the ligaments often exists before pain develops, and there may be actual deformity without pain. As the condition progresses, coldness and occasionally numbness of the feet indicate definite impairment of the circulation. Outward rotation of the feet and legs is common; this lessens the strain upon the sensitive plantar ligaments. If the condition persists, there may be much stiffness, peroneal muscle spasm, and fixed eversion of the foot.

Continued eversion of the foot and depression of the arches are followed by the development of secondary symptoms as a result of pressure.
Tenderness about the medial side of the heel and under the first metatarsophalangeal joint, together with callosities, is likely to be present. If
relaxation of the longitudinal arch is marked, the pressure may cause
development of a callus beneath the prominent scaphoid bone. The
gait becomes slouchy and awkward and is sometimes marked by a swaying of the body from side to side.

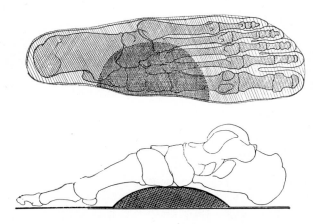

Fig. 166.—Longitudinal arch support.

In certain persons, particularly in Negroes, there may be all of the
classical signs of flatfoot without pain or disability. Flat feet are a
racial characteristic of the Negro and, in fact, of all races except the white.

Diagnosis.—Careful differentiation should be made between static
disturbances of the foot and other conditions such as arthritis, circulatory
insufficiency, and congenital malformation.

Prognosis.—In younger individuals the pain can always be relieved
by proper treatment, but in adults, and especially in those of neurasthenic
type, the prognosis is less favorable. In heavy individuals with small
feet or weak muscles the outlook is unfavorable, particularly if the
patient's occupation requires prolonged standing.

Treatment.—Pain and impaired function are the only indications
for treatment of the flat foot in adults. In the treatment of disabilities of

the feet it is essential to remember that not only must the deformity be corrected, but normal joint motion and normal muscle power must always be restored as completely as possible.

The objects of the treatment of static disability of the foot are (1) to establish normal mechanical relationships in the foot and ankle and (2) to maintain the corrected position by improving the muscle strength and tone. The pressure symptoms will usually subside and the callosities will disappear when the deformity is successfully treated.

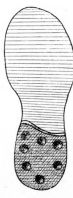

Fig. 167.—Thomas or "orthopaedic" heel. The medial border of the heel is extended forward.

When the foot has been recently affected and is acutely painful, the patient should be upon it as little as possible. It is important that the longitudinal arch be supported. This is best accomplished by means of a felt or sponge rubber pad (Fig. 166) and adhesive strapping. Physical therapy, consisting of massage following whirlpool baths, hot soaks, or baking, should then be employed. Corrective foot exercises should be begun as soon as possible in order to develop the muscles which adduct and invert the foot.

For the chronically painful flatfoot of gradual onset, the alignment of the shoe is most important. It is often wise to elevate the medial border of the heel ¼ inch and to apply a Thomas or "orthopaedic" heel, the medial border of which is prolonged forward about ¾ inch (Fig. 167). The size and shape of the shoe should provide sufficient room for the toes; the heel should be broad and low; and the front portion of the shoe is preferably turned medially. The sole should correspond as nearly as possible with the shape of the foot and should be relatively thick. Heat, massage, and corrective exercises of the foot are important and should be used regularly. Contrast baths of hot and cold water are especially useful in the treatment of foot disabilities in older people. If the patient is overweight, a reducing diet should be prescribed and insisted upon. Activity should be restricted, overuse of the feet being avoided until the pain has subsided. The patient should be taught to walk in as nearly physiologic a manner as possible. It is often desirable for the patient to take corrective exercises in the altered shoes. It may be necessary to fit longitudinal arch pads into the shoes. These supports should be of the nonrigid type and preferably made of felt, sponge rubber, or similar material. The pads can be attached to special leather insoles which slip conveniently into the shoe, or they can be glued to the proper area of the lining of the shoe.

For adequate support of the arches in large, heavy individuals it may be necessary to use spring steel or rigid metal foot plates. In general these are not recommended by the author and are used only in selected cases when satisfactory support cannot be obtained by other means. In many clinics, however, foot plates are advised routinely for depressed longitudinal arches. Sometimes a curved steel strip inserted between the outer and inner soles of the shoe will suffice to support the arch. The *Whitman plate* of rigid steel, which has an inner flange fitted under the longitudinal arch and an outer flange against the heel, is employed with success in many clinics. This type of foot plate is used for from three months to a year, depending upon the condition of the arch.

B. In Children

Any abnormality of the child's feet should be carefully appraised and treated in an effort to prevent disability when he becomes an adult. In children flat feet are usually associated with relaxation of the ligaments of the knees and with knock-knee. Children with flat feet appear awkward and insecure, turn their feet outward when walking, and wear down the medial margin of the soles of their shoes. The stability of the ankles may seem impaired. In the older child there is often a marked eversion of the feet with prominence of the internal malleoli. In such a case there is seldom much pain or disability, but occasionally the child complains of excessive fatigue after exercise and even cries at night from pain in his feet. Occasionally a synovitis of the knees may develop.

Treatment.—The treatment should include the use of corrective shoes which have built-in long arch supports, turned-in toes, and elevation of the medial side of the heels. A felt or sponge rubber support for the longitudinal arch may be used in ordinary shoes to hold the foot in an inverted position. Corrective exercises should be employed as soon as the child is old enough to cooperate. In older children with flat feet and persistent pain, it occasionally may be necessary to carry out an operative correction. The arthrodeses of Hoke, Miller, and White have often been productive of excellent structural and satisfactory functional results. If an accessory scaphoid bone is present, the Kidner operation (see page 494) may be indicated.

The Foot of the Normal Child

When a child first begins to stand and walk, there is a natural tendency for the long arches to flatten, the feet to pronate, the legs and feet to rotate out, and the knees to show a slight valgus deformity. As the child grows and muscle power develops, the feet usually lose this pronation, and good long arches are present on weight-bearing; the legs become straight. Occasionally, however, because of obesity, rapid growth, or nutritional deficiency, these static deformities do not correct themselves with normal growth and development. They may increase and lead to a functional decompensation of the feet and legs with complete flattening of the longitudinal arch on weight-bearing. As this early condition is often extremely disturbing to the parents, they must be given assurance that their child will not grow up deformed.

Treatment.—The treatment should be, first, preventive and, second, corrective. If there is an underlying medical etiologic factor, it should be treated. The prevention of further deformity of the feet as well as the correction of existing deformity can sometimes be accomplished with special corrective shoes.

Certain points regarding infants' and children's shoes should be noted. These are as follows:

The *sole* should be firm enough to protect against hard, uneven surfaces but pliable enough in the forefoot to allow motion of the toes. The *counter* should grip the heel firmly and prevent pronation. The *heel* should be very slightly elevated (from ⅛ to ³⁄₁₆ inch) from the time walking is started until three to four years of age, and then raised slightly higher (to about ⅜ inch). A medial elevation of the heel of ⅛ to ³⁄₁₆ inch to prevent pronation is sometimes desirable. The *shank,* which supports the longitudinal arch, should be firm and hold its shape. Many orthopaedic surgeons recommend a Thomas heel (Fig. 167) to reinforce the shank. Metallic supports for the long arch are contraindicated unless placed between the leather layers of the sole and the heel.

Patronage of only the best shoe stores, specializing in children's shoes and careful fitting, is mandatory for good results. Under such circumstances the results are gratifying in the great majority of cases. The parents should be extremely careful that the shoes are not too short. Children's shoes should be examined as to size and fit every three to six months. In the child short shoes can very quickly produce contracted or hammer toes, corns, calluses, and even hallux valgus. The author prefers for all children and especially the younger group to go without shoes for all or part of the summer months, particularly at the seashore. Going barefooted definitely allows muscle development which the use of shoes restricts.

Spastic Flatfoot

The spastic flatfoot is held firmly in a position of eversion. It may be a sequel of an untreated flexible flatfoot and is seen at times in association with obesity or chronic arthritis. In the early stages the foot is extremely painful. There is often tenderness over the peroneal tendons, and attempts to invert the foot cause sharp pain. There is sometimes an accompanying swelling of the foot. The extremity may be held in marked external rotation. In acute stages every step is painful and the patient walks with an extremely awkward shuffling gait. Later the foot may become rigid from the development of secondary bone changes with proliferation about the joint margins where there is abnormal pressure and strain (Fig. 164, *C*).

Many rigid, everted flat feet have a congenital synostosis or synchondrosis between the anterior end of the os calcis and the scaphoid bone (*calcaneonavicular bar*), which may be seen in oblique roentgenograms. A less common type of tarsal coalition is union of the astragalus and the os calcis by a bridge of bone situated behind the sustentaculum tali (*talocalcaneal bridge*), which appears in posterior oblique roentgenograms of the heel. In the presence of either of these anomalies, pain in the partially rigid foot may develop at or shortly before puberty.

Treatment.—In the early stages correction may be accomplished by the use of casts which are wedged gradually into inversion. If there is no roentgenographic evidence of bony anomalies, forcible overcorrection under anesthesia, followed by immobilization in plaster, is often advisable. Heat, massage, corrective foot exercises, and a support under the longitudinal arch should then be employed. It is often advisable to allow the patient to walk while the cast holds the foot in the inverted position. Some orthopaedic surgeons, believing that foci of infection play a part in producing the peroneal muscle spasm which may be the cause of spastic flatfoot, recommend attempts to eradicate all infectious foci which may be present. If it is impossible to correct the deformity by manipulation alone, a lengthening of the peroneal tendons may be indicated. Occasionally it is necessary to lengthen also the Achilles tendon. After operation a well-moulded plaster cast should be applied with the heel sharply inverted and the anterior part of the foot adducted and slightly pronated. Occasionally in severe cases with pain, arthrodesis of the subastragalar and mediotarsal joints is indicated. This operation is usually followed by complete relief of the pain.

In rigid flatfoot, operations for reshaping the longitudinal arch are seldom to be recommended. Operative resection of a congenital bony bridge is not followed, as a rule, by increased mobility and is not advised.

Shortening of the Achilles Tendon

Shortening of the Achilles tendon, especially in the weak or everted foot, leads to the development of foot strain. In adults shortening of the Achilles tendon may be due either to a congenital structural change or to reflex muscular spasm from irritation caused by the disturbed mechanics of the foot. In the reflex type there is discomfort which may be associated with tenderness and sharp pain and spasm on attempting to dorsiflex the foot.

Treatment.—In cases of the reflex type, raising the heel of the shoe may lead to relief of the symptoms. In the structural type an attempt should be made to stretch the Achilles tendon by wedged plaster casts or by special stretching exercises. Experience has shown that operative lengthening of the Achilles tendon weakens this type of foot and should be discouraged. In women pain in the feet is sometimes caused by shortening of the Achilles tendon from wearing shoes with very high heels. In such cases the heels should be gradually lowered and stretching exercises should be carried out. Sudden change from high-heel to low-heel shoes often produces much discomfort in the legs from pull upon the gastrocnemius and soleus muscles.

Claw Foot

The typical claw foot has an abnormally high longitudinal arch, a depression of the metatarsal arch, and dorsal contractures of the toes (Fig. 168). The plantar fascia is contracted, the anterior half of the foot drawn downward and sometimes inward, and the Achilles tendon may be shortened. Excessive height of the longitudinal arch is termed *cavus* deformity. It is often seen in the absence of the other deformities of claw foot and usually causes few symptoms.

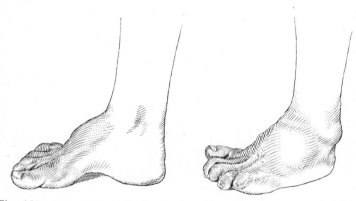

Fig. 168.—Claw foot of moderate degree in young adult. Note high longitudinal arch, dorsal contracture of the toes, and adduction of the forefoot.

The deformities of claw foot may be slight or severe. In most instances they show a gradual progression. With the muscular contractures which are associated with claw foot, there is a loss of the normal elasticity of the arches. Shaffer has applied the term "nondeforming clubfoot" to the type of foot which shows clawing of the toes, a high longitudinal arch, and a short Achilles tendon.

Etiology.—In some cases the deformity of claw foot is the result of an inherited tendency. It may be associated also with the wearing of high heels, which produces a postural equinus, or with excessive use of the leg muscles, as in professional dancers. After infantile paralysis it sometimes develops in the unparalyzed foot. The deformity may occur also in the course of progressive lesions of the central nervous system, such as Friedreich's ataxia and peroneal muscular atrophy. Frequently claw foot has been found in association with spina bifida occulta. It may follow conditions such as cellulitis, fibrositis, rheumatoid arthritis, and the like, and is sometimes seen after compound fractures of the tibia which have been immobilized in poor position or have received inadequate after-care. Most commonly, however, claw foot can be ascribed to no specific etiologic factor, and is then spoken of as "idiopathic claw foot." Idiopathic claw foot is a progressive deformity and may be unilateral or bilateral.

Symptoms.—Although considerable deformity may be present without causing symptoms, the patient usually complains of tender calluses beneath the metatarsal heads and over the proximal interphalangeal joints.

Treatment and Prognosis.—In the milder cases the treatment may consist of simple stretching of the plantar fascia and Achilles tendon and the wearing of proper shoes. The shoes should be fitted with metatarsal pads or bars to relieve strain upon the anterior portion of the foot.

For claw foot of moderate degree it may be necessary to carry out a plantar fasciotomy and to stretch the foot under anesthesia. Occasionally transplantation of one or more of the extensor tendons of the toes to the distal portion of the metatarsal bones or to the flexor tendons is indicated.

In more severe cases it is sometimes advisable to strip the plantar fascia from its attachment to the os calcis, section all the flexor and extensor tendons of the toes, and lengthen the Achilles tendon.

In still more advanced cases dorsal wedge osteotomy combined with subastragalar arthrodesis is the only procedure which will effect satisfactory correction of the deformity. In extreme cases it may be necessary also to excise the astragalus and the metatarsal heads.

In the paralytic type of claw foot no recurrence of the deformity after operative correction is to be anticipated. In the idiopathic type, however, there may be a return of the deformity, especially if the operative procedure has been of conservative nature. All of these deformed feet should be fitted with proper shoes and with supports for both the anterior and longitudinal arches. Corrective foot exercises and physical therapy should be begun early. The results are often satisfactory when the treatment is properly selected and is followed by observation of the patient over a period of years.

Köhler's Disease (Avascular Necrosis or Osteochondritis of the Tarsal Scaphoid Bone)

Osteochondritis of the tarsal scaphoid bone is an uncommon affection which begins insidiously in childhood, causes considerable local discomfort and limping, and tends toward gradual spontaneous recovery. The etiology is not established, but the affection seems to fall into the group of localized and self-limited bone diseases of youth which are ascribed to ischemic degenerative changes. Trauma sometimes appears to be a contributing factor. Clinically there are tenderness and slight thickening over the affected scaphoid bone. The roentgenographic appearance of the scaphoid is pathognomonic, the bone being small, dense, and of irregular outline and disordered internal structure as though it had been crushed (Fig. 169A). Microscopic sections of such bones have shown massive necrosis, which is followed by organization, resorption of dead bone, and the formation of new bone.

Treatment and Prognosis.—Protection of the diseased bone from excessive traumatization is essential. Support of the longitudinal arch and restriction of activity may suffice. If there is much pain on weight-bearing, however, it is preferable to immobilize the foot in slight inversion by means of a plaster cast for a period of six to ten weeks. The results are usually satisfactory, there being little or no permanent disability.

Anterior Metatarsalgia

Etiology.—A painful metatarsal arch often occurs in (1) the everted or abducted foot, (2) the foot with a short Achilles tendon, and (3) the foot with a high longitudinal arch, such as the claw foot. Disturbances of the metatarsal arch are most common in individuals over thirty years of age and occur more often in females than in males. The affection is a result of muscular weakness which allows downward displacement of the metatarsal heads. Tight, short, high-heel shoes play an important part in the pathogenesis. A short and tight shoe compresses the anterior part of the foot, elevates the head of the fifth metatarsal bone and throws weight upon the fourth metatarsal, causing pain about its head. Undoubtedly weakness of the longitudinal arch contributes also to depression of the anterior arch.

Clinical Picture.—Often the first sympton is a burning, cramping pain in the anterior part of the foot, usually under the middle metatarsal heads. Occasionally the pain is preceded by the feeling, experienced on

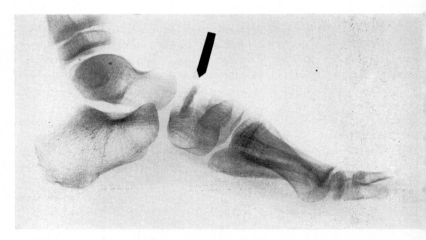

Fig. 169*A*.—Lateral roentgenogram showing Köhler's Disease (osteochondritis of the tarsal scaphoid) in a six-year-old boy. Note thin scaphoid of irregular shape and density.

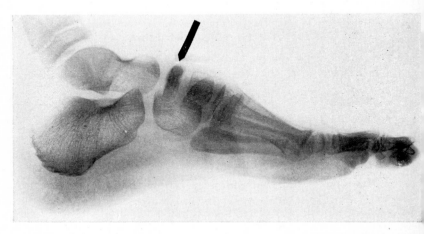

Fig. 169*B*.—Lateral roentgenogram of same case as Fig. 169*A*, five months later. Note almost complete disappearance of irregular density and return to normal shape.

standing or walking, that a bone has slipped out of place. Pain on standing and walking may become so severe as to be quite disabling. At times the pain radiates to the end of the toe, up into the foot, and even into the leg. The pain is seldom experienced with the shoe off. Tenderness is most often found beneath the fourth metatarsal head, although it may be present also beneath the head of the second or third metatarsal. A painful callus, in which there may be a plantar wart which adds to the discomfort, frequently develops under the metatarsal heads.

Examination of the foot often shows depression of the metatarsal arch even when the foot is bearing no weight. The most characteristic features, however, are the tenderness and the calluses which are present beneath the metatarsal heads. The deformity is associated with marked relaxation of the ligaments of the anterior arch. In severe cases there is usually dorsal contracture of the toes and restriction of their motion. It is impossible to flex the toes fully, and any attempt to do so produces pain in the tender areas. Swelling and acute inflammatory reaction are seldom present. Anterior metatarsalgia may occur in association with hallux valgus or hallux rigidus.

Treatment.—The basic objects of treatment are (1) relief of the pain by arch supports and (2) strengthening of the muscles of the foot and ankle by corrective exercises.

The patient should wear a shoe which has a thick sole, adequate width at the toes, a supporting longitudinal arch, and a narrow counter. A small felt or rubber pad, placed immediately behind the metatarsal heads and held in place with circular adhesive strapping, will usually relieve the acute symptoms (Fig. 170A). Various types of supports made of leather, felt, rubber, cork, or metal, and designed to elevate the metatarsal arch, may be fitted into the shoe. A transverse bar posterior to the metatarsal heads, made of leather and attached to the outside of the shoe (the *metatarsal bar,* Fig. 170B), or placed between the inner and outer soles (the *Cook anterior heel*), will often relieve the symptoms of metatarsal strain. All patients should be instructed regarding hot soaks, contrast baths, massage, and corrective foot exercises. The exercises should be continued for several weeks. With gradual improvement of the muscle strength the affection may be completely relieved.

Occasionally a sensitive plantar wart may be the source of severe pain. Warts are best treated by roentgen therapy or excision. Relieving the pressure upon a sensitive wart by means of proper pads or supports, however, will sometimes lead to its disappearance. Manipulation to loosen up adhesions in the anterior part of the foot is occasionally indicated in metatarsalgia. In resistant cases associated with malposition of the bones, resection of the metatarsal head in the area of tenderness is occasionally necessary. After such a resection it is necessary for the patient to wear a well-fitted support under the metatarsal arch.

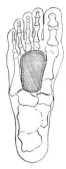

Fig. 170*A*.—Metatarsal arch support. Note position just behind the metatarsal heads. (After Lewin.)

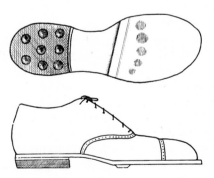

Fig. 170*B*.—Shoe with metatarsal bar. Note that bar is fixed·to sole just behind the metatarsal heads.

Morton's Toe (Plantar Neuroma)

In 1876 T. G. Morton described a type of metatarsalgia characterized by sudden attacks of sharp pain usually localized to a single toe. The fourth toe is most commonly involved. The condition is usually unilateral; women are affected more commonly than men. In the early stages there is a burning sensation in the region of the metatarsal head which may radiate into the toes and be accompanied by paresthesia and numbness. The characteristic pain, however, is sharp and lancinating; it is often so intense as to demand immediate removal of the shoe and manipulation of the toes. After these sudden attacks tenderness may persist for several days and be followed by numbness of the toes.

As a rule the appearance of the foot is normal. A small area of exquisite tenderness may usually be located by firm palpation of the third web space, and a small tender nodule can occasionally be palpated. In late cases it is sometimes possible to elicit crepitation together with characteristic pain by careful palpation with one hand while the other squeezes the metatarsal heads together.

In recent years it has been demonstrated that the pain is associated with a localized thickening of the third common digital plantar nerve at its bifurcation in the web space. The enlargement or neuroma is presumably a result of repeated traumatization of the nerve trunk by the metatarsal heads.

Treatment.—The symptoms can sometimes be relieved by a metatarsal arch support. Excision of the enlarged segment of the digital nerve is a safe and effective procedure, produces little loss of sensation, and is the treatment of choice in most cases. Sometimes exploration discloses a bursa which also should be completely excised.

Stress Fracture of a Metatarsal Bone (March or Fatigue Fracture)

Fracture of a metatarsal shaft, usually the second or third, may result from the stress associated with weight-bearing after prolonged walking has exhausted the muscular and tendinous support of the foot (Figs. 171A and 171B). A congenital shortening of the first metatarsal bone, *metatarsus atavicus,* which throws an increased leverage on the shaft of the second metatarsal, is frequently a predisposing factor. Symptoms may be completely absent at the instant of fracture, beginning a week or more later as exuberant callus forms. The pain and swelling which appear at this time may lead to an erroneous diagnosis of malignant tumor. Stress fractures are especially common in army recruits during their basic training. Fractures of similar nature have been reported as occurring in bones other than the metatarsals.

Treatment.—Extensive experience in the Armed Forces has demonstrated that rest, adhesive strapping, and the use of an anterior arch pad constitute the most effective form of treatment. Sometimes, however, a plaster cast is necessary for a period of from three to four weeks. After the cast has been removed, the patient's shoe should be fitted with an anterior arch pad or a metatarsal bar and he should not engage in excessive walking for several months.

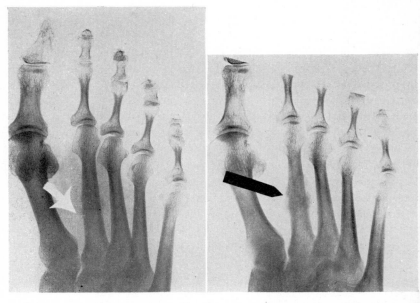

Fig. 171*A*.—Roentgenogram showing stress fracture of second metatarsal (march fracture). Note the fine fracture line with beginning callus formation in the middle of the shaft of the second metatarsal.

Fig. 171*B*.—Roentgenogram showing stress fracture of second metatarsal in same case as Fig. 171*A*, six months later. Note complete disappearance of thin fracture line and exuberant callus formation.

Freiberg's Disease (Avascular Necrosis or Osteochondritis of the Second Metatarsal Head)

Freiberg's disease is characterized by the gradual development of degenerative changes in the head of the second metatarsal bone (Fig. 172) or, rarely, in other metatarsal heads. The affection is uncommon; it occurs usually in adolescent children but is often seen in adults. The etiology is believed to be a disturbance of the circulation which results in a localized aseptic necrosis. Trauma is possibly a contributing factor. The roentgenograms show bone absorption and irregularity, with thickening of the distal half of the affected bone. Clinically there are pain on weight-bearing and thickening and tenderness of the affected metatarsal head.

Treatment.—In the acute stage of the affection, treatment by means of a plaster boot or anterior arch pad is usually sufficient. Occasionally in late cases it is necessary to resect the excess bone or to excise the deformed metatarsal head in order to relieve the pain and discomfort. After such operations the use of an anterior arch support is advisable.

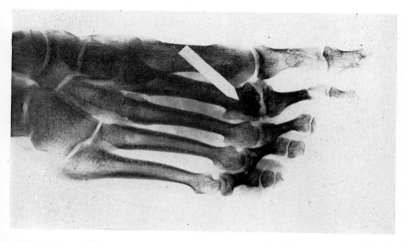

Fig. 172.—Oblique roentgenogram showing Freiberg's Disease (osteochondritis of head of second metatarsal). Note the flattening, irregularity, and bone production about the head of the second metatarsal. The patient was forty years of age.

Hallux Valgus

Hallux valgus is a lateral angulation of the great toe at its metatarsophalangeal joint. There is usually an associated enlargement of the medial side of the head of the first metatarsal bone, together with the formation of a bursa and callus over this area (Fig. 173). The bony prominence and its overlying bursa constitute the so-called "bunion."

Etiology and Pathology.—Narrow, pointed, and short shoes are the chief causative factor. The first metatarsal bone is usually adducted, or in the varus position, while the toe is abducted; in extreme cases all of the metatarsals may be adducted and all of the toes abducted. There are usually an associated widening of the anterior part of the

foot and a depression of the anterior arch. Contracture of the flexor
and extensor hallucis longus muscles is associated with a lateral displacement of the extensor tendons. Occasionally the malalignment and the
symptoms are aggravated by arthritis. The pain of hallux valgus is due
to traumatic arthritis, to pressure upon the digital nerve, and often to
compression and inflammation of the bursa overlying the metatarsal
exostosis. Atrophy of the articular cartilage may be extensive.

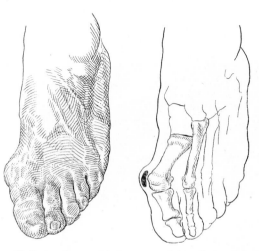

Fig. 173.—Hallux valgus, with bursa overlying the metatarsal head.

Treatment and Prognosis.—In mild cases, properly fitting shoes
and repeated overcorrection by stretching may prevent progression of
the deformity and afford relief of the discomfort. The patient should
sleep with a pad or special toe separator between the first and second
toes. The depression of the metatarsal arch should be corrected by a
supportive pad and exercises. In acute infection of the bursa, rest and
hot compresses are indicated.

When considerable deformity is accompanied by disabling pain, operative treatment is indicated. It is the only available method of correcting
the deformity and so relieving the pain. Many different operative procedures for the treatment of bunions have been described. The simplest
of these is removal of the exostosis and the bursa. In addition, the ligaments on the medial side may be reefed, the capsule on the opposite side
divided, and the extensor proprius hallucis tendon sectioned or lengthened

(*Silver operation*). Transplantation of the adductor hallucis tendon from phalanx to metatarsal, described by McBride, is frequently advisable.

Resection of the proximal half of the first phalanx (*Keller* or *Schanz operation*) is often the procedure of choice for the correction of severe deformity. An alternative procedure is to excise the metatarsal head and transplant a flap of soft tissue around the smoothed metatarsal neck (*Mayo operation*). Motion should be started in two weeks and weight-bearing in three weeks. The shoe should be fitted with an anterior arch support. In the absence of arthritic changes, a wedge osteotomy of the proximal end of the first metatarsal bone, after removal of the exostosis and bursa, may be the operation of choice; it corrects the varus deformity of the first metatarsal bone, which is an important contributing factor in hallux valgus.

After all operations for hallux valgus, the great toe should be held in an overcorrected position, either by a splint or by a soft cushion pad placed between the first and second toes, until it is certain that the deformity will not recur. Hot soaks, massage, and corrective foot exercises should be employed as long as tenderness and stiffness persist. Some patients recover rapidly from operations for hallux valgus and are permanently relieved of pain, especially those who have had the minimum of surgery performed and who can be relatively inactive in their occupations. Others experience pain for several months afterward. The patient should be observed periodically in an effort to forestall recurrence of the deformity.

Hallux Rigidus (Hallux Flexus)

Hallux rigidus is characterized by restriction of motion in the first metatarsophalangeal joint, occasioned usually by trauma, osteoarthritis, or disuse associated with chronic foot strain. Burning and throbbing pain occurs in the affected part of the foot after standing or walking.

Treatment.—In mild cases the treatment consists of (1) wearing a thick inflexible sole on the shoe or (2) having a long steel strip inserted between inner and outer soles of the shoe in order to prevent motion in the affected metatarsophalangeal joint. The use of a metatarsal bar is sometimes helpful. Occasionally slight elevation of the medial side of the sole of the shoe will abolish the pain. If the symptoms cannot be relieved in this way, operative removal of the proximal half of the first phalanx or the head of the first metatarsal bone is indicated. After excision of the metatarsal head, support must be afforded by means of a pad placed within the shoe and located beneath the shaft of the first metatarsal bone.

Hammer Toe

Hammer toe is characterized by dorsiflexion of the metatarsophalangeal joint and plantar flexion and rigidity of the interphalangeal joints (Fig. 174). Any toe may be so affected, but the second toe is most frequently involved. Tender corns and calluses are usually present on the toe. The deformity is due to the pressure of a short, narrow shoe upon the end of a long toe. The deformities begin in early childhood and are often found in association with bunions.

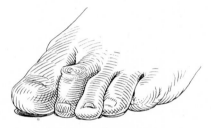

Fig. 174.—Hammer toe.

Treatment.—In early cases simple manipulation and splinting of the affected toe may suffice to relieve the moderate discomfort. In older cases arthrodesis of the proximal interphalangeal joint in extension is indicated. Sometimes complete excision of the first phalanx yields a very satisfactory result.

Overlapping or Displacement of the Toes

This condition most often involves the little toe. It may be of developmental origin or may arise from wearing tight shoes. The toe may become very painful because of corns or callus formation.

Treatment.—In infants and younger children manipulation and splinting of the toe may correct the deformity. Tenotomy or transplantation of the extensor tendon may be necessary. When this treatment fails to produce satisfactory relief of the symptoms, resection of the proximal phalanx or amputation of the toe may be indicated.

Pigeon-Toe

Pigeon-toe is an habitual turning in of the feet on walking and may be encountered in association with flexible flatfoot in small children. It is a physical sign rather than a disease entity and is often found together with hallux varus, metatarsus varus, bowlegs, medial torsion of the tibia, congenital contracture of the internal rotators of the hip, or relapsed clubfeet.

Treatment.—The deformity is usually corrected spontaneously as the child grows older. Raising the outer border of the soles of the shoes ⅛ to ¼ inch may improve the gait. The child should be instructed to walk with the toes pointed out. If torsion is present in the tibia or the femur, the use of a Denis Browne night splint to hold the lower extremities in wide external rotation may be very helpful. For older children, roller skating provides excellent corrective exercise.

Affections of the Heel

1. *Injury and Inflammation About the Insertion of the Achilles Tendon.*—These affections are evidenced by pain behind the heel and are of the following types:

a. *Tenosynovitis.*—Swelling is usually noticeable in the region of the Achilles tendon, and fine crepitus on motion is often unmistakable. The affection is usually marked by acute local tenderness and considerable disability. The treatment consists of rest, avoidance of pressure, and the application of heat to the tender area. When it is necessary for the patient to walk, a pad should be placed in the shoe to elevate the heel and so lessen the excursion of the tendon. In chronic Achilles tenosynovitis, rest, contrast baths, and massage are indicated.

b. *Bursitis.*—Inflammation of the *retrocalcaneal bursa*, which is situated between the Achilles tendon and the os calcis (Fig. 175), causes local tenderness and pain upon motion. The disorder is treated by rest, heat, and elevation of the heel by means of a pad. If the symptoms do not subside with this type of therapy, the bursa should be excised. The irritation of a tight shoe sometimes causes a bursa (the *superficial calcaneal* or *posterior Achilles bursa*) to form between the Achilles tendon and the skin. In inflammation of this bursa, relief of pressure and application of heat are indicated. Occasionally, when the bursa becomes frankly infected, it should be incised or resected.

c. *Periostitis.*—Discomfort is sometimes caused by inflammation of the periosteum at the attachment of the Achilles tendon. The treatment is similar to that of bursitis.

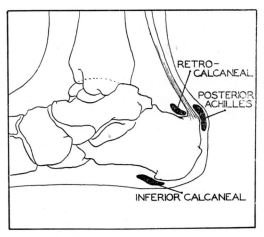

Fig. 175.—Most commonly affected bursae about the os calcis. Note the inferior calcaneal spur.

d. *Calcaneal Apophysitis or Epiphysitis.*—This condition is a somewhat uncommon affection of children, occurring most often in boys between nine and fourteen years of age. Calcaneal epiphysitis is a low-grade inflammatory reaction, occurring in the posterior calcaneal epiphysis and ascribed to chronic pressure or strain. Roentgenograms may show the epiphysis to be irregular or segmented, with areas of increased density. The affection is best treated by rest and relief of the strain and pressure. The heel of the shoe should be elevated ½ inch or more. It is occasionally advisable to apply a plaster cast in order to secure complete rest of the affected area.

e. *Partial and Complete Ruptures of the Achilles Tendon.*—Incomplete ruptures of the Achilles tendon may be followed by the formation of small irregular masses of fibrous consistency. Occasionally calcification similar to that of myositis ossificans occurs in these masses; when pain is persistent in such cases, the calcified area should be excised. Complete rupture of the Achilles tendon by indirect violence is of fairly common occurrence, especially in athletic individuals of stocky build. The power of voluntary plantar flexion is greatly diminished, and the rupture is evident on palpation. Recent ruptures should be treated by immediate exploration and suture. Rupture of the plantaris tendon, evidenced by a sudden sharp pain like the sting of a whip, may occur frequently, although clinical differentiation from incomplete rupture of the Achilles tendon is questionable. The treatment consists of rest, adhesive strapping, and support of the heel. Ruptures of other tendons of the ankle and foot are quite rare.

2. *Spurs, Periostitis, and Bursitis Under the Os Calcis.*—Extensive spur formation beneath the os calcis may take place without producing symptoms (Fig. 175). If a bursal sac develops and becomes inflamed, however, pain and tenderness may be severe. Hemorrhage beneath the os calcis, resulting from a fall or blow, may cause extreme discomfort. Bursitis and periostitis under the os calcis are sometimes spoken of as "policeman's heel."

Treatment.—In mild cases complete relief can sometimes be obtained by the use of (1) a soft rubber heel pad with a hole cut in its center to relieve pressure upon the tender area, (2) a cupped metal plate to eliminate pressure in this area, (3) a special heel which is shaped to bear all of the weight at its posterior margin, or (4) a high longitudinal arch pad. Rest, hot applications, and massage should also be used. An injection of procaine into the bursal sac or tender area may be followed by relief of the symptoms. Any obvious focus of infection should be treated. If the pain persists, it may be necessary to excise the bursa and the underlying spur. A long U-shaped incision around the heel provides the best exposure, but in most cases an incision along the medial side of the heel is sufficient. It is advisable to remove a thin slice of cortical bone from the inferior surface of the os calcis, together with the adherent soft tissue. Even after this type of operation the resumption of weight-bearing is sometimes followed by recurrence of the symptoms.

Exostoses of the Bones of the Foot

There are certain points in the foot at which pressure from shoes is likely to cause chronic irritation and the resultant formation of exostoses and bursae. The lateral side of the fifth metatarsal head sometimes develops such changes, which are similar to those of a bunion and have been called a "bunionette." Other sites are the medial and upper aspects of the scaphoid bone, the dorsum of the first cuneiform, the plantar aspect of the os calcis, and the posterior surface of the os calcis at or above the attachment of the Achilles tendon. Occasionally an exostosis forms beneath a toenail; such localized proliferation is termed a *sub-ungual exostosis* and is seen with greatest frequency in the great toe.

Treatment.—If removal of the causative pressure cannot be accomplished satisfactorily, the exostosis and bursa should be excised. Subungual exostosis is treated by excision of the nail and of the under-lying phalangeal exostosis.

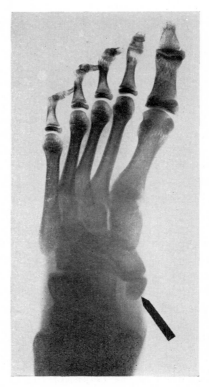

Fig. 176.—Anteroposterior roentgenogram showing accessory scaphoid of the foot (os tibiale externum). Note well-demarcated, small bone adjacent to medial border of scaphoid.

Accessory Bones of the Foot

Twenty-one accessory bones of the foot have been described. This number includes the *sesamoid bones,* which are embedded in tendons. Two sesamoid bones are found constantly under the base of the great toe. Sometimes these bones are the site of pain and tenderness following local trauma. In such cases the symptoms may be completely relieved by excision of the sesamoids. These small bones are sometimes bipartite, and this developmental variation must be distinguished from fracture. Painful bursae which sometimes occur in association with the sesamoid bones may require excision.

The most common of the abnormal accessory bones are the *os trigonum,* which is found posterior to the astragalus; the *os tibiale externum* or *accessory scaphoid,* located at the medial aspect of the scaphoid bone (Fig. 176); and the *os peroneale,* lying in the peroneal tendons on the lateral side of the foot. These bones are often mistaken for fracture fragments and in obscure injuries of the foot should be carefully differentiated. They can usually be recognized without difficulty by means of their typical size, shape, position, and smoothly rounded outline. A large accessory scaphoid bone may be associated with local tenderness from pressure of the shoe and with pain and weakness in the longitudinal arch; in such cases excision of the accessory scaphoid and fixation of the posterior tibial tendon into a groove well beneath the scaphoid bone (Kidner operation) is frequently indicated. The results of this procedure are usually good.

Displacement of the Peroneal Tendons

Occasionally an abnormal mobility of the tendon sheaths and laxity of the ligaments behind the lateral malleolus allows one or both of the peroneal tendons to become displaced from their groove and to slip anteriorly over the malleolus. The displacement usually occurs on active dorsiflexion and eversion; it is sometimes accompanied by severe pain. Occasionally this affection is of developmental origin but more commonly it is a sequel of trauma.

Treatment.—If the diagnosis is made immediately after the displacement has occurred, manipulative reposition and immobilization by means of a plaster boot may effect a cure. Increasing the height of the heel will help to prevent recurrence of the displacement. In some cases the displacement will recur unless a brace is worn to prevent inversion and active eversion of the foot. In chronic recurrent cases operation yields the most satisfactory results since it affords permanent cure. The tendon sheaths may be sutured firmly into their normal position, the depth of the peroneal groove may be increased, or a strip of the Achilles tendon may be used to form a stabilizing loop.

Tender Swellings About the Ankle

Localized areas of swelling and tenderness about the ankle sometimes occur in association with weak feet. A bursa is often found in the region of the lateral malleolus, and there is associated proliferation of fatty and connective tissue. The patient may complain of weakness and discomfort in the swollen areas.

Treatment.—The discomfort should be relieved by physical therapy, and the mechanics of the foot should be corrected by arch supports. Dietary reduction of the obesity is important. In obstinate cases operative removal of the redundant and sensitive tissue is indicated.

CHAPTER XXIII

AFFECTIONS OF THE NECK AND SHOULDER

In this chapter are grouped (1) the most frequently observed ortho-paedic affections peculiar to the neck, *i.e.*, torticollis and cervical rib, and (2) the most common affections of the shoulder, *i.e.*, minor injuries including traumatic synovitis, strains, and sprains; subacromial and sub-coracoid bursitis; rupture of the supraspinatus tendon and tears of the musculotendinous cuff; rupture of the biceps brachii; snapping shoulder; recurrent and old dislocations of the shoulder; and old dislocations of the acromial and sternal ends of the clavicle.

PART I. AFFECTIONS OF THE NECK

Torticollis (Wry Neck)

Torticollis is a deformity of the neck which, as a rule, includes elements both of rotation and of flexion. In most cases one sternocleido-mastoid muscle is shortened. This shortening results in flexion of the neck toward the affected side and rotation of the chin toward the opposite side. Torticollis may be congenital or acquired.

CONGENITAL TORTICOLLIS

Etiology and Pathology.—The term *congenital torticollis* includes all cases in which the deformity is evident at birth. Occasionally torticollis is caused by a primary congenital defect in the vertebrae of the cervical spine. Far more commonly, however, it is due to secondary congenital changes, such as abnormal position of the head in utero or injury of the sternocleidomastoid muscle during birth. It has been thought by some observers that the pathogenesis is rupture of many of the muscle fibers during birth, with the formation of a hematoma and subsequent replace-ment of part of the muscle by scar tissue. A nontender, cylindrical enlargement of the sternocleidomastoid muscle is sometimes observed in the newborn infant; it usually regresses slowly in from three to six months. Incomplete regression may be followed by the development of a contracture of the sternocleidomastoid muscle.

The shortening of the sternocleidomastoid muscle is associated with an increased amount of fibrous tissue in its substance. A secondary contracture develops in the adjacent tissues of the neck.

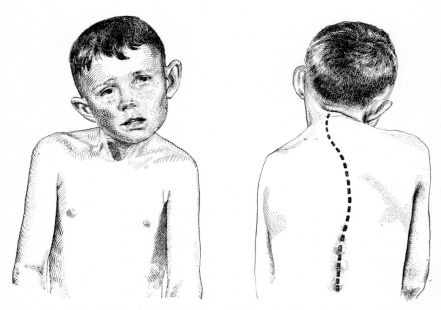

Fig. 177.—Congenital torticollis. Note asymmetrical development of face, prominence of the right sternocleidomastoid muscle, and lateral curvature of the cervicodorsal spine.

Clinical Picture.—Congenital torticollis is seen more commonly in females than in males, and on the left side more often than the right. At first the deformity is slight. It may not be noticed until the child is able to sit or stand. In other cases, however, the deformity may be severe, with a characteristic flattening and shortening of the face on the side to which the head is tilted. The facial asymmetry develops within the first three months and is thought to be due to impairment of the blood supply to the depressed side of the head. When correction of the torticollis is accomplished, a gradual decrease of the asymmetry will take place. The chin is rotated away from the side of the shortened muscle, and the head is displaced and tilted toward the side of the shortening (Fig. 177). The shoulder on the affected side may be elevated. Rotation and lateral bending of the neck are restricted, while flexion and extension are usually of normal range. Attempts to correct the deformity cause the affected muscle to tighten. There is often an associated cervicodorsal scoliosis. Eyestrain from ocular imbalance secondary to the deformity is frequent. In the rare affection of double torticollis the chin is elevated in the midline.

Diagnosis.—Tuberculosis of the cervical spine presents the greatest difficulty in differential diagnosis; in tuberculosis, however, the chin usually points toward the tight sternocleidomastoid muscle instead of away from it. Dislocations and fractures are to be differentiated, as well as osteomyelitis, acute myositis, and adenitis. Acute ocular and oral diseases sometimes cause a similar deformity. Of great differential value is the history of painless deformity since birth. The clinical diagnosis should always be supplemented by roentgenographic examination.

Prognosis.—There is little hope of improvement without treatment. Proper treatment in infants and children often results in complete cure. Following correction of the torticollis, the asymmetry of the face gradually becomes less noticeable. In cases corrected before the age of three or four years, the facial deformity may completely disappear.

Treatment.—The fundamental principle of treatment is overcorrection of the shortened sternocleidomastoid muscle. The treatment should be started as soon as the deformity is recognized.

Nonoperative Treatment.—Early cases with slight deformity may often be corrected by simple stretching of the head and neck into the overcorrected position and by exercises to strengthen the weak muscles. Rarely it may be wise to stretch the contracted structures under anesthesia and to follow this by fixation in a special brace or plaster cast; this may be necessary on several occasions from two to four weeks apart. The corrected position should be maintained until the weakened muscles have regained strength sufficient to hold the head and neck straight. Continued observation is most important. In the milder cases the results of nonoperative methods are good.

Operative Treatment.—All cases of moderate or severe deformity and all late cases require operative treatment, which in brief consists of section of the sternocleidomastoid muscle; maintenance of overcorrection of the deformity, which may be accomplished by means of plaster cast, brace or traction; and finally a program of exercises for training the muscles to maintain the correction permanently. In some clinics good results have been reported without the use of a postoperative support. A subcutaneous myotomy of the contracted muscle is occasionally performed; the open operation, however, is safer and more satisfactory. The muscle can be divided either at its origin from the sternum and clavicle or at its insertion into the mastoid process; however, division at the lower end is the easier operation and avoids the danger of injuring the spinal accessory nerve. All tight fascial structures, which may include the platysma muscle, should also be sectioned. After operation corrective exercises should be started and continued until there is no tendency toward recurrence, which may be for as long as six months. Many surgeons prefer to use a corrective brace during this period. There is always danger of a recurrence of the deformity; this should be explained to the parents before treatment is started.

ACQUIRED TORTICOLLIS

Eighty per cent of the cases of acquired torticollis occur in the first ten years of life. Acquired torticollis, unlike congenital torticollis, is often accompanied by pain.

The following types of acquired torticollis are most frequently observed:

1. *Acute,* caused by direct irritation of the muscles from injury or by an inflammatory reaction of the muscles (myositis) or of the cervical lymph nodes (lymphadenitis).

2. *Spasmodic,* in which rhythmic convulsive spasms of the muscles take place as a result of an organic disorder of the central nervous system. This will be discussed separately.

3. *Hysterical,* due to psychogenic inability of the patient to control the muscles of the neck.

In addition, torticollis may be associated with tuberculosis, osteomyelitis, arthritis, and injuries of the cervical spine, with contracture of scar tissue in the neck following a burn, with paralysis of the sternocleidomastoid muscle, with scoliosis of the cervical spine, and with meningitis and ocular defects.

Treatment.—The treatment of acquired torticollis should be directed toward the removal of local and general causes. Acute traumatic or inflammatory torticollis is sometimes relieved by hot applications and gentle massage and stretching of the neck. If severe contractures of the sternocleidomastoid muscle and the surrounding tissues persist after the causative process has subsided, they should be divided and after-care as described for congenital torticollis should be given.

Spasmodic Torticollis

Etiology.—Spasmodic torticollis is thought to be due either to (1) an organic lesion of the central nervous system or (2) reflex contractions from irritation of the cervical nerve roots by arthritic changes. It seems to occur most often, however, in individuals with a psychoneurotic tendency and in those who have been through periods of strain with mental anxiety and overwork.

Clinical Picture.—The deformity comes on gradually in adult life. The first symptoms are usually stiffness and discomfort of the muscles of one side of the neck. These are followed by a drawing sensation and a momentary twitching or slight contraction which pulls the head toward the affected side. The symptoms slowly become more marked until a convulsive spasm of the muscles develops and draws the head forcibly to one side. The spasm may exhibit either an irregular or a regular rhythm, is independent of voluntary control, and becomes especially marked when the patient grows excited. It may be associated with severe neuralgic pain throughout the head and neck. It is interesting to note that often the convulsive spasms can be inhibited by the light pressure of a finger against the head.

Prognosis.—There is little tendency toward spontaneous recovery. The results of operative treatment are sometimes good.

Treatment.—Occasionally conservative methods, consisting of psychotherapy, muscle training, and prolonged mechanical support of the neck with a well-fitting brace or plaster cast, lead to relief. Operative measures, however, are usually necessary. A resection of the spinal accessory nerve may relieve the spasmodic jerkings, or it may be necessary to remove the posterior branches of the upper cervical nerve roots as well as to divide the affected muscles.

Cervical Rib and Scalenus Anticus Syndrome

Cervical ribs are congenital anomalies consisting of supernumerary, independent units of growth similar to the first dorsal ribs. The extra ribs are attached most often to the seventh cervical vertebra but may be attached to the sixth. Cervical ribs are usually bilateral; when this is the case, one rib is always higher and presents a more advanced stage of development than the other.

Four types of cervical rib are found:

1. An exaggeration of the transverse process of the seventh cervical vertebra, with a fibrous band connecting it with the first rib (Fig. 178).

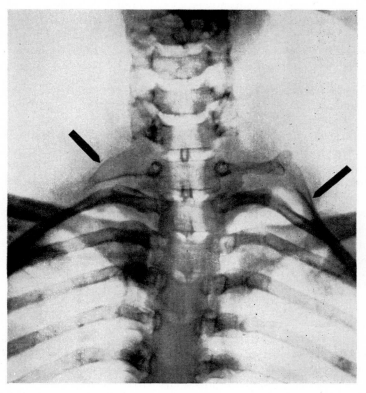

Fig. 178.—Anteroposterior roentgenogram showing left cervical rib and enlarged right transverse process of seventh cervical vertebra.

2. An incomplete rib attached to the seventh cervical vertebra with a band running to the first rib.

3. A complete rib which articulates with the first rib (Fig. 178).

4. A complete rib which is fused with the first rib anteriorly.

The lower roots of the brachial plexus are in close approximation to the anomalous ribs. The seventh cervical trunk crosses over the transverse process of the seventh cervical vertebra, and the eighth cervical trunk crosses over either the extra rib or the fibrous band. The subclavian vessels also are quite close. The artery lies in front of the rib and often presents at this point a localized dilatation which causes an increased pulsation in the neck. The subclavian vein lies a considerable distance below and in front of the artery and is seldom pressed upon or affected by the cervical rib. The scalenus anticus muscle is attached to the first rib in front of the inferior and middle trunks of the brachial plexus and the subclavian artery.

Frequently spasm can be demonstrated in the scalenus anticus muscle. It may cause pressure upon the underlying vessels and nerves. Since many observers believe spasm of the scalenus anticus to be the primary cause of the symptoms, the condition has been termed *scalenus anticus syndrome.*

Clinical Picture.—Although cervical ribs may be present without causing symptoms, a characteristic clinical picture frequently develops. The symptoms usually appear in adult life, most often at the age of about thirty years. They occur much more commonly in women than in men.

Locally there may be a tumor in the neck which may be both palpable and visible. It is most frequently found as a firm, rounded, immovable mass, 2 to 3 centimeters above the middle of the clavicle. Above this there is usually a palpable pulsation which is caused by the subclavian artery. About this area lies the brachial plexus. As postural changes result in gradual stretching of the middle and lower portions of the brachial plexus over the rib, friction takes place with use of the shoulder and arm. At first there is no pain, but repeated trauma finally produces a definite brachial neuritis. This may be followed by weakness and atrophy, starting in the intrinsic muscles of the hand and involving finally the entire extremity. Occasionally a claw hand deformity develops (Fig. 109). Paresthesia of the arm and forearm, especially of the part supplied by the ulnar nerve, is sometimes present and may be accompanied by radiating pain. Tingling and numbness are often the first symptoms, but later, as the pressure becomes more severe, anesthesia and paralysis may develop. At first, relief can be secured by changing the position of the arm. As the condition progresses, however, change of position no longer relieves the pain. Pallor, coldness, and cyanosis may appear in the fingers. There may be diminution of the volume of the radial pulse. Some observers believe that these changes are due to the action of the affected sympathetic nerve fibers in the lower part of the brachial plexus, while others believe that they are caused by direct mechanical pressure upon the subclavian artery. In advanced cases thrombosis of the subclavian artery may take place, giving rise to gangrene, which starts in the fingers. Gradually a collateral circulation may be established, however, which will compensate for the circulatory impairment. Occasionally the patient presents a scoliosis of the cervical spine with its convexity toward the side of the cervical rib.

Clinical manifestations similar to those of cervical ribs are sometimes encountered in the absence of demonstrable bony abnormality at the base of the neck. In such patients compression of the brachial plexus and the subclavian artery may be caused by spasm of the scalenus anticus muscle, the nerves and artery being pressed against the first rib by the tense muscle. Some observers believe that even in the presence of a cervical rib, spasm of the scalenus anticus muscle may be entirely responsible for the clinical picture by compressing the brachial plexus and subclavian artery against the extra rib.

Differential Diagnosis.—Because of the weakness and atrophy of the smaller muscles of the hand, the presence of a cervical rib is sometimes confused with syringomyelia, progressive muscular atrophy, injury of the spinal cord, or ulnar palsy. The factor of pain down the arm may confuse the diagnosis with that of arthritis of the cervical spine or infectious neuritis. Subacromial bursitis must occasionally be excluded. Occupational neuroses which give similar neuralgic symptoms must be differentiated. Rupture and protrusion of a cervical intervertebral disk must be considered; it can often be differentiated by the localization of symptoms and signs to a single nerve root. Any patient whose symptoms fail to respond to conservative orthopaedic measures, however, should receive neurosurgical consultation concerning the possibility of a cervical disk protrusion.

Treatment.—Conservative measures may be tried, especially in cases which seem to be improved by rest. Injection of procaine into the scalenus anticus muscle often produces temporary relief. To relieve the strain upon the lower brachial plexus and roots, the shoulder should be brought upward and backward with the use of a sling or brace. Hot baths, massage, and active exercises for the shoulder and arm should be given. Emphasis should be placed upon exercises for strengthening the trapezius and levator scapulae muscles. In some cases change to an occupation which does not put a strain upon the shoulder or arm will result in complete relief of the symptoms.

In cases in which the diagnosis is firmly established, surgical removal of the cervical rib may be followed by complete relief of the symptoms. However, the symptoms can often be cured by tenotomy of the scalenus anticus muscle, which may be compressing the subclavian artery and irritating the inferior and middle trunks of the brachial plexus. Tenotomy of the scalenus anticus, because of its technical ease and safety, is the operation of choice, and always should be done before a surgical removal of a cervical rib.

PART II. AFFECTIONS OF THE SHOULDER

Introduction.—The shoulder possesses less stability and less mechanical protection than any other large joint of the body. The glenoid fossa of the scapula is shallow, presenting only a slight concavity for the large globe of the humeral head. The concavity is disposed vertically, moreover, and gravity, instead of increasing the joint stability as in the case of hip or knee, exerts through the entire weight of the arm a constant force tending to produce a shearing strain. Not only does the bony configuration of the shoulder joint afford little stability, but the capsular ligaments, necessarily long and loose to permit the wide range of shoulder motion, oppose little strength to any force tending to cause a subluxation. It is therefore to be expected that the muscles and tendons about the shoulder play a relatively important part in maintaining joint stability. They form, in fact, a strong and flexible protective covering closely investing the entire joint, and in part the tendons are actually fused with the capsule. To provide for motion with a minimum of friction, the shoulder bursae (Fig. 179) are important, and these structures are in close relationship with the tendons and with the capsule.

These anatomic considerations are of significance in the interpretation of common clinical findings in affections of the shoulder. The intimate association of synovial membrane, ligaments, tendons, and bursae makes multiple involvement likely when the shoulder is injured, renders specific diagnostic analysis difficult, and leads to a confused terminology of shoulder affections. That any acute injury of the shoulder is likely to clear up slowly and incompletely, leading to symptoms of chronic nature, is a common clinical observation. Increasing the likelihood of a chronic disability are the constant drag of the unsupported arm on the shoulder joint and also the fact that in adduction, the position in which the injured joint is most conveniently held, contractures and atrophy quickly develop and decrease the range of painless motion.

Minor Injuries: Traumatic Synovitis, Sprain, and Strain

Clinical Picture.—After most shoulder injuries pain is severe; it is sometimes felt not only about the joint itself but throughout the arm, particularly on its lateral aspect about the insertion of the deltoid muscle. Tenderness also may be generalized. There is usually pain on motion, especially on abduction or external rotation, which results in the arm's being held closely against the side of the thorax. If the arm is allowed to remain in this position, a vicious circle is set up; adhesions, contractures, and atrophy develop and further increase the disability.

Differentiation of the various types of injury at the shoulder is essential to treatment. *Acute traumatic synovitis* undoubtedly is of common occurrence but is relatively of less importance than in the weight-bearing joints; it is associated usually with injury of one or more of the surrounding structures. Shoulder *sprain,* or stretching or slight tearing of the capsular ligaments, accompanied by extravasation of blood, is a common athletic injury characterized clinically by tenderness over the joint capsule, pain on motion, and slow recovery. Muscular *strain* about the shoulder is suspected when particular pain is elicited by contraction of a specific muscle against resistance and when localized tenderness is present over the muscle or its tendon.

Treatment.—The first essential in the treatment of any acute injury of the shoulder is rest. This may be facilitated by the use of a sling, often in conjunction with a shoulder cap of adhesive plaster. In the more severe cases some surgeons believe that it is preferable to support the joint in abduction, which is the position of physiologic rest and the one in which adhesions and contractures are least likely to occur. If the shoulder is seen within the first few hours after injury, application of cold by means of an ice cap may retard extravasation of blood. Afterward heat is applied constantly to relieve pain and to hasten absorption of the extravasated blood. However, rest must not be continued for too long a time. Massage, followed by gradually increasing active exercise, should be started as soon as the acute symptoms have begun definitely to subside.

Subacromial Bursitis

The subacromial or subdeltoid bursa is a large, flat, thin-walled sac covering laterally the upper end of the humerus and the shoulder joint

(Fig. 179). It consists of an upper or subacromial portion which overlies the tendon insertions into the shoulder capsule and the greater tuberosity of the humerus and which is in turn covered by the acromion process, and a lower or subdeltoid portion which overlies the humeral tuberosity and is covered by the belly of the deltoid muscle. The two portions are occasionally separated by a thin membrane; they never communicate with the cavity of the shoulder joint. In opening the normal shoulder the bursa is scarcely recognizable as a definite structure, but in common inflammatory states it may be so distended and thickened as to be palpable even through the deltoid muscle.

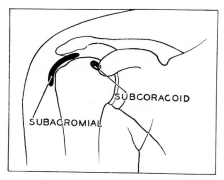

Fig. 179.—Two most commonly affected bursae about the shoulder.

Subacromial bursitis is commonly accepted as a disease entity, although clinically it often cannot be differentiated with certainty from lesions of other closely related structures about the shoulder joint. Its etiology may be infectious or traumatic.

Pyogenic infection with accumulation of pus within the bursa and without purulent involvement of the shoulder joint rarely occurs. The diagnosis is suspected from local acute signs without the severe joint and systemic reaction of a septic arthritis and is confirmed by aspiration. The treatment, like that of the analogous purulent prepatellar bursitis, consists of rest, heat, and systemic antibiotic therapy.

In the majority of cases of subacromial bursitis, however, there is no frank local infection, and foci of infection elsewhere and single injuries or repeated trauma are to be weighed carefully as causative factors. Clinically the patient with acute bursitis experiences severe pain in the shoulder, sometimes referred down the entire arm as well. This pain may permit the arm to be swung in the sagittal plane but sharply limits any rotation or abduction. Often when abduction is carried out passively an angle can be identified at which pressure of the inflamed sac beneath the acromion process causes a sudden increase in the intensity of the pain. Tenderness may be generalized over the shoulder joint but is often most marked over the central portion of the bursa just beneath the acromion process. In more chronic cases the signs are much less definite, and, since in such cases there must almost surely be associated pathologic changes in other structures about the joint and contiguous to the bursa, the term *periarthritis* is often applied to them. In such cases an old tear of the musculotendinous cuff of the shoulder joint or degenerative changes in the tendon of the long head of the biceps may be present. Long-standing cases, in addition to the signs already mentioned, frequently present disabling adduction contracture, limitation of rotation, and severe muscle weakness and atrophy. A roentgenogram is indicated to investigate the possible presence of calcification within the bursa or the supraspinatus tendon (Fig. 180) and of arthritic changes in the shoulder joint.

Treatment.—The first essential in the treatment of *acute bursitis* is rest and support, preferably in bed and with the arm in as much abduction as can be secured. Pillows or splints may be used. A simple Velpeau dressing may give sufficient immobilization to relieve the pain, but the position of adduction must not be long maintained. Frequently, light adhesive traction gives the best combination of immobilization, support, and gentle corrective force acting to lessen the muscle spasm. Heat is indicated and may afford full relief of the pain. It is best applied by the use of compresses, poultices, electric pad, or diathermy. Diathermy treatments are said by some to be extremely effective in relief of the acute symptoms. In some cases, however, the application of ice packs is very effective. Procaine block of the suprascapular nerve, which carries a large part of the sensory supply of the shoulder joint, is often most helpful. Block of the stellate ganglion may afford relief but is technically hazardous. Injection of a weak solution of procaine into the inflamed bursal sac sometimes leads to instant relief of the pain. If this form of therapy is employed, the bursa should be punctured by numerous needle holes from different directions. Sometimes it is possible to irrigate the bursa with normal saline by placing two needles from different angles into the sac. Roentgen therapy often affords satisfactory relief. If the severe pain of an acute bursitis fails to respond satisfactorily to these measures, excision of the bursa may be indicated.

As the discomfort and tenderness become less acute, massage and exercise of the shoulder should be started. Any definite foci of infection, particularly in the mouth, nose, and throat, should be eradicated after the acute stage of the bursitis has passed.

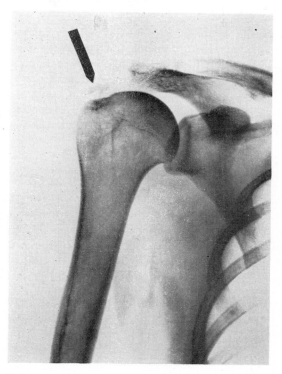

Fig. 180.—Roentgenogram showing calcification near subacromial bursa in a patient forty years of age.

If, in addition to the bursitis, a *chronic periarthritis* is present, gentle manipulation of the shoulder under anesthesia is occasionally indicated to release painful adhesions and increase the range of joint motion. Manipulation should not be done, however, unless traction in abduction and prolonged physical therapy have proved ineffectual. Manipulation must always be carried out with the greatest caution in order to avoid fracture of the atrophic humerus at its surgical neck. It should never be done in the presence of active arthritis. It should be followed by physical therapy including active exercises to develop the abductors of the shoulder. An abduction splint is sometimes indicated.

In chronic or recurrent cases irrigation of the subacromial bursa sometimes relieves the pain. Excision of the bursa often affords complete relief. Operation is inadvisable unless more conservative measures have failed to alleviate the symptoms.

Excision of the small calcified bodies or soft calcareous materials which in the roentgenogram are sometimes visible near the floor of the bursa (Fig. 180) and which are occasionally even palpable, may be carried out when their presence is associated with obstinate pain and tenderness. Otherwise their removal is not indicated, since they have frequently been observed to undergo resorption under roentgen or diathermy treatment or after needling, or even to disappear spontaneously.

Subcoracoid Bursitis

Inflammation of the subcoracoid bursa, which lies between the capsule of the shoulder joint and the coracoid process of the scapula, arises when the shoulder is allowed to droop forward, causing the lesser tuberosity of the humerus to impinge against the coracoid process. The pain is always well localized and accompanied by a limitation of rotation and abduction of the shoulder. Subcoracoid bursitis is sometimes difficult to differentiate from laceration of the capsule of the shoulder joint.

Treatment.—The treatment is similar to that of subacromial bursitis, and, in addition, postural exercises to correct the shoulder girdle deformity are useful.

Rupture of the Supraspinatus Tendon and Tears of the Musculotendinous Cuff

Rupture of the supraspinatus tendon is a common and important cause of shoulder disability. In severe cases the tear may be extensive, involving not only the supraspinatus tendon but almost the entire musculotendinous cuff of the shoulder.

Pathology.—The flattened tendon of the supraspinatus muscle, after blending intimately with the adjacent infraspinatus tendon and the capsule of the shoulder joint, inserts into the highest facet of the greater tuberosity of the humerus. The supraspinatus tendon thus forms both the roof of the shoulder joint and the floor of the subacromial bursa.

Rupture of the supraspinatus tendon usually occurs near its insertion (Fig. 181). Retraction of the muscle after extensive tears leaves a direct opening between the subacromial bursa and the shoulder joint. Minor lacerations are probably common in later adult years and have been found in a large percentage of routine postmortem examinations. At times a small fragment of the greater tuberosity of the humerus is torn away together with avulsion of the tendon near its insertion.

With time the pathologic changes accompanying complete rupture become more pronounced. Progressive retraction of the muscle widens the rent in the joint capsule. The distal stub of the tendon, at first a sharply outlined mass, becomes atrophic and may disappear, while the edge of the tuberosity gradually becomes rounded and smooth.

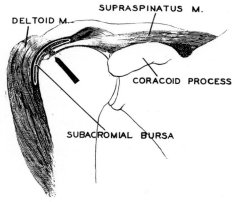

Fig. 181.—Rupture of the supraspinatus tendon. Arrow points to rupture.

Etiology.—There is almost always a history of considerable trauma, and at times the rupture accompanies an anterior dislocation of the shoulder. The mechanism is presumably an indirect violence associated with sudden powerful elevation of the arm in an attempt to regain balance or to cushion a fall. The presence of a heavy object in the hand increases the likelihood of rupture. It is not infrequently caused by the throwing of a ball.

Clinical Picture.—Rupture of the supraspinatus tendon is most common in laborers past the age of forty years. The rupture is accompanied by a transient sharp pain in the shoulder, and a few hours later there begins a steady ache which may last for several days.

Examination with the humerus adducted discloses a tender point below the acromion process, and a sulcus between acromion and tendon insertion may be palpable. As a rule, the ability to initiate and maintain abduction of the shoulder is not lost when the supraspinatus tendon alone is ruptured, but is absent in complete or massive avulsions of the cuff.

When the arm is carried into abduction, there is transient pain and slight crepitus as the torn insertion of the tendon passes under the edge of the acromion process; the same pain is felt at the corresponding angle as the arm is again lowered.

Subsequently the patient may experience severe shoulder pain for months. This is often most marked at night and is so aggravated after exertion during the day that any type of active work becomes impossible. In late cases atrophy of the supraspinatus and infraspinatus muscles is a constant sign.

Treatment.—For complete rupture of the supraspinatus tendon and extensive tears of the musculotendinous cuff, operative repair is indicated. When the diagnosis is in doubt, exploration may be carried out through a short vertical incision. For the repair a wide exposure is necessary and may be gained by extending the incision posteriorly with osteotomy of the acromion process, exposing the whole roof of the shoulder joint. It is often advisable to divide the coraco-acromial ligament. Temporary use of an abduction brace after operation is sometimes helpful. Chief reliance, however, is placed upon active exercises of the shoulder. These are started two weeks after operation, increased gradually, and continued until maximum function has been regained.

Rupture of the Biceps Brachii

Rupture of the biceps brachii is of infrequent occurrence. The long head may rupture at or near its origin from the glenoid tubercle, at some point within the bicipital groove, or at the musculotendinous junction. Rupture may also occur within the muscle belly of one or both heads, or at their insertion into the tubercle of the radius.

Etiology.—Rupture of the biceps is ordinarily a result of sudden indirect violence, usually without direct injury of the overlying tissues. Rupture of the long head as it traverses the bicipital groove is said to be associated always with a previous weakening of the tendon by changes due to occupational trauma or chronic arthritis. In the aged such ruptures may follow violence of trivial degree.

Clinical Picture.—At the moment of rupture there is usually sharp pain and occasionally an audible snap. The most characteristic physical finding is a sharply convex bulge near the middle of the arm (Fig. 182). There may be slight local tenderness, and weakness of flexion of the elbow and supination of the forearm as compared with these motions in the normal arm. The roentgenogram sometimes shows a small avulsion fracture of the glenoid rim. Rupture of the long head is sometimes difficult to differentiate clinically from dislocation of this tendon out of the bicipital groove.

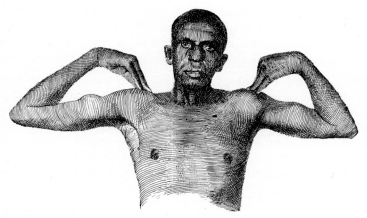

Fig. 182.—Rupture of the long head of the right biceps muscle. (After Conwell.)

Treatment.—Early cases should be treated by immediate exploration and suture. When separation from the glenoid tubercle or rupture of the tendon of the long head has occurred, the proximal portion of the tendon may be excised and its distal portion fixed to the coracoid process or into the floor of the bicipital groove. Adequate postoperative immobilization should be followed by a program of graded exercise.

Snapping Shoulder

A shoulder in which an audible click or snap can be elicited by appropriate muscular contractions is occasionally observed. This condition is known as snapping shoulder and sometimes becomes habitual or involuntary, especially if the patient learns how to cause the snap and elicits it repeatedly. The sound is produced by an incomplete luxation of the joint or by the slipping of a taut tendon over a bony prominence. Rarely a structural change, such as the presence of an anomalous group of muscle fibers, has been demonstrated at exploratory operation. As a rule the symptoms are trivial and no treatment is required.

Recurrent Dislocation of the Shoulder

Traumatic anterior dislocation of the shoulder joint, even when treated according to accepted principles, is sometimes followed by repeated dislocations. These cases of recurrent dislocation, while few in contrast to the large number of primary traumatic displacements, are common enough to form an important clinical entity, especially in the military services. Recurrent posterior dislocation is rarely encountered.

Etiology and Pathology.—Factors which may facilitate repeated dislocation are incompletely healed tears or relaxation of the capsular ligaments, weakness of the surrounding musculature, and congenital or acquired changes in the contour of the humeral head or of the glenoid fossa. In most cases, however, avulsion of the glenoid labrum from the anterior rim of the glenoid cavity seems to be of chief importance, together with erosion of the glenoid rim and a defect of the postero-lateral aspect of the head of the humerus.

Clinical Picture.—The majority of patients are young adults. The condition is seen with especial frequency in athletes and in persons subject to the trauma of epileptic seizures. At first the dislocation occurs only after severe trauma, but successive recurrences require less and less causative force, and finally dislocation may follow any movement, however trivial, which involves abduction of the shoulder. With successive recurrences, reduction of the displacement becomes correspondingly easier. The pain attending dislocation similarly decreases, but the disability remains extreme, and the patient may feel a constant dread of impending displacement. Atrophy of the muscles of the shoulder girdle sometimes occurs, and rarely signs of involvement of the brachial plexus develop.

Treatment.—The nonoperative treatment of recurrent dislocation consists of preventing the displacement by limiting abduction of the arm and of carrying out resistive exercises to strengthen the muscles which internally rotate the shoulder. The displacement may be prevented by strapping the arm to the thorax, by pinning the sleeve to the coat, or by the application of a chest belt and an arm band connected by a short flexible strap. Such devices are inconvenient and annoying.

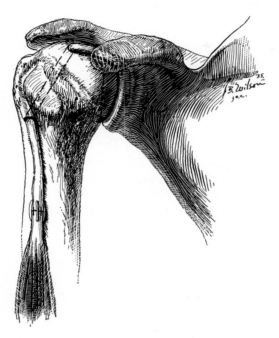

Fig. 183.—Nicola operation for recurrent dislocation of the shoulder. The tendon of the long head of the biceps muscle has been removed from the bicipital groove and passed through a tunnel in the upper end of the humerus. (After Nicola.)

The treatment of choice is surgical. A wide variety of procedures has been devised by different operators. Bankart's suture of the capsule to the glenoid rim, a difficult but highly effective procedure, is the operation of choice of many surgeons. In the Nicola operation the tendon of the long head of the biceps, sometimes reinforced by a strip of the joint capsule, is placed in a tunnel through the humeral head to act as a suspensory ligament (Fig. 183). This operation is popular but is not always successful in preventing redislocation. Henderson has had very good results from suspension of the humeral head to the acromion process by a loop of peroneal tendon. In recent years the Putti-Platt operation, the principle of which is to limit external rotation of the shoulder, has become popular in many clinics. In this operation the subscapular tendon and the capsule are divided one inch from their humeral attachment, the cut end of the lateral portion is sutured to the anterior rim of the glenoid fossa, and the cut end of the medial portion is attached to the tendinous cuff over the greater tuberosity of the humerus; thus, the medial portion of the tendon overlaps the lateral. There have been many modifications of these procedures.

After all operations for recurrent dislocation of the shoulder, carefully graded exercises should be carried out for many months, with precautions against strenuous exercise requiring abduction of the shoulder.

Old Dislocation of the Shoulder

Cases of unreduced shoulder dislocation of long standing are occasionally met with and present a difficult therapeutic problem. Such patients show an obvious deformity and on attempting to use the affected shoulder have considerable pain and disability. The nerves of the brachial plexus are sometimes affected (see page 288).

Pathology.—When the humeral head remains displaced from the glenoid cavity a series of pathologic changes occurs and makes reduction more and more difficult as time goes on. The glenoid cavity fills with granulation tissue, and the torn capsule contracts. The head of the humerus becomes bound down by scar tissue, and the muscles about the joint become shortened and fibrotic. Atrophy of the humerus itself develops rapidly and may constitute a formidable obstacle to manipulation.

Treatment.—If the dislocation has been present for not more than eight weeks it can occasionally be reduced by closed manipulation. In order to provide adequate relaxation, the anesthetic agent may be supplemented with curare. Care must be taken not to employ sudden or excessive force which might injure the brachial plexus, rupture the axillary vessels, or fracture the humerus at its surgical neck. After reduction the arm may be bandaged to the side or may be immobilized in plaster in slight abduction and flexion. Two weeks later a program of daily physical therapy, including active exercise, is started.

For older dislocations and those which previously have failed to be reduced by a closed manipulation, operation is indicated. A wide exposure is necessary. After reduction the arm is immobilized at the side by a plaster or adhesive dressing. Again the after-treatment consists of the prolonged use of daily physical therapy.

Occasionally it is advisable to excise the head of the humerus. The functional result is sometimes satisfactory. In a few cases, because of the patient's age or poor general condition, the excessive duration of the dislocation, or the absence of significant pain or limitation of motion, strenuous efforts to effect replacement are not to be advised.

Old Acromioclavicular Dislocation

Dislocation of the acromioclavicular joint is a common injury. It occurs frequently in football players as a consequence of falls or blows upon the point of the shoulder, and the resulting disability when the arm is elevated makes it impossible to pass the ball effectively. The diagnosis is usually evident upon inspection and palpation but should be supported by roentgenographic examination to exclude the possibility of fracture of the acromial end of the clavicle. The roentgenogram should always be taken with the patient standing and the arm unsupported or carrying a weight, because often in the supine position the dislocation becomes spontaneously reduced and the instability will not be evident. Unless carefully treated, acromioclavicular dislocations are likely to become chronic, since the weight of the dependent extremity tends to maintain the dislocation.

Pathology.—The usual displacement is a dropping of the acromion downward and forward because of the weight of the arm; the acromial end of the clavicle thereby acquires undue upward prominence and mobility. More important than the tearing of the articular capsule and rupture of the acromioclavicular ligaments is rupture of the powerful coracoclavicular ligaments (Fig. 184,A) which normally prevent upward displacement of the lateral end of the clavicle.

Treatment and Prognosis.—In many cases of old acromioclavicular dislocation the disability is negligible and no treatment is indicated other than a program of active exercises for the shoulder. If the symptoms are disabling, however, they can be satisfactorily relieved by operation although a slight prominence of the lateral end of the clavicle frequently recurs. The strongest repair is secured by tying the clavicle down to the coracoid process as well as to the acromion; this may be done effectively by constructing new coracoclavicular and acromioclavicular ligaments of fascia lata (Fig. 184,B). After operation the position of reduction must be maintained for eight weeks by means of temporary internal fixation with wire, an ample adhesive dressing, or a plaster jacket incorporating support of the arm. Lifting of heavy objects should be avoided for an additional eight weeks.

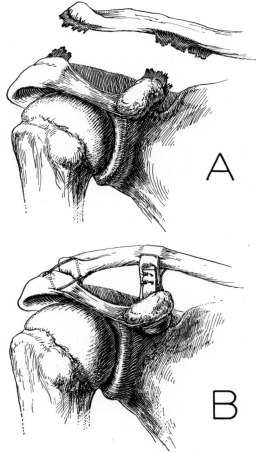

Fig. 184.—Acromioclavicular dislocation. *A,* Note rupture of acromioclavic-ular and coracoclavicular ligaments which accompanies the dislocation; *B,* operative reduction of the dislocation and construction of new ligaments. (After Henry.)

An alternative procedure, consisting of excision of the lateral end of the clavicle, has been described by Mumford and by Gurd and apparently produces satisfactory functional results. Fusion of the acromioclavicular joint limits mobility of the shoulder and is therefore inadvisable.

Old Sternoclavicular Dislocation

Dislocation of the sternal end of the clavicle occurs much less frequently than acromioclavicular dislocation. Sternoclavicular dislocation may result from a violent fall or blow upon the shoulder, in which case the sternoclavicular ligaments are ruptured and the intra-articular fibrocartilage remains attached usually to the clavicle. The displacement tends to persist unless corrected by treatment. In debilitated individuals chronic or recurrent dislocation is sometimes found without history of acute trauma. The dislocation also may develop gradually when there is a paralysis of the pectoral muscles. In sternoclavicular dislocation the end of the clavicle is ordinarily displaced anteriorly, and the deformity is usually evident upon inspection and palpation.

Treatment.—Surgical treatment is indicated only if the deformity is accompanied by pain. The most effective treatment is to suture the end of the clavicle to the sternum or the first rib with fascia lata. After operation the corrected position must be maintained for six to eight weeks by means of a pressure pad and a strong adhesive dressing. The lifting of heavy objects should be avoided for an additional period of several weeks.

CHAPTER XXIV

AFFECTIONS OF THE ELBOW, WRIST, HAND, AND JAW

PART I. AFFECTIONS OF THE ELBOW

The elbow is a hinge joint with a range of motion of from 180 to 30 degrees. Pronation and supination are made possible by rotation of the head of the radius on the capitellum of the humerus. Despite the wide extent of elbow motion, stability is well maintained by the fitting of the trochlear process of the humerus deeply into the greater sigmoid fossa of the ulna, by powerful muscular and tendinous supports, and by strong lateral ligaments. Stability of the radiohumeral joint is not due to bony configuration, since the head of the radius presents only a shallow concavity for articulation with the capitellum, but rather to the strong annular ligament which holds the radial head in approximation with the lesser sigmoid fossa of the ulna.

The wide range of motion in the elbow region renders its structures peculiarly liable to strains and sprains. Because of its tendinous investment and its exposed position, the elbow may suffer attacks of bursitis, and, because of the proximity of important structures on its anterior aspect, injuries of the elbow occasionally lead to important circulatory and neurologic complications.

Strains and Sprains

Muscular strains about the elbow are common results of isolated episodes of slight trauma or of unaccustomed repeated trauma of minor degree.

Diagnosis.—An effort should always be made to allocate the lesion to one muscle or muscle group; this is best done by careful localization of the maximum pain and tenderness and by analysis of the type of resisted active motion which causes most discomfort. In differential diagnosis ligamentous sprain, bursitis, and minor fractures must be kept in mind. In youth epiphyseal separations in the elbow region are particularly important because of the large number of epiphyses and the wide range in the time of their consolidation; the first of these epiphyses makes its roentgenographic appearance at seventeen months, and the last union is not complete before the age of twenty years. It is advisable to examine the elbow roentgenographically after any considerable injury, and in children a film of the normal elbow is valuable for detailed comparison with the traumatized area.

Treatment.—Strain is treated by temporary immobilization of the affected muscle in a position of relaxation by means of removable plaster splints, adhesive plaster, or sling. Physical therapy consisting of heat and massage is started at once and is followed by graded active exercise.

Ligamentous sprain, while resembling muscle strain in causation, symptomatology, and treatment, may be slower in subsiding. Sprain of the external lateral ligament occurs fairly commonly among baseball, tennis, and golf players.

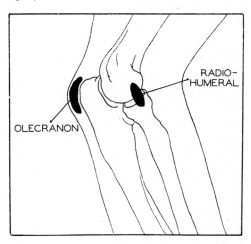

Fig. 185.—Most commonly affected bursae about the elbow.

Olecranon Bursitis

About the elbow joint as many as ten bursae have been described, but most of these are inconstant and of little clinical significance. The *olecranon bursa* (Fig. 185), situated between the tip of the olecranon process and the skin, is frequently involved by inflammatory changes.

A single episode of local injury may produce olecranon bursitis, but continued traumatization of slight degree is a more common cause. The diagnosis is usually evident from the history of injury, from the localization of pain, swelling, and tenderness posteriorly only, and from the slight restriction of flexion by pain as the inflamed structure is placed under tension.

Treatment.—The type of therapy varies with the acuteness of the individual case. Purulent bursitis is uncommon; its treatment includes rest, heat, aspirations, antibiotics, and sometimes incision and drainage. The more frequent nonspecific inflammation may usually be cured by aspiration of the fluid, application of a compression bandage and local heat, and care to prevent repetition of the causative trauma. In chronic cases the bursal sac may become greatly thickened; this condition is sometimes caller *miner's elbow*. The sac sometimes contains many small loose bodies. Such chronic changes indicate excision of the bursa. It is occasionally necessary to remove in addition to the bursa a small bony spur which may lie at the tip of the olecranon process and may extend for a short distance into the triceps tendon.

Radiohumeral Bursitis (Tennis Elbow)

The common disorder often termed radiohumeral bursitis exhibits typical clinical characteristics; its cause, however, has not been established. In some instances irritation of bursal tissue overlying the radiohumeral joint capsule (Fig. 185) seems to be responsible. However, at operation a definite bursal sac is seldom found. Many observers believe that the usual lesion is a partial rupture of the origin of the extensor muscles with a secondary traumatic periostitis at the external epicondyle.

Clinical Picture.—The usual onset is a gradually increasing discomfort following continued slight traumatization in the region of the radiohumeral joint. Tennis playing, which requires repeated pronation and supination of the forearm with extension of the elbow, is a common cause. The disorder is frequent among athletes, butchers, carpenters, motormen, and the like. Pain is experienced in the lateral aspect of the elbow, particularly when the patient reaches forward to pick up an object or to turn a doorknob, and the discomfort may spread down the entire forearm and be very persistent and annoying. Examination shows a small area of tenderness over the lateral condyle of the humerus and the radiohumeral joint. The grip may be weak. Passive motion of the elbow is unaffected, while active extension against resistance may cause intense discomfort. Roentgenograms are usually negative.

Treatment.—Radiohumeral bursitis may be treated nonoperatively or operatively. Temporary immobilization of the elbow with a sling, adhesive dressing, or plaster cast and the use of heat and massage will usually produce relief. The application of a dorsiflexion splint to the wrist, which relaxes the extensor tendons, is often helpful. The tender area may be injected with procaine. Excellent results from manipulation of the elbow with or without anesthesia have been reported. Roentgen therapy is often followed by relief. In cases which fail to respond to these measures, operation is indicated. The common extensor origin should be released from the epicondyle; any bursal tissue found between the common extensor tendon and the joint capsule should be excised.

Bicipitoradial Bursitis

Occasionally discomfort and tenderness in the region of the bicipito-radial bursa, together with increased local pain on resisted flexion-supination of the elbow, follow violent use of the biceps with the forearm pronated, as in the pitching of a baseball. Treatment consisting of rest, heat, and massage is indicated.

Radiohumeral Subluxation In Children

A common and sometimes unrecognized occurrence in young children is subluxation of the proximal end of the radius on the capitellum of the humerus. This condition has been termed "nursemaid's elbow" because of the mechanism by which it is produced: a sudden, direct pull on the elevated extremity, which may occur when a child falls while its hand is being held by an adult. The diagnosis is made on the history together with characteristic physical findings. The child refuses to use the arm, and the elbow is held slightly flexed. All movements are of essentially normal range except supination. The forearm is held in neutral position as regards rotation, and attempts to supinate cause pain and a sensation of mechanical blocking.

Treatment.—A very brief manipulation without anesthesia is indicated. With the child's elbow flexed to a right angle, the forearm is supinated forcibly while pressure is exerted on the radial head by the operator's thumb. As the point of obstruction is passed a definite click is usually felt; following this the child almost immediately resumes use of the arm. If for any reason prompt reduction is not carried out, the subluxation will usually undergo spontaneous reduction in a few days.

Old Dislocation of the Elbow

Old unreduced posterior dislocation of the radius and ulna on the humerus is occasionally encountered and presents a characteristic clinical picture. The deformity is usually obvious to inspection and palpation, the olecranon and the triceps tendon appearing abnormally prominent posteriorly. There may be severe pain on resisted motion, and the range of mobility is much restricted, particularly in flexion.

Treatment.—When the dislocation has been present for as long as two or three weeks, an open reduction is usually necessary, since forced manipulation is likely to damage the soft tissues or to fracture the humeral condyles. A wide operative exposure is essential and is often gained by the posterior route with division of the triceps tendon. Care must be exercised to avoid unnecessary injury of the soft tissues and in particular of the ulnar nerve. After reduction, suture of the tendon, and closure, the elbow is immobilized in flexion. In the after-treatment physical therapy is of value but must be carefully supervised and should not include passive stretching.

Volkmann's Ischemic Contracture

This very disabling contracture of the fingers and wrist, first described in 1875 by von Volkmann, is an occasional complication of injuries of the upper extremities and particularly of fractures about the elbow joint. An analogous condition is sometimes observed in the lower extremities. The muscles of the forearm are indurated and rigid, the joints present unsightly contracture deformities, and the hand often becomes almost completely useless (Fig. 186).

Etiology and Pathology.—The cause of the contracture is thought to be a severe ischemia resulting from spasm of the brachial artery with reflex spasm of the collateral vessels. Early exploration at the site of injury may show a severe segmental spasm of the brachial artery extending down into the radial and ulnar branches, narrowing them to the size of a string and obliterating their lumens. A visible lesion of the vessel itself may or may not be present.

The muscle bellies, which require a great deal of blood, are rapidly and profoundly affected by the ischemia. Microscopically, evidence of widespread degeneration and necrosis of the muscle fibers is quickly followed by round cell infiltration and by the extensive formation of fibrous tissue which later undergoes progressive contraction. Nerves to the forearm and hand may be damaged by the original injury or by the subsequent ischemia.

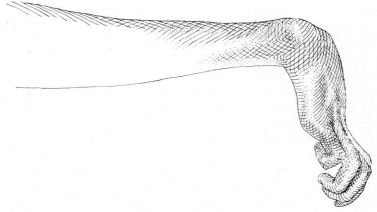

Fig. 186.—Volkmann's ischemic contracture. Note contractures of the wrist and fingers and atrophy of the forearm.

Clinical Picture.—Ischemic contracture occurs most commonly after supracondylar fractures of the humerus. Severe pain should at once suggest the onset of this complication but is not always present. The most important clinical sign is absence of the radial pulse. The hand may quickly become cyanotic, slightly swollen, and cold, and the fingers may be insensitive and powerless. Ischemia of forty-eight hours' duration usually results ultimately in a severe degree of contracture. As fibrosis proceeds, the forearm becomes hardened and shrunken, and the hand develops severe claw deformity (Fig. 186) and extreme disability. Examination may show also a paralysis which has resulted from damage of one or more nerve trunks.

Treatment.—The early treatment of Volkmann's contracture is exceedingly important and in each case should be instituted as soon as possible. Prophylactic treatment should begin immediately after the original injury. If at this time there are no signs of circulatory embarrassment in the forearm and hand, reduction of the fracture may be carried out at once or may be started by the application of adhesive traction. If reduction by manipulation is elected, several precautions are to be observed. Flexion should never be forced against resistance and must never be carried to the point of affecting the strength of the radial pulse. When at the original manipulation sufficient flexion cannot be obtained to maintain satisfactory alignment, a second or third closed reduction can be carried out in the following few days, the elbow being splinted in increasing flexion as the edema and hemorrhage in the antecubital fossa subside. After gentle manipulation, immobilization is secured by a posterior splint of plaster applied with care to avoid circular constriction. Observation during the next few days must be frequent and critical, and if severe pain or the signs of circulatory obstruction appear, immediate loosening or removal of the bandages is obligatory.

In borderline cases in which ischemia appears imminent, the safest treatment is to regard the fracture as of decidedly secondary importance and to concentrate all efforts upon improving the circulation. Procaine block of the brachial plexus may avert a catastrophe. Sympathicolytic drugs, which produce vasodilation, may prove most useful. Elevation of the arm by means of traction with the elbow in partial flexion, and the application of cold are indicated until there is sufficient circulatory improvement to permit of a closed reduction. Skeletal traction by means of a Kirschner wire inserted through the olecranon process may be helpful, but skin traction is usually effective.

When a condition of acute severe ischemia is manifest, immediate operative intervention is indicated. Experience has shown that in such cases closed reduction is inadequate treatment and is likely to be followed by disastrous consequences. The hematoma should be evacuated through an anterior incision. The artery must be exposed at the level of injury, care being taken to avoid damage of any of its branches. If warm saline applications, gentle massage of the vessel, and the intravenous injection of papaverine fail to restore the radial pulse, or if a lesion of the arterial wall is manifest, the constricted segment should be resected between ligatures. Collateral vessels, thus freed of reflex spasm, will in most cases maintain an adequate circulation. The fracture may be reduced gently before the wound is closed. In the next few days, repeated procaine block of the brachial plexus or the stellate and cervical sympathetic ganglia may be indicated. A sympathicolytic drug may be used. The wrist and fingers should be splinted in functional position to forestall contractures.

Treatment of the late case is frequently unsatisfactory. Moderate improvement of the deformity and recovery of power often follow gradual stretching of the contracted muscles. This may be accomplished by means of a banjo splint fitted with elastic finger traction and hinged for progressive extension of the wrist, or by the gradual wedging of a well-molded plaster cast. Intensive physical therapy is essential. When conservative measures prove ineffective, surgery is indicated. Many of the earlier operative procedures have not proved worth while and have been abandoned. Tendon lengthening is occasionally necessary. The muscle-sliding operation of Page, in which the attachment of the flexor muscles at the elbow is cut and pulled distally by hyperextension of the fingers and wrist, has in some hands produced good results. Arthrodesis of the wrist is occasionally indicated. When there is definite involvement of a nerve trunk, as after imperfect reduction of the original fracture, exploration for the purpose of freeing the nerve may be of benefit.

Traumatic Myositis Ossificans

Another important complication of injuries about the elbow, seen also in other parts of the body at times, is the formation of excessive amounts of new bone which may restrict the range of joint motion. Such new bone may be the result of any of several related pathologic processes. Excessive bone formation resulting simply from an active healing process and limited in area to the actual site of bony or periosteal injury is called *exuberant callus*. Bone produced by the organization and ossification of a hematoma, a process directly analogous to callus formation, may be found beneath the periosteum or extending out into the muscle or other soft tissues and is called *ossifying hematoma* (Fig. 187). The condition of intramuscular ossification following local injury is known as *traumatic myositis ossificans*. It is not to be confused with *myositis ossificans progressiva*, a rare constitutional disease described on page 106.

Traumatic myositis ossificans may result either from repeated slight injuries or from a single episode of more severe trauma. Examples of the chronic type are the *rider's bone*, which forms within the thigh adductors of horsemen, and the ossification within the pectoralis major which in soldiers sometimes follows the habitual firing of a rifle. Intramuscular ossification following a single injury may occur in various regions of the body but is most frequent in the thigh, in the upper part of the arm, and about the elbow joint (Fig. 187). Ossification in and about the elbow is of particular importance because it may cause a serious limitation of joint motion.

Etiology and Pathology.—The exact genesis of the new bone is uncertain. Osteoblasts from the adjacent injured periosteum undoubtedly play a part, while in many cases a metaplasia of local fibroblasts into bone-forming cells seems to take place. Some observers have attributed importance to a constitutional factor predisposing to ossification.

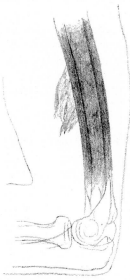

Fig. 187.—Ossifying hematoma. (Drawing from roentgenogram.)

The new bone forms commonly in the lower portion of the belly of the brachialis muscle, anterior to the elbow joint. It may appear first as minute osteocartilaginous spicules which lie parallel to the muscle fibers; these later coalesce forming an irregular bony mass which gradually becomes more rounded, homogeneous, and dense. Rarely a complete bridge of bone may develop, forming a spontaneous extra-articular arthrodesis. Usually the bone formation ceases within three to six months. The bony mass may be connected to the shaft by an osseous pedicle or a fibrous septum or may lie entirely separate from it. Spontaneous regression of the mass occurs frequently and may result in its complete disappearance.

Clinical Picture.—Traumatic myositis ossificans is seen most frequently in patients between the ages of fifteen and thirty years. In the case of the elbow joint, the antecedent injury is most often a posterior dislocation or a fracture of the lower end of the humerus, but the condition may follow an uncomplicated strain or contusion. The diagnosis is to be suspected when tenderness, swelling, limitation of elbow motion, or pain on motion fails to clear up within the usual period, or when after an initial improvement these signs begin to become more marked. The area of ossification is usually palpable and is demonstrable in the roentgenogram after three or four weeks. Early osteogenic sarcoma must be considered in the differential diagnosis but can as a rule be definitely excluded by the roentgenogram.

Treatment.—The stage at which the process is encountered determines the treatment. Since vigorous physical therapy is believed to stimulate the ossification, massage and strenuous exercise are to be avoided after elbow injuries; this is not likely to lead to contractures since in the elbow, and particularly in young individuals, motion may be readily regained after immobilization. When a diagnosis of myositis ossificans in the region of the elbow has been made, prolonged rest of the elbow is indicated. Although guarded active motion may do no harm, the most certain method of treatment is immobilization. This is best obtained by means of a light, well-fitting plaster cast, extending from the upper arm to the metacarpal heads, with the elbow at an angle of from 90 to 100 degrees and the forearm in a midposition of rotation. Immobilization should be continued until arrest of the process of ossification is definitely demonstrable in the roentgenograms. Active motion may then be gradually restored, but massage and passive stretching should be avoided.

Operation is contraindicated in the early stages of the ossification, as additional trauma will usually be followed by an increased formation of bone. When, despite an adequate period of waiting, which should be at least six to twelve months, the bony tumor has failed to be absorbed and is causing limitation of joint motion, or serious discomfort, operative intervention is indicated. Thorough excision of the bony mass must be carried out with care to avoid unnecessary trauma and to control carefully all hemorrhage. Immobilization for a period of from one to two weeks after operation is advisable.

Traumatic myositis ossificans in other parts of the body presents essentially the same clinical picture and is treated in the same way.

PART II. AFFECTIONS OF THE WRIST AND HAND

Introduction.—The wrist joint is of double hinge type, permitting approximately 180 degrees of motion in the anteroposterior plane and approximately 80 degrees in the lateral. A small part of the anteroposterior motion takes place in the intercarpal joints but they do not contribute to lateral movement. The stability of the wrist is maintained not by bony configuration but by ligaments and the numerous tough fibrous tendon sheaths which closely invest them. One of the chief functions of the complicated bony structure of the carpus is to provide a certain elasticity which minimizes the traumatic effect of falls on the hands.

The hand may be conveniently regarded as a structural and functional whole made up of carpus, metacarpus, and digits. The carpal and metacarpal bones form a protective double arch in which, bridged over in front by the strong palmar fascia, lie the nerves, vessels, and tendons which supply the ultimate functional units of the fingers.

Disabilities of the wrist and hand, in addition to being extremely common, are of particular functional and economic importance. They fall largely into two major groups: (1) traumatic lesions and (2) infections. Many of the traumatic disorders are important not so much because of their immediate symptomatology as because of their disabling sequelae. Acute infections of the hand require surgical treatment based upon exhaustive anatomical and clinical study; for reference the works of Kanavel and of Bunnell are excellent. In addition to frank traumatic and infectious lesions, the wrist and hand are subject to a number of affections of chronic type, the causes of which are less well known.

Tenosynovitis

Inflammation of the tendon sheaths about the wrist may be of infectious, toxic, or traumatic origin. *Acute suppurative tenosynovitis,* due to the staphylococcus or streptococcus, is one of the most important types of acute infection of the hand and requires immediate treatment as a major surgical condition. Purulent synovitis occurs rarely from hematogenous gonococcus or pneumococcus infection; the treatment is rest in functional position, elevation, heat, and antibiotic therapy; surgical drainage may be necessary. Tenosynovitis of less specific type may occur in association with various foci of infection and, like certain cases of bursal and joint inflammation, is generally considered to be of toxic origin. *Tuberculous tenosynovitis* is encountered as a diffuse granulomatous and often purulent involvement of the tendon sheath or as a cystic expansion of the sheath containing particles of fibrin known as *rice bodies;* its treatment varies with the individual case but in general consists of excision of the pathologic tissue and temporary immobilization of the wrist. The postoperative result is usually satisfactory. Streptomycin is indicated as a most helpful adjuvant to surgery, and in some cases excellent results have been reported from its use alone. It may be accompanied by para-aminosalicylic acid to decrease the likelihood that the organisms will become steptomycin-resistant. *Traumatic tenosynovitis* is a frequent clinical entity following minor occupational injury of the wrist region and, because of its importance in differential diagnosis, warrants further description here. Traumatic tenosynovitis also occurs frequently in the sheaths of the anterior and posterior tibial and the Achilles tendons.

Etiology and Pathology.—Traumatic tenosynovitis is usually a result of strenuous, oft repeated, or unaccustomed use of the adjacent joint. Serous or fibrinous fluid may accumulate in the affected tendon sheath, sometimes resulting later in chronic sclerosing changes and stenosis.

Clinical Picture.—Pain on motion of the affected tendon is the presenting symptom. Swelling usually occurs but may not be conspicuous, and redness is usually absent. Tenderness on pressure over the tendon sheath is a constant finding. On motion of the affected tendon unmistakable crepitation can usually be elicited. Disability of marked degree may develop rapidly.

Diagnosis.—In differential diagnosis other lesions resulting from minor trauma in the affected region must be excluded. *Muscular strain* and *ligamentous sprain* are usually preceded by a single traumatic episode and are accompanied by pain and tenderness limited to the structure involved. At the wrist, fractures with little displacement are common, and, when the history is at all suggestive, fracture must be ruled out by roentgenographic examination, including oblique projections to visualize the scaphoid bone.

Treatment.—Acute traumatic tenosynovitis often responds quickly to complete immobilization. In the wrist and forearm an elastic bandage, adhesive strapping, or a leather cuff may be used, but in most cases it is far preferable to begin the treatment with the more complete immobilization obtained with well-fitting anterior and posterior plaster splints. In the ankle and lower leg, strapping or plaster immobilization is usually indicated. The application of heat is often a helpful adjunct. Complete immobilization should be continued until all tenderness has subsided, when carefully graded activity is to be resumed.

Chronic sclerosing tenosynovitis, first described by de Quervain in 1895 and sometimes called *de Quervain's tenosynovitis,* commonly affects the abductor pollicis longus and extensor pollicis brevis, producing a stenosis of their sheaths in their common osseofibrous canal. The patient complains of disabling pain which is most severe near the styloid process of the radius. Localized tenderness and pain on stretching the affected tendons are constantly present. The involvement is frequently bilateral. Release of the constriction by longitudinal incision or by partial resection of the sheath is usually curative. The operation should include search for anomalous tendons, which are common in this region.

Old Dislocation of the Semilunar Bone

Two lesions of the carpus are frequently seen following episodes of moderate or severe trauma: (1) fracture of the scaphoid bone and (2) anterior dislocation of the semilunar bone. Cases of neglected scaphoid injuries are discussed on page 353, in the chapter on Fracture Deformities. Unreduced dislocation of the semilunar bone is an important entity since it results in an extreme disability of the hand.

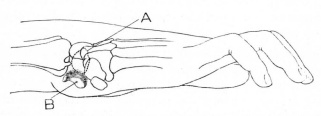

Fig. 188.—Anterior dislocation of the semilunar bone. *A,* Normal position of semilunar bone; *B,* position after dislocation. (Drawing from roentgenogram.)

Pathology.—When, by a fall upon the hyperextended hand, the semilunar bone has been squeezed from its position between the radius and the os magnum, it lies anteriorly with its concave distal surface rotated forward (Fig. 188). In this position the semilunar is located immediately beneath the structures crossing the volar aspect of the wrist and is likely to cause involvement of the flexor tendons by friction and of the median nerve by pressure.

Clinical Picture.—Enlargement of the anterior aspect of the wrist is usually obvious, and in some cases the displaced bone is palpable. There may be noticeable atrophy of the muscles of the hand. The wrist and fingers are held slightly flexed, extension is limited and painful, and the grip is markedly weakened. In a large proportion of the cases the characteristic anesthesia and paralysis which result from involvement of the median nerve will be found.

Treatment.—In late cases the displaced semilunar bone should be excised, and following its removal a plaster splint or cast should be applied for immobilization. Physical therapy is begun after a week and must usually be employed daily for an extended period.

Old posterior dislocation of the semilunar bone is seen only rarely; the treatment, like that of unreduced anterior dislocation, is excision of the semilunar followed by splinting and physical therapy.

Rupture of the Extensor Pollicis Longus Tendon

The tendon of the extensor pollicis longus muscle is occasionally ruptured as a late effect of either of two conditions: (1) occupational trauma, as frequently observed in kettledrummers, and (2) fracture of the lower end of the radius. In either case the rupture is preceded by chronic degenerative changes in the tendon; these may result from friction against irregularities in the groove in the radius, from impairment of the blood supply, or from direct laceration of the tendon itself.

Clinical Picture.—Unlike the rupture of a normal tendon, the separation may occur without pain or sensation of snapping. Following fracture of the radius, the rupture often takes place on exertion from one to three months after the original trauma. The diagnostic signs are inability to extend the distal phalanx of the thumb against resistance and absence of the subcutaneous "bowstring" formed by the normal tendon when the thumb is actively extended.

Treatment.—Exploration, followed by tendon suture, graft, or transplantation, is indicated. Cautious early mobilization is to be employed postoperatively.

Ganglion

The wrist is the commonest site of the *ganglion* of joint or tendon sheath, a frequently seen but little understood lesion of benign character.

Pathology and Etiology.—The typical ganglion is a small, smooth, cystic structure containing a thick, clear, mucinous fluid. It is usually connected to the capsule of an adjacent joint or to a tendon sheath by a narrow pedicle without a lumen; sometimes no pedicle is demonstrable. Ganglions may reach considerable dimensions and may be multilocular or multiple.

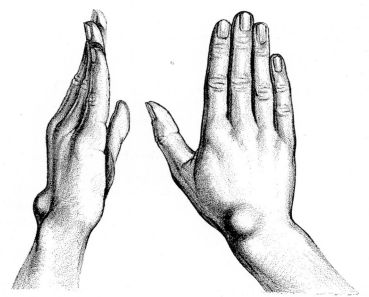

Fig. 189.—Ganglion of wrist. Note smooth, well-demarcated swelling on radial side of wrist.

The etiology is obscure. It was formerly thought that these cysts resulted from herniation of the lining membrane of a joint or tendon sheath. Recent observations have led to the belief that they are produced by a colloid degeneration which occurs locally in the connective tissue and which may be related to ischemic changes. It has also been suggested that the cyst formation is possibly analogous to the developmental process which leads, in tissue of similar origin, to the formation of the normal joint cavities.

Clinical Picture.—Ganglions occur most commonly in patients between the ages of fifteen and thirty-five years. At the wrist they are most frequent on the dorsum (Fig. 189), but are found also on the volar aspect. Small ganglions near the joints of the fingers are common. About the knee, ganglions may appear in the popliteal space, laterally in front of the tendon of the biceps, or anteriorly beneath the patellar ligament. The front of the ankle and dorsum of the foot are other common sites.

The swelling is of slow growth and causes few symptoms. Occasionally there is discomfort in the adjacent joint or tendons, particularly after overuse or strain. The swelling is rounded, nontender, tense or fluctuant, and unattached to the skin. It often varies in prominence with motion of the adjacent joint. Ganglions frequently regress or disappear spontaneously. In differential diagnosis ganglions must be distinguished from benign soft tissue tumors such as fibromas and lipomas, from bursitis, and from tuberculous tenosynovitis.

Treatment.—The old treatment of rupturing the cyst by trauma or pressure is painful and likely to be followed by recurrence. The combination of aspiration, chemical cauterization, and the application of a pressure bandage is sometimes employed. Many cases seem to respond satisfactorily to roentgen therapy. The most successful results, however, are obtained from surgical excision. The operation must be planned with the expectation that the ganglion will be found to arise not from a superficial structure but from the articular capsule itself.

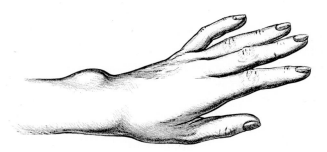

Fig. 190.—Madelung's deformity. Note dorsal prominence caused by posterior subluxation of distal end of ulna.

Madelung's Deformity

Madelung's deformity is an uncommon affection of the wrist, characterized by dorsal prominence of the lower end of the ulna (Fig. 190), instability of the distal radio-ulnar articulation, and local changes in the conformation of the radius and ulna.

Etiology.—The cause has not been definitely established but is apparently a local nutritional or growth disturbance resulting from changes which are due to congenital abnormality or occupational trauma.

Clinical Picture.—The condition is most often seen in adolescents and is not infrequently bilateral. The patient complains of deformity of the wrist and of a feeling of weakness and insecurity. The wrist may appear enlarged, and on palpation there may be demonstrable instability of the radio-ulnar joint. The end of the radius is displaced anteriorly, carrying with it the carpus and hand. There is a resulting dorsal prominence of the lower end of the ulna and an abnormal limitation of dorsiflexion. In severe cases the range of supination and pronation may be decreased.

Treatment.—In all except the most advanced cases a trial of non-operative treatment is indicated. The wrist is immobilized by a dressing which incorporates a short dorsiflexion splint and a pressure pad over the prominent ulnar head. Graded exercises may be given to strengthen the local musculature. Excision of the distal end of the ulna is sometimes helpful. In advanced cases it may be advisable to perform an open operation to reinforce the ligaments at the distal radio-ulnar joint, and in severe late lesions osteotomy of the radius or ulna may be necessary in order to correct the deformity.

Avascular Necrosis of the Carpal Bones

This rare and little understood affection of one or more of the bones of the carpus is characterized by the gradual development of pain and disability in the wrist, associated with typical roentgenographic changes. A history of antecedent injury is often obtainable, and the condition is sometimes termed *traumatic osteitis* or *osteoporosis*. The etiologic mechanism is usually considered to be a local nutritive disturbance dependent upon circulatory changes induced by trauma. The pathologic changes are those of avascular necrosis. Involvement of the semilunar bone is often known as *Kienböck's disease,* and of the scaphoid bone as *Preiser's disease.*

Clinical Picture.—The majority of patients are men between the ages of twenty and forty years. The original trauma may be trivial or severe and may cause pain and swelling which persist for several days or weeks. A period of months or even years then elapses in which no symptoms are present. Thereafter a gradual development of aching pain takes place, at first felt only on jarring or on exertion but later persistent and severe. Local swelling and tenderness appear, dorsiflexion becomes limited, and the disability may become extreme. When the semilunar bone is severely affected, the head of the third metacarpal may lose its normal dorsal prominence because of a proximal displacement of the entire bone, and longitudinal thrusts upon the metacarpal in a proximal direction will cause pain. The range of wrist motion often becomes restricted.

Roentgenographic Picture.—In early films there may be no definite changes, but, as the condition advances, characteristic alterations of the affected bone appear. It becomes flattened and may be abnormally dense. In some cases irregular areas of rarefaction are conspicuous, suggesting fragmentation. In adjacent bones, changes suggesting an early osteoarthritis often develop.

Treatment.—Nonoperative treatment is usually indicated. The wrist is immobilized in a short dorsiflexion splint, which is removed daily for diathermy and massage. If after several months the improvement is found to be unsatisfactory, excision of the affected bone or bones is indicated; postoperatively the wrist should be immobilized for one month, after which exercise is gradually resumed. In late cases with advanced arthritic changes, arthrodesis of the wrist is sometimes indicated.

Accessory Bones of the Hand

According to the findings of comparative anatomy and embryology, a large variety of supernumerary bones may occur in the carpal region. Clinically, however, accessory bones of the hand are much less frequent and less important than those of the foot.

Of chief diagnostic significance is the rare *divided scaphoid,* resulting from failure of radial and ulnar anlagen of the scaphoid bone to fuse. Roentgenographically this condition resembles an ununited fracture, but most authorities agree that it is of purely developmental origin. It is possible that imperfect fusion is a predisposing factor in traumatic fractures of the scaphoid. The unciform process of the unciform bone may develop separately, and the ulnar styloid process may fail to unite with the distal end of the ulna. In differential diagnosis it must be remembered, however, that these developmental variations are extremely uncommon.

Developmental fusion of one or more adjacent carpals sometimes occurs. An accessory epiphysis is rarely seen at the proximal end of the second or the fifth metacarpal bone.

Dupuytren's Contracture

This not infrequent affection, first analyzed and described by Dupuytren in 1832, is a slowly progressive contracture of the palmar fascia, occurring most often in males past middle life and as a rule involving the ring finger, little finger, or both (Fig. 191).

Pathology.—The essential morbid process is a very chronic inflammation of the palmar fascia with progressive fibrosis and contracture. In advanced cases the skin is secondarily involved. Changes in flexor tendons and digital joints are slight and occur only in late and extreme cases.

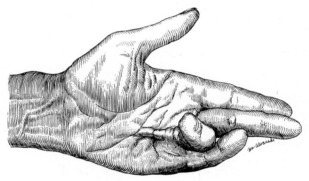

Fig. 191.—Dupuytren's contracture of fourth finger. Note flexion deformity of fourth finger and prominent band caused by localized contracture of the palmar fascia. (After Colonna.)

Etiology.—The cause is unknown. The possible etiologic rôle of chronic trauma has not been established by analysis of statistics. In some cases there is a definite hereditary factor. In all probability some degree of toxicity associated with chronic infectious or metabolic disorders is nearly always present; its etiologic significance, however, is questionable.

Clinical Picture.—The contracture is first evidenced by the appearance of a small nodular thickening in the palmar fascia overlying a flexor tendon in the region of a metacarpophalangeal joint, often associated with a dimpling of the skin at this point. A thickened longitudinal band is gradually formed and flexion contracture of the finger progressively increases. The metacarpophalangeal and adjacent interphalangeal joints become flexed, while the distal interphalangeal joint, controlled by no prolongations of the palmar fascia, retains a normal range of extension.

In extreme cases the tip of the finger may be drawn into constant contact with the palm. As a rule there is little pain or tenderness. Frequently both hands are involved; usually the affection appears much earlier, however, in one hand than in the other. In some cases the plantar fascia shows small nodular thickenings similar to those in the palmar fascia.

Differential Diagnosis.—Flexion contractures secondary to congenital malformation, spasticity, trauma, and infection must be excluded. The insidious and painless onset, the presence of flexion at the metacarpophalangeal level, and the inability to extend the proximal interphalangeal joint even when the wrist is flexed, are characteristic of Dupuytren's contracture. It should be remembered that in some instances the microscopic appearance of the lesion in its early stage may simulate that of fibrosarcoma.

Treatment.—Any obvious focus of infection should be removed. Nonoperative treatment is indicated only in the earliest cases, in which frequent forced extension may be of some value. For all other cases the only effective treatment is operative. Frequently the procedure of choice is a careful and thorough excision of the abnormal palmar fascia. Exposure is obtained by wide freeing and retraction of the skin, and the fascia and its longitudinal bands are dissected out as completely as possible. At times a full-thickness skin graft, with or without resection of a portion of the palmar skin, may be indicated. Postoperatively a splint is worn for a few days, but active and passive motion must be begun as soon as healing of the skin permits. Excision of the fascia obviates, as a rule, the danger of recurrence. However, it is a major procedure. The simple operation of multiple subcutaneous divisions of contracted fascial bands with the tenotomy knife is sometimes preferred, particularly for cases in which the contracture is well localized. For satisfactory results all of the constricting bands must be divided, and the postoperative treatment, including the use of an extension splint at night in addition to exercises, must be prolonged in an effort to prevent recurrence of the contracture.

Snapping Finger

Occasionally a finger or thumb is seen which at a single constant angle shows a partial obstruction of the movement of flexion or of extension. Motion past the angle of obstruction, which usually must be accomplished passively, may be accompanied by a definite sensation of snapping. This affection, called also *trigger finger,* is usually of gradual and painless development. The pathologic changes consist of a localized stenosis of the flexor tendon sheath, located usually near the metacarpophalangeal joint, or a nodular thickening of the tendon itself. Usually a small mass is palpable clinically.

Treatment.—A trial of nonoperative treatment, consisting of complete immobilization of the digit in extension for several weeks, may be made. In adults an exploratory operation is usually indicated. Sometimes simple longitudinal section of the sheath at the point of constriction will afford complete relief. In the author's experience this has been particularly true in infants and young children. Any localized thickening of the tendon should be removed, care being taken to avoid a complete section. After operation active motion should be started at once.

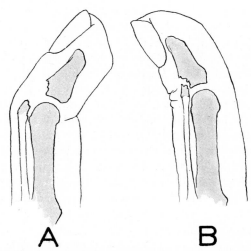

Fig. 192.—Mallet finger. *A,* Typical deformity due to avulsion of tendon together with a small fragment of bone. *B,* Position of reduction.

Mallet Finger (Baseball or Dropped Finger)

Sudden forcible flexion of a distal phalanx may cause an avulsion of the extensor tendon at its insertion. A small portion of the posterior lip of the phalangeal base is often torn away with the tendon. The injury is common among athletes and has been called *baseball, mallet,* or *dropped finger.*

Clinical Picture.—The history of injury together with inability to extend actively the distal phalanx is diagnostic. In early cases swelling and tenderness may obscure the loss of power in the finger. Roentgenographic examination should always be made.

Treatment.—The distal interphalangeal joint should be held constantly in hyperextension for from four to six weeks while the proximal interphalangeal joint is held flexed (Fig. 192). This can best be done with plaster or a small metal splint bent to fit the finger. The results of adequate treatment are usually good. In late cases resort may be had to suture of the tendon or of the bone fragment to the phalanx, but the results are often imperfect.

PART III.   AFFECTIONS OF THE JAW

Disability of the temporomandibular joint, while forming a relatively uncommon condition in orthopaedic surgery, may nevertheless represent to the individual patient an affliction of peculiarly distressing nature. Two clinical entities of fairly frequent occurrence, *snapping jaw* and *ankylosis of the jaw,* can be efficiently relieved by resort to the methods of joint surgery.

Snapping Jaw

The term snapping jaw is applied to a common clinical condition which is characterized by a clicking sensation in the temporomandibular joint on opening and closing the mouth. Usually the symptoms are trivial, but a few patients experience severe pain or locking of the jaw and require careful investigation and treatment.

Pathology.—Except for an occasional case attributable to malocclusion of the teeth, intractable snapping of the jaw is caused by one of two distinct pathologic entities: (1) mechanical derangement of the interarticular fibrocartilage or (2) recurrent dislocation of the temporomandibular joint with irregularity of the joint surfaces. In the etiology both developmental and traumatic factors are presumably concerned. Derangements of the interarticular disk are in some respects analogous to disorders of the semilunar cartilages of the knee. In dislocation of the jaw the condyle of the mandible, which slips forward when the mouth is opened, reaches a position anterior to the eminentia articularis of the temporal bone.

Clinical Picture.—The condition of snapping jaw is usually of gradual onset during adolescence or early adult life, occurring most commonly in young women. The slipping may at first take place only when the mouth is opened widely, as in yawning, but often becomes increasingly frequent and troublesome and in some cases leads to intense discomfort. The diagnosis may be evident from the history and physical findings but should be further investigated with roentgenograms of the temporomandibular joints taken with the mouth in open and in closed positions.

Treatment.—Early cases may be treated with heat and massage daily over a period of several weeks, combined with a soft diet and avoidance of any unnecessary motion of the jaw in talking. Partial rest secured by the use of the Barton bandage or Thomas collar may be helpful. Complete rest of the jaws, obtained by wiring the teeth for several weeks, is often curative. In some cases, however, operation becomes necessary, the type of procedure depending upon the pathologic changes demonstrated at exploration. For lesions of the fibrocartilage, simple excision of the disk has given satisfactory results. Reefing of the joint capsule is sometimes indicated. Recurrent dislocation may be treated effectively by the creation of a bone block as described by Mayer.

Ankylosis of the Jaw

Loss of motion in the temporomandibular joint constitutes a deforming and extremely disabling affection which can be relieved by surgical measures.

Etiology.—Ankylosis of the jaw is most frequently seen as the late result of a local traumatic lesion. It is at times a sequel of osteomyelitis of the temporal bone following infection of the middle ear. In other cases the ankylosis may result from rheumatoid arthritis of the temporomandibular joint.

Treatment.—The operation of choice is an arthroplastic procedure in which the head of the mandible and the upper portion of the ramus are resected. A layer of fascia may be placed around the end of the ramus but is by no means essential to a good clinical result.

BIBLIOGRAPHY

The following textbooks contain excellent reference material:

American Academy of Orthopaedic Surgeons: Instructional Course Lectures, Vols. 1-9 — Ann Arbor, J. W. Edwards, 1943-1952.

American Academy of Orthopaedic Surgeons, Office of the Surgeon General of the United States Army and the Veterans Administration: Orthopaedic Appliances Atlas, Vol. 1 — Ann Arbor, J. W. Edwards, 1952.

Bancroft, F. W., and Marble, H. C., Editors: Surgical Treatment of the Motor-Skeletal System, 2nd Edition — Philadelphia, J. B. Lippincott Co., 1951.

Bankart, A. S. B.: Manipulative Surgery — London, Constable, 1932.

Brailsford, J. F.: The Radiology of Bones and Joints, 4th Edition — London, J. & A. Churchill Ltd., 1948.

Brittain, H. A.: Architectural Principles in Arthrodesis — Baltimore, The Williams & Wilkins Co., 1942.

Campbell, W. C.: Operative Orthopedics, 2nd Edition — St. Louis, The C. V. Mosby Co., 1949.

Charnley, J.: Closed Treatment of Common Fractures — Edinburgh, E. & S. Livingstone Ltd., 1950.

Colonna, P. C.: Regional Orthopaedic Surgery — Philadelphia, W. B. Saunders Co., 1950.

Compere, E. L., and Banks, S. W.: Pictorial Handbook of Fracture Treatment — Chicago, The Year Book Publishers, Inc., 1952.

Cozen, L.: Office Orthopaedics — Philadelphia, Lea & Febiger, 1950.

Fairbank, H. A. T.: Atlas of General Affections of Skeleton — Edinburgh, E. & S. Livingstone Ltd., 1951.

Ferguson, A. B.: Roentgen Diagnosis of the Extremities and Spine, Enlarged 2nd Edition — New York, Paul B. Hoeber, Inc., 1949.

Fisher, A. G. T.: Treatment by Manipulation in General and Consulting Practice, 5th Edition — New York, Paul B. Hoeber, Inc., 1948.

Geckeler, E. O.: Plaster of Paris Technic, 2nd Edition — Baltimore, The Williams & Wilkins Co., 1948.

Henry, A. K.: Extensile Exposure Applied to Limb Surgery — Baltimore, The Williams & Wilkins Co., 1948.

Homans, J.: A Textbook of Surgery, 6th Edition — Springfield, Ill., Charles C. Thomas, 1945.

543

Howorth, M. B.:	Textbook of Orthopaedic Surgery	Philadelphia, W. B. Saunders Co., 1952.
Jones, R., and Lovett, R. W.:	Orthopedic Surgery, 2nd Edition	New York, William Wood & Co., 1929.
Kendall, H. O., and Kendall, F. P.:	Muscles: Testing and Function	Baltimore, The Williams & Wilkins Co., 1949.
Key, J. A., and Conwell, H. E.:	The Management of Fractures, Dislocations, and Sprains, 5th Edition	St. Louis, The C. V Mosby Co., 1951.
Lacroix, P.:	Organization of Bones	London, J. & A. Churchill Ltd., 1951.
deLorimier, A. A.:	The Arthropathies: Handbook of Roentgen Diagnosis, 2nd Edition	Chicago, The Year Book Publishers, Inc., 1949.
Luck, J. V.:	Bone and Joint Diseases: Pathology Correlated With Roentgenological and Clinical Features	Springfield, Ill., Charles C. Thomas, 1950.
Magnuson, P. B., and Stack, J. K.:	Fractures, 5th Edition	Philadelphia, J. B. Lippincott Co., 1949.
McBride, E. D.:	Disability Evaluation. Principles of Treatment of Compensable Injuries, 4th Edition, Revised	Philadelphia, J. B. Lippincott Co., 1948.
McMurray, T. P.:	A Practice of Orthopaedic Surgery, 3rd Edition	Baltimore, The Williams & Wilkins Co., 1949.
Mennell, J.:	Science and Art of Joint Manipulation, Vol. I, 2nd Edition	Philadelphia, The Blakiston Co., 1949.
Mercer, W.:	Orthopaedic Surgery, 4th Edition	Baltimore, The Williams & Wilkins Co., 1950.
Nangle, E. J.:	Instruments and Apparatus in Orthopaedic Surgery	Oxford, Blackwell Scientific Publications, 1951
Nicola, T.:	Atlas of Surgical Approaches to Bones and Joints	New York, The Macmillan Co., 1945.
Platt, Sir H., Editor:	Modern Trends in Orthopaedics	New York, Paul B. Hoeber, Inc., 1950.
Quigley, T. B.:	Plaster of Paris Technique in the Treatment of Fractures and Other Injuries	New York, The Macmillan Co., 1945.
Raney, R. B.:	The Prevention of Deformity in Childhood	Elyria, Ohio, National Society for Crippled Children, 1941.
Sever, J. W.:	Principles of Orthopaedic Surgery, 3rd Edition	New York, The Macmillan Co., 1940.

Shafer, S. J., and Compere, E. L.: — Basic Sciences for Orthopaedics (Veterans Administration) — Washington, D. C., Superintendent of Documents, U. S. Government Printing Office, 1948.

Slocum, D. B.: — Amputations — St. Louis, The C. V. Mosby Co., 1949.

Snapper, I.: — Medical Clinics on Bone Diseases. A Text and Atlas, 2nd Edition — New York, Interscience Publishers, Inc., 1949.

Steindler, A.: — Orthopedic Operations: Indications, Technique, and End Results (4th Printing) — Springfield, Ill., Charles C. Thomas, 1947.

Post-graduate Lectures on Orthopaedic Diagnosis and Indications, Vols. I, II, and III — Springfield, Ill., Charles C. Thomas, 1950, 1951, 1952.

Watson-Jones, R.: — Fractures and Joint Injuries, 4th Edition (Reprint) — Baltimore, The Williams & Wilkins Co., 1952.

Weinmann, J. P., and Sicher, H.: — Bone and Bones: Fundamentals of Bone Biology — St. Louis, The C. V. Mosby Co., 1947.

Wiles, P.: — Essentials of Orthopaedics — Philadelphia, The Blakiston Co., London, J. & A. Churchill, 1949.

Chapter I

Introduction

Allison, N., and Ghormley, R. K.: — Diagnosis in Joint Disease — New York, William Wood & Co., 1931.

Andry, N.: — Orthopaedia: or the Art of Correcting and Preventing Deformities in Children — London, 1743.

Angevine, D. M., and Ash, J. E.: — Atlas of Orthopaedic Pathology — Washington, D. C., The Army Medical Museum, 1943.

Beekman, F.: — Hospital for the Ruptured and Crippled. A Historical Sketch Written on the Occasion of the Seventy-Fifth Anniversary of the Hospital — Privately printed in New York, 1939.

Bick, E. M.: — Source Book of Orthopaedics, 2nd Edition — Baltimore, The Williams & Wilkins Co., 1948.

Surgical Pathology of Synovial Tissue — J. Bone & Joint Surg. 12: 33 (Jan.) 1930.

Cave, E. F., and Roberts, S. M.: — A Method for Measuring and Recording Joint Function — J. Bone & Joint Surg. 18: 455 (April) 1936.

Collins, D. H.: | The Pathology of Articular and Spinal Diseases | Baltimore, The Williams & Wilkins Co., 1950.

Colonna, P. C., Friedenberg, Z. B., and Moore, J. S.: | The Normal and Abnormal Response of Bone Tissue, in Monographs on Surgery, 1950, 411-438. | New York, Thos. Nelson & Sons, 1950.

Davies, D. V.: | Synovial Membrane and Synovial Fluid in Joints | Lancet **2**: 815 (Dec. 7) 1946.

Ghormley, J. W.: | Hip Motions | Am. J. Surg. **66**: 24 (Oct.) 1944.

Ghormley, R. K.: | Specialization in Medicine; What Is Orthopaedic Surgery? | J. Bone & Joint Surg. **31A**: 459-463 (July) 1949.

Gilfillan, C. W.: | Notes in Orthopedic Pathology | Los Angeles, College of Medical Evangelists, 1949.

Inman, V. T., and Saunders, J. B. deC. M.: | Referred Pain from Skeletal Structures | J. Nerv. & Ment. Dis. **99**: 660-667 (May) 1944.

Kahlstrom, S. C., Burton, C. C., and Phemister, D. B.: | Aseptic Necrosis of Bone | Surg., Gynec. & Obst. **68**: 129, 631 (Feb. & March) 1939.

Keith, A.: | The Menders of the Maimed | London, Oxford University Press, 1919, and Philadelphia, J. B. Lippincott Co., 1951.

Kendall, H. O., and Kendall, F. P.: | Normal Flexibility According to Age Groups | J. Bone & Joint Surg. **30A**: 690-694 (July) 1948.

King, E. S. J.: | Localized Rarefying Conditions of Bone | Baltimore, William Wood & Co., 1925.

Knaggs, R. L.: | The Inflammatory and Toxic Diseases of Bone | New York, William Wood & Co., 1925.

Little, E. M.: | Orthopaedics Before Stromeyer | The Robert Jones Birthday Volume, New York, Oxford University Press, 1928.

MacConaill, M. A.: | Movements of Bones and Joints: Fundamental Principles With Particular Reference to Rotation Movement | J. Bone & Joint Surg. **30B**: 322-326 (May) 1948.

| Movements of Bones and Joints: Function of Musculature | J. Bone & Joint Surg. **31B**: 100-104 (Feb.) 1949.

| Movements of Bones and Joints: Synovial Fluid | J. Bone & Joint Surg. **32B**: 244-252 (May) 1950.

| Movements of Bones and Joints | J. Bone & Joint Surg. **33B**: 251-257 (May) 1951.

Moore, J. R., and Nicholson, J. T.: — Deformities, Congenital, in Cyclopedia of Medicine, Surgery, Specialties, Vol. 4, 397-451. — Philadelphia, F. A. Davis Co., 1950.

Murray, P. D. F.: — Bones, A Study of the Development and Structure of the Vertebrate Skeleton — London, Cambridge University Press, 1936.

New York Number: — Basic Sciences in Surgery — S. Clin. North America (April), 1952.

New York Orthopaedic Hospital: — Outlines for Examinations of Patients in the New York Orthopaedic Dispensary and Hospital — Printed by the New York Orthopaedic Hospital.

Osgood, R. B.: — The Evolution of Orthopaedic Surgery — St. Louis, The C. V. Mosby Co., 1925.

Phemister, D. B.: — Fractures of Neck of Femur, Dislocations of Hip, and Obscure Vascular Disturbances Producing Aseptic Necrosis of Head of Femur — Surg., Gynec. & Obst. 59: 415 (Sept.) 1934.

Raney, R. B.: — Andry and the Orthopaedia — J. Bone & Joint Surg. 31A: 675-682 (July) 1949.

Shephard, E.: — Tarsal Movements — J. Bone & Joint Surg. 33B: 258-264 (May) 1951.

Weichec, F. J., and Krusen, F. H.: — A New Method of Joint Measurement and a Review of the Literature — Am. J. Surg. 43: 659 (March) 1939.

Chapter II

Congenital Deformities

Congenital Clubfoot

Blumenfeld, I., Nathan, K., and Hicks, E. O.: — The Conservative Treatment of Congenital Talipes Equinovarus — J. Bone & Joint Surg. 28: 765 (Oct.) 1946.

Bohm, M.: — The Embryologic Origin of Club-Foot — J. Bone & Joint Surg. 11: 229 (April) 1929.

Brockman, E. P.: — Congenital Club-Foot — New York, William Wood & Co., 1930.

Modern Methods of Treatment of Club-Foot — Brit. M. J. 2: 572 (Sept. 18) 1937.

Browne, D.: — Talipes Equino-varus — Lancet 2: 969-974 (Nov. 3) 1934.

Kite, J. H.: | Non-Operative Treatment of Congenital Club-feet: A Review of 100 Cases | South. M. J. **23**: 337 (April) 1930.

Principles Involved in the Treatment of Congenital Club-Foot | J. Bone & Joint Surg. **21**: 595 (July) 1939.

Stewart, S. F.: | Club Foot: Its Incidence, Cause, and Treatment | J. Bone & Joint Surg. **33A**: 577-590 (July) 1951.

Thomson, S. A.: | Treatment of Congenital Clubfoot | J. Bone & Joint Surg. **31A**: 431-434 (April) 1949.

Other Congenital Deformities

Barenberg, L. H., and Greenberg, B.: | Intrauterine Amputations and Constricting Bands; Report of Case With Anesthesia Below Constriction | Am. J. Dis. Child. **64**: 87 (July) 1942.

Barsky, A. J.: | Congenital Anomalies of Hand | J. Bone & Joint Surg. **33A**: 35 - 64 (Jan.) 1951.

Davis, J. S., and German, W. J.: | Syndactylism | Arch. Surg. **21**: 32 (July) 1930.

Fahlstrom, S.: | Radio-Ulnar Synostosis; Historical Review and Case Report | J. Bone & Joint Surg. **14**: 395 (April) 1932.

Freund, E.: | Congenital Defects of Femur, Fibula and Tibia | Arch. Surg. **33**: 349 (Sept.) 1936.

Harmon, P. H., and Fahey, J. J.: | The Syndrome of Congenital Absence of the Fibula; Report of 3 Cases With Special Reference to Pathogenesis and Treatment | Surg., Gynec. & Obst. **64**: 876 (May) 1937.

Heyman, C. H., and Herndon, C. H.: | Congenital Posterior Angulation of Tibia | J. Bone & Joint Surg. **31A**: 571-580 (July) 1949.

Katzeff, M.: | Arthrogryposis Multiplex Congenita | Arch. Surg. **46**: 673 (May) 1943.

Kiskadden, W. S., Schechtman, A. M., and Brock, C.: | Theories of Etiology of Congenital Deformities | Internat. Abstr. Surg. **88**: 1-14 (Jan.) 1949.

Kite, J. H.: | Congenital Metatarsus Varus; Report of 300 Cases | J. Bone & Joint Surg. **32A**: 500-506 (July) 1950.

Lyons, C. G., and Sawyer, J. G.: | Cleidocranial Dysostosis | Am. J. Roentgenol. **51**: 215 (Feb.) 1944.

McCauley, J. C., Jr.: | Surgical Treatment of Clubfeet | S. Clin. North America, 561-573 (April) 1951.

McCormick, D. W., and Blount, W. P.: | Metatarsus Adductovarus, "Skewfoot" | J. A. M. A. **141**: 449-453 (Oct. 15) 1949.

Meyerding, H. W., and Dickson, D. D.:	Correction of Congenital Deformations of the Hand	Am. J. Surg. **44**: 218-223 (April) 1939.
Miles, P. W.:	Cleidocranial Dysostosis: Survey of Six New Cases and One Hundred and Twenty-Six From Literature	J. Kansas M. Soc. **41**: 462 (Nov.) 1940.
Mitchell, H. S.:	The Klippel-Feil Syndrome (Congenital Webbed Neck)	Arch. Dis. Childhood **9**: 213 (Aug.) 1934.
Moore, B. H.:	Peripheral Nerve Changes Associated With Congenital Deformities	J. Bone & Joint Surg. **26**: 282 (April) 1944.
Murphy, D. P.:	Congenital Malformations. A Study of Parental Characteristics With Special Reference to the Reproductive Process	Philadelphia, University of Pennsylvania Press, 1940.
Ollerenshaw, R.:	Congenital Defects of the Long Bones of the Lower Limb; A Contribution to the Study of Their Causes, Effects and Treatment	J. Bone & Joint Surg. **7**: 528 (July) 1925.
Peabody, C. W.:	Hemihypertrophy and Hemiatrophy; Congenital Total Unilateral Somatic Asymmetry	J. Bone & Joint Surg. **18**: 466 (April) 1936.
Peabody, C. W., and Muro, F.:	Congenital Metatarsus Varus	J. Bone & Joint Surg. **15**: 171 (Jan.) 1933.
Rechtman, A. M., and Horwitz, M. T.:	Congenital Synostosis of the Cervicothoracic Vertebrae (Klippel-Feil Syndrome)	Am. J. Roentgenol. **43**: 66 (Jan.) 1940.
Schrock, R. D.:	Congenital Elevation of the Scapula	J. Bone & Joint Surg. **8**: 207 (Jan.) 1926, and Nelson's New Loose Leaf Surgery, New York, 1935.
Smith, A. DeF.:	Congenital Elevation of Scapula	Arch. Surg. **42**: 529 (March) 1941.
Soule, A. B., Jr.:	Mutational Dysostosis (Cleidocranial Dysostosis)	J. Bone & Joint Surg. **28**: 81 (Jan.) 1946.
Starr, D. E.:	Congenital Absence of the Radius; A Method of Surgical Correction	J. Bone & Joint Surg. **27**: 572 (Oct.) 1945.
Streeter, G. L.:	Focal Deficiencies in Fetal Tissues and Their Relation to Intra-Uterine Amputation	Contributions to Embryology, No. 126, Publication No. 414, Carnegie Institution, Washington, 1930.

Chapter III

Congenital Deformities

Congenital Dislocation of the Hip

Anderson, M. E., and Bickel, W. H.: — Shelf Operation for Congenital Subluxation and Dislocation of Hip — J. Bone & Joint Surg. **33A:** 87-102 (Jan.) 1951.

Badgley, C. E.: — Correlation of Clinical and Anatomical Facts Leading to Conception of Etiology of Congenital Hip Dysplasias — J. Bone & Joint Surg. **25:** 503 (July) 1943.

Etiology of Congenital Dislocation of Hip — J. Bone & Joint Surg. **31A:** 341-356 (April) 1949.

Bost, F. C., Hagey, H., Schottstaedt, E. R., and Larsen, L. J.: — Results of Treatment of Congenital Dislocation of Hip in Infancy — J. Bone & Joint Surg. **30A:** 454-468 (April) 1948.

Colonna, P. C.: — Congenital Dislocation of the Hip in Older Subjects; Based on a Study of 66 Open Operations — J. Bone & Joint Surg. **14:** 277 (April) 1932.

Arthroplasty for Congenital Dislocation of the Hip: Late Follow-Up Report — J. Bone & Joint Surg. **24:** 812 (Oct.) 1942.

Arthroplasty of the Hip for Congenital Dislocation in Children — J. Bone & Joint Surg. **29:** 711-722 (July) 1947.

Crego, C. H.: — The Use of Skeletal Traction as a Preliminary Procedure in the Treatment of Early Congenital Dislocation of the Hip — J. Bone & Joint Surg. **21:** 353 (April) 1939.

Crego, C. H., and Schwartzmann, J. R.: — Follow-up Study of Early Treatment of Congenital Dislocation of Hip — J. Bone & Joint Surg. **30A:** 428-442 (April) 1948.

Fairbank, H. A. T.: — Congenital Dislocation of the Hip: With Special Reference to the Anatomy — Brit. J. Surg. **17:** 380 (Jan.) 1930.

Freiberg, J. A.: — Early Diagnosis and Treatment of Congenital Dislocation of the Hip — J. A. M. A. **102:** 89 (Jan. 13) 1934.

Galloway, H. P. H.: — The Open Operation for Congenital Dislocation of the Hip; Special Reference to Results — J. Bone & Joint Surg. **8:** 539 (July) 1926.

Gill, A. B.: — Operation for Old or Irreducible Congenital Dislocation of the Hip — J. Bone & Joint Surg. **10:** 696 (Oct.) 1928.

Gill, A. B.: | Plastic Construction of Acetabulum in Congenital Dislocation of the Hip — The Shelf Operation | J. Bone & Joint Surg. **17**: 48 (Jan.) 1935.

End Results of Early Treatment of Congenital Dislocation of Hip | J. Bone & Joint Surg. **30A**: 442-453 (April) 1948.

Hart, V. L.: | Primary Genetic Dysplasia of Hip With and Without Classical Dislocation | J. Bone & Joint Surg. **24**: 753 (Oct.) 1942.

Congenital Dysplasia of Hip Joint | J. Bone & Joint Surg. **31A**: 357-372 (April) 1949.

Congenital Dysplasia of the Hip Joint and Sequelae | Springfield, Ill., Charles C Thomas, 1952.

Hass, J.: | Congenital Dislocation of the Hip | Springfield, Ill., Charles C Thomas, 1951.

Kreuz, F. P. and Shands, A. R., Jr.: | Some Congenital and Developmental Problems of the Hip Joint in Infancy and Childhood, in Monographs on Surgery for 1951, 327-392. | New York, Thos. Nelson & Sons, 1951.

Krida, A.: | Congenital Dislocation of the Hip; The Effect of Anterior Distortion; A Procedure for Its Correction | J. Bone & Joint Surg. **10**: 594 (July) 1928.

Massie, W. K.: | Vascular Epiphyseal Changes in Congenital Dislocation of Hip | J. Bone & Joint Surg. **33A**: 284-306 (April) 1951.

Massie, W. K., and Howorth, M. B.: | Congenital Dislocation of Hip, Part I, Method of Grading Results | J. Bone & Joint Surg. **32A**: 519-531 (July) 1950.

Massie, W. K., and Howorth, M. B.: | Congenital Dislocation of Hip, Results of Open Reduction as Seen in Early Adult Period | J. Bone & Joint Surg. **33A**: 171-198 (Jan.) 1951.

McCarroll, H. R.: | Primary Anterior Congenital Dislocation of Hip | J. Bone & Joint Surg. **30A**: 416-421 (April) 1948.

Platt, H.: | Congenital Dislocation of Hip | Brit. J. Surg. **30**: 291 (April) 1943.

Putti, V.: | Early Treatment of Congenital Dislocation of the Hip | J. Bone & Joint Surg. **11**: 798 (Oct.) 1929.

Severin, E.: | Contribution to the Knowledge of Congenital Dislocation of the Hip Joint. Late Results of Closed Reduction and Arthrographic Studies of Recent Cases | Acta Chir. Scandinav. **84**: Suppl. 63, 1941.

Severin, E.:   Congenital Dislocation of   J. Bone & Joint Surg.
                                the Hip; Development   **32A:** 507-518 (July)
                                of the J o i n t After   1950.
                                Closed Reduction

Other Congenital Dislocations

Boorstein, S. W.:   Congenital   Backward   Am. J. Dis. Child **38:** 107
                                Dislocation of the Knee   (July) 1929.
Cozen, L.:   Congenital Dislocation of   Arch. Surg. **35:**   956
                                the Shoulder and Other   (Nov.) 1937.
                                Anomalies. Report of a
                                Case and Review of the
                                Literature
McFarland, B. L.:   Congenital Dislocation of   J. Bone & Joint Surg. **11:**
                                the Knee   281 (Apr.) 1929.

Chapter IV

Affections of Growing Bone

Albright, F., Burnett,   Osteomalacia and Late   Medicine **25:** 399 (Dec.)
C. H., Parson, W.,   Rickets   1946.
Reifenstein, E. C., Jr.,
and Roos, A.:
Arkin, A. M. and   Aseptic N e c r o s i s in   J. Bone & Joint Surg.
Schein, A. J.:   Gaucher's Disease   **30A:** 631-641 (July)
                                                                 1948.
Baker, L. D., and   Osteopathia Condensans   J. Bone & Joint Surg. **23:**
Jones, H. A.:   Disseminata,   Osteo-   164 (Jan.) 1941.
                                poikilosis (S p o t t e d
                                Bones) : Report of Case
Bickel, W. H., Ghormley,   Osteogenesis Imperfecta   Radiology **40:**145 (Feb.)
R. K., and Camp,   1943.
J. D.:
Bloom, A. R.:   Osteopoecilia   Am. J. Surg. **22:** 239
                                                                 (Nov.) 1933.
Blount, W. P.:   Tibia Vara: Osteochon-   J. Bone & Joint Surg. **19:**
                                drosis D e f o r m a n s   1 (Jan.) 1937.
                                Tibiae
Bradlow, P. A. and   Infantile Cortical Hyper-   J. Bone & Joint Surg.
Steinberg, S. H.:   ostosis   **32A:** 677-681 (July)
                                                                 1950.
Bromer, R. S.:   The Roentgen-Ray Diag-   Am. J. Roentgenol. **19:**
                                nosis of I n f a n t i l e   112 (Feb.) 1928.
                                Scurvy

                                Osteochondritis Luetica;   New England J. Med.
                                Comparison with Ana-   **200:** 524 (Mar. 14)
                                logous Zones in Rickets   1929.
                                and Infantile Scurvy
Caffey, J.:   Infantile Cortical Hyper-   J. Pediat. **29:** 541-559
                                ostoses   (Nov.) 1946.

Chown, B.: — Renal Rickets and Dwarfism: A Pituitary Disease — Brit. J. Surg. **23:** 552 (Jan.) 1936.

Clifton, W. M., Frank, A., and Freeman, S.: — Osteopetrosis (Marble Bones) — Am. J. Dis. Child. **56:** 1020 (Nov.) 1938.

Cohen, J.: — Osteopetrosis: Case Report, Autopsy Findings, and Pathological Interpretation: Failure of Treatment With Vitamin A — J. Bone & Joint Surg. **33A:** 923-939 (Oct.) 1951.

Davis, P. G., and Rossen, J. A.: — Renal Rickets — J. Pediat. **18:** 103 (Jan.) 1941.

Fairbank, H. A. T.: — Osteogenesis Imperfecta — J. Bone & Joint Surg. **30B:** 164-186 (Feb.) 1948.

— Osteopetrosis — J. Bone & Joint Surg. **30B:** 339-356 (May) 1948.

— Myositis Ossificans Progressiva — J. Bone & Joint Surg. **32B:** 108-116 (Feb.) 1950.

— Osteopathia Striata — J. Bone & Joint Surg. **32B:** 117-125 (Feb.) 1950.

Finkelstein, H.: — The Correction of Rachitic Deformities by Preliminary Decalcification — J. Bone & Joint Surg. **17:** 780 (July) 1935.

Green, W. T., and Farber, S.: — "Eosinophilic or Solitary Granuloma" of Bone — J. Bone & Joint Surg. **24:** 499 (July) 1942.

Haas, S. L.: — Nutritional and Growth Disturbances of Bone, in Cyclopedia of Medicine, Surgery, Specialties, Vol. 10, 1-37 — Philadelphia, F. A. Davis Co., 1951.

Hainberg, A. E.: — Skeletal Changes in Sickle Cell Anemia; Report of Unusual Case — J. Bone & Joint Surg. **32A:** 893-900 (Oct.) 1950.

Harris, H. A.: — Bone Growth in Health and Disease — London, Oxford University Press, 1933.

Hess, W. E., and Street, D. M.: — Melorheostosis — J. Bone & Joint Surg. **32A:** 422-427 (April) 1950.

Hodgen, J. T. and Frantz, C. H.: — Arrest of Growth of the Epiphyses — Arch. Surg. **53:** 664 (Dec.) 1946.

Hume, J. B.: — The Causation of Multiple Exostoses — Brit. J. Surg. **17:** 236 (Oct.) 1929.

Hutter, C. G., and Scott, W.: — Tibial Torsion — J. Bone & Joint Surg. **31A:** 511-518 (July) 1949.

554 BIBLIOGRAPHY

Jansen, M.:	Dissociation of Bone Growth	The Robert Jones Birthday Volume, London, Oxford University Press, 1928.
Jenkinson, E. L., and Lewin, P.:	Bone Diseases in Infancy and Childhood	Am. J. Roentgenol. **17:** 201 (Feb.) 1927.
Key, J. A., Elzinga, E., and Fischer, F.:	Local Atrophy of Bone; Effect of Immobilization and of Operative Procedures	Arch. Surg. **28:** 936 (May) 1934.
Kraft, E.:	The Pathology of Monomelic Flowing Hyperostosis or Melorheostosis	Radiology **20:** 47 (Jan.) 1933.
Lichtenstein, L.:	Polyostotic Fibrous Dysplasia	Arch. Surg. **36:** 874 (May) 1938.
Macewen, W.:	The Growth of Bone	Glasgow, Jas. Maclehose & Sons, 1912.
Mahorner, H. R.:	Dyschondroplasia	J. Pediat. **10:** 1 (Jan.) 1937.
McCune, D. J., and Bradley, C.:	Osteopetrosis (Marble Bones) in an Infant: Review of Literature and Report of Case	Am. J. Dis. Child. **48:** 949 (Nov.) 1934.
McCune, D. J., and Bruch, H.:	Osteodystrophia Fibrosa	Am. J. Dis. Child. **54:** 806 (Oct.) 1937.
Moore, J. J., and de Lorimier, A. A.:	Melorheostosis Leri	Am. J. Roentgenol. **29:** 161 (Feb.) 1933.
Pedersen, H. E., and McCarroll, H. R.:	Vitamin-Resistant Rickets	J. Bone & Joint Surg. **33A:** 203-220 (Jan.) 1951.
Platt, J. L., and Eisenberg, R. B.:	Eosinophilic Granuloma of Bone, Report of Six Cases	J. Bone & Joint Surg. **30A:** 761-768 (July) 1948.
Ponseti, I.:	Bone Lesions in Eosinophilic Granuloma, Hand - Schüller - Christian Disease, and Letterer-Siwe's Disease	J. Bone & Joint Surg. **30A:** 811-833 (Oct.) 1948.
Price, N. L., and Davie, T. B.:	Renal Rickets	Brit. J. Surg. **24:** 548 (Jan.) 1937.
Ray, R. B., and Kellner, A.:	Eosinophilic Granuloma of Bone	J. Bone & Joint Surg. **28:** 629 (July) 1946.
Rowland, R. S.:	Xanthomatosis and the Reticulo-Endothelial System	Arch. Int. Med. **42:** 611 (Nov.) 1928.
	Schüller-Christian's Disease	Am. J. Roentgenol. **30:** 649 (Nov.) 1933.
Sosman, M. C.:	Xanthomatosis (Schüller-Christian's Disease; Lipoid Histiocytosis)	J. A. M. A. **98:** 110 (Jan. 9) 1932.

Strong, R. A.: Xanthomatosis (Schüller-Christian's Disease) J. A. M. A. **107:** 422 (Aug. 8) 1936.

Stronge, R. F., and McDowell, H. B.: Case of Engelmann's Disease J. Bone & Joint Surg. **32B:** 38-39 (Feb.) 1950.

Thoman, W. S., and Murphy, R. E.: Infantile Cortical Hyperostoses Radiology **54:** 735-740 (May) 1950.

Tutunjian, K. H., and Kegerreis, R.: Myositis Ossificans Progressiva With Report of a Case J. Bone & Joint Surg. **19:** 503 (April) 1937.

Vanzant, B. T., and Vanzant, F. R.: Hereditary Deforming Chondrodysplasia J. A. M. A. **119:** 786 (July 4) 1942.

Wolbach, S. B.: Vitamin A Deficiency and Excess in Relation to Skeletal Growth J. Bone & Joint Surg. **29:** 171-192 (Jan.) 1947.

Chapter V

Affections of Adult Bone

Albright, F.: Osteoporosis Ann. Int. Med. **27:** 861-882 (Dec.) 1947.

Albright, F., Aub, J. C., and Bauer, W.: Hyperparathyroidism: A Common and Polymorphic Condition as Illustrated by 17 Proved Cases From One Clinic J. A. M. A. **102:** 1276 (Apr. 21) 1934.

Albright, F., and Reifenstein, E. C.: The Parathyroid Glands and Metabolic Bone Disease: Selected Studies Baltimore, The Williams & Wilkins Co., 1948.

Ballin, M.: Skeletal Pathology of Endocrine Origin Ann. Surg. **98:** 868 (Nov.) 1933.

Behrend, Albert: Albright's Syndrome Am. J. Surg. **121:** 245-252 (Feb.) 1945.

Camp, J. D.: Osseous Changes in Hyperparathyroidism; A Roentgenologic Study J. A. M. A. **99:** 1913 (Dec. 3) 1932.

Camp, J. D., and Scanlan, R. L.: Chronic Idiopathic Hypertrophic Osteo-Arthropathy Radiology **50:** 581-594 (May) 1948.

Cushing, H.: The Pituitary Body and Its Disorders Philadelphia, J. B. Lippincott Co., 1912.

Acromegaly From a Surgical Standpoint Brit. M. J. **2:** 1 (July 2) 1927.

de Takats, G., and Miller, D. S.: Post-Traumatic Dystrophy of the Extremities: A Chronic Vasodilator Mechanism Arch. Surg. **46:** 469 (April) 1943.

Fairbank, H. A. T.: Paget's Disease J. Bone & Joint Surg. **32B:** 253-265 (May) 1950.

Goldenberg, R. R.: — Skull in Paget's Disease — J. Bone & Joint Surg. **33A:** 911-923 (Oct.) 1951.

Gutman, A. B., Swenson, P. C., and Parsons, W. B.: — The Differential Diagnosis of Hyperparathyroidism — J. A. M. A. **103:** 87 (July 14) 1934.

Jaffe, H. L.: — Primary and Secondary (Renal) Hyperparathyroidism — S. Clin. North America **22:** 621 (April) 1942.

Lake, M.: — Studies of Paget's Disease (Osteitis Deformans) — J. Bone & Joint Surg. **33B:** 323-335 (Aug.) 1951.

McClure, R. D., and Lam, C. R.: — End-Results in the Treatment of Hyperparathyroidism — Ann. Surg. **121:** 454-469 (April) 1945.

Moehlig, R. C.: — Paget's Disease (Osteitis Deformans) and Osteoporosis — Surg., Gynec. & Obst. **62:** 815 (May) 1936.

Moehlig, R. C., and Adler, S.: — Carbohydrate Metabolism Disturbance in Osteoporosis and Paget's Disease — Surg., Gynec. & Obst. **64:** 747 (April) 1937.

Moore, S.: — Osteitis Deformans: Theory of Its Etiology — J. Bone & Joint Surg. **33A:** 421-430 (April) 1951.

Newman, F. W.: — Paget's Disease, A Statistical Study of 82 Cases — J. Bone & Joint Surg. **28:** 798-804 (Oct.) 1946.

Pritchard, J. E.: — Fibrous Dysplasia of Bones — Am. J. M. Sc. **222:** 313-332 (Sept.) 1951.

Proffitt, J. N., McSwain, B., and Kalmon, E. H., Jr.: — Fibrous Dysplasia of Bone — Ann. Surg. **130:** 881-895 (Nov.) 1949.

Reifenstein, E. C., Jr., and Albright, F.: — Paget's Disease: Its Pathologic Physiology and the Importance of This in the Complications Arising From Fracture and Immobilization — New England J. Med. **231:** 343 (Sept. 7) 1944.

Russell, L. W., and Chandler, F. A.: — Fibrous Dysplasia of Bone — J. Bone & Joint Surg. **32A:** 323-337 (April) 1950.

Sherman, M. S.: — Osteomalacia — J. Bone & Joint Surg. **32A:** 193-206 (Jan.) 1950.

Strassburger, P., Garber, C. Z., and Hallock, H.: — Fibrous Dysplasia of Bone — J. Bone & Joint Surg. **33A:** 407-421 (April) 1951.

Sugarbaker, E. D.: — Osteitis Deformans (Paget's Disease of Bones): Review of Fifty-One Cases — Am. J. Surg. **48:** 414 (May) 1940.

Sweetapple, H. A.: — Sudeck's Atrophy — M. J. Australia **2:** 581 (Oct. 26) 1946.

Thannhauser, S. J.:	Neurofibromatosis (von Recklinghausen) and Osteitis Fibrosa Cystica Localisata et Disseminata (von Recklinghausen)	Medicine **23**: 105-149 (May) 1944.
Volls, J., Polak, M., and Schajowicz, F.:	F i b r o u s Dysplasia of Bone	J. Bone & Joint Surg. **32A**: 311-322 (April) 1950.
Wakeley, C. P. G., and Atkinson, F. R. B.:	Acromegaly, A Detailed Report on Two Cases	Surgery **3**: 8 (Jan.) 1938.
Warrick, C. K.:	Polyostotic Fibrous Dysplasia—Albright's Syndrone	J. Bone & Joint Surg. **31B**: 175-183 (May) 1949.
Wyatt, G. M., and Randall, W. S.:	Monostotic Fibrous Dysplasia	Am. J. Roentgenol **61**: 354-365 (Mar.) 1949.

Chapter VI

Infections of Bone (Exclusive of Tuberculosis)

Pyogenic Infections of Bone

Ackman, D., and Smith, F.:	The Role of Chemotherapy in Wounds and Surgical Infections. 1. Clinical and Bacteriologic Studies	Ann. Surg. **123**: 70-95 (Jan.) 1946.
Altemeier, W. A.:	Treatment of Acute Hematogenous Osteomyelitis With Penicillin	Ohio State M. J. **42**: 489 (May) 1946.
Altemeier, W. A., and Wadsworth, C. L.	Evaluation of Penicillin T h e r a p y in Acute Hematogenous Osteomyelitis.	J. Bone & Joint Surg. **30A**: 657-673 (July) 1948.
Badgley, C. E.:	Osteomyelitis of the Ilium	Arch. Surg. **28**: 83 (Jan.) 1934.
Baer, W. S.:	The Treatment of Chronic Osteomyelitis With the Maggot (Larva of the Blow Fly)	J. Bone & Joint Surg. **13**: 438 (July) 1931.
Baker, L. D., and Shands, A. R., Jr.:	Acute Osteomyelitis With Staphylococcemia	J. A. M. A. **113**: 2119 (Dec.) 1939.
Baker, L. D., Schaubel, H. J., and Kuhn, H. H.:	Open Versus Closed Treatment of Acute Osteomyelitis: Clinical Report on Use of Antitoxin and Sulfonamide Drugs With and Without Early Drainage	J. Bone & Joint Surg. **26**: 345-349 (April) 1944.
Blanche, D. W.:	Osteomyelitis in Infants	J. Bone & Joint Surg. **34A**: 71-86 (Jan.) 1952.

Brailsford, J. T.: | Brodie's Abscess and Its Differential Diagnosis | Brit. M. J. **2**: 119 (July 16) 1938.

Brown, H. P., Jr.: | Acute Hematogenous Osteomyelitis of the Long Bones | Ann. Surg. **109**: 596 (April) 1939.

Caldwell, G. A.: | Repair of Bony Defects Associated With Osteomyelitis | Ann. Surg. **123**: 698-704 (April) 1946.

Caldwell, G. A., and Wickstrom, J. K.: | Osteomyelitis, in Cyclopedia of Medicine, Surgery, Specialties, Vol. 9, 977-999 | Philadelphia, F. A. Davis Co., 1951.

Capener, N., and Pierce, K. C.: | Pathological Fractures in Osteomyelitis | J. Bone & Joint Surg. **14**: 501 (July) 1932.

Dickson, F. D.: | The Clinical Diagnosis, Prognosis and Treatment of Acute Hematogenous Osteomyelitis | J. A. M. A. **127**: 212 (Jan. 27) 1945.

Downey, J. W., and Simon, H. E.: | Brodie's Abscess. Two Case Reports | Am. J. Surg. **70**: 86-94 (Oct.) 1945.

Fett, H. C., O'Connor, J. J., and Johnson, J. A.: | Experiences in Treatment of Traumatic Cavitation in the Upper Tibia | Am. J. Surg. **73**: 11 (Jan.) 1947.

Green, W. T., and Shannon, J. G.: | Osteomyelitis of Infants. A Disease Different From Osteomyelitis of Older Children | Arch. Surg. **32**: 462 (March) 1936.

Hebb, H. D.: | The Role of Penicillin in the Treatment of Chronic Osteomyelitis | Canad. M. A. J. **54**: 446 (May) 1946.

Horwitz, T., and Lambert, R. G.: | Chronic Osteomyelitis Complicating War Compound Fractures: An Evaluation of 125 Patients Treated by Early Secondary Closure | Surg., Gynec. & Obst. **82**: 573-578 (May) 1946.

Howard, L. G., Anderson, D. G., Christophe, K., Potter, T. A., and Moore, R. L.: | Treatment of Chronic Osteomyelitis With Penicillin and Primary Closure of Operative Wounds. | Arch. Surg. **60**: 112-124 (Jan.) 1950.

Kerwein, G. A., and Capps, R. B.: | Typhoid Osteomyelitis: Case Report | Am. J. Surg. **60**: 433 (June) 1943.

Knight, M. P., and Wood, G. O. | Surgical Obliteration of Bone Cavities Following Traumatic Osteomyelitis | J. Bone & Joint Surg. **27**: 547 (Oct.) 1945.

Kulowski, J.: | Pyogenic Osteomyelitis of the Spine: An Analysis and Discussion of 102 Cases | J. Bone & Joint Surg. **18**: 343-364 (April) 1936.

Meyerding, H. W.: — Chronic Sclerosing Osteitis (Sclerosing Non-Suppurative Osteomyelitis of Garré); Differential Diagnosis — S. Clin. North America **24:** 762-779 (Aug.) 1944.

Nathan, P. W.: — Differential Diagnosis and the Treatment of Acute Osteomyelitis of the Upper End of the Femur, Involving the Hip Joint — Surg., Gynec. & Obst. **54:** 52 (Jan.) 1932.

Orr, H. W.: — Osteomyelitis and Compound Fractures and Other Infected Wounds — St. Louis, The C. V. Mosby Co., 1929.

Phemister, D. B.: — Pyogenic Osteomyelitis — Nelson's Surgery **3:** 695 1935.

Reynolds, F. C., and Zeapfel, F.: — Management of Chronic Osteomyelitis Secondary to Compound Fractures — J. Bone & Joint Surg. **30B:** 331-338 (April) 1948.

Robertson, D. E.: — Acute Hematogenous Osteomyelitis — J. Bone & Joint Surg. **20:** 35 (Jan.) 1938.

Toumey, J. W.: — Sclerosing Osteitis of Garré — S. Clin. North America **20:** 857-861 (June) 1940.

Turner, P.: — Acute Infective Osteomyelitis of the Spine — Brit. J. Surg. **26:** 71 (July) 1938.

Wagner, L. C., and Hanby, J. E.: — Brodie's Abscess: Pain Distribution, Occurrence and Diagnosis — Am. J. Surg. **39:** 135 (Jan.) 1938.

Zadek, I.: — Acute Osteomyelitis of the Long Bones of Adults — Arch. Surg. **37:** 531 (Oct.) 1938.

Other Infections of Bone

Alfred, K. S., and Harbin, M.: — Blastomycosis and Coccidioidomycosis of Bone, Report of Case of Blastomycosis — J. Bone & Joint Surg. **32A:** 887-892 (Oct.) 1950.

Benninghoven, D., and Miller, E. R.: — Coccidioidal Infection in Bone — Radiology **38:** 663 (June) 1942.

Colonna, P. C., and Gucker, T., III: — Blastomycosis of the Skeletal System: A Summary of Sixty-Seven Recorded Cases and a Case Report — J. Bone & Joint Surg. **26:** 322 (April) 1944.

Cope, V. Z.: — Actinomycosis of Bone With Special Reference to Infection of Vertebral Column — J. Bone & Joint Surg. **33B:** 205-214 (May) 1951.

Coventry, M. B., Ivins, J. C., Nichols, D. R., and Weed, L A.: — Infection of the Hip by Brucella Suis — J. A. M. A. **141:** 320-325 (Oct. 1), 1949.

Cullen, C. H., and Sharp, M. E.:	Infections of Wounds With Actinomyces	J. Bone & Joint Surg. **33B:** 221-227 (May) 1951.
Evans, W. A., Jr.:	Syphilis of Bones in Infancy: Some Possible Errors in Roentgen Diagnosis	J. A. M. A. **115:** 197 (July 20) 1940.
Faget, G. H., and Mayeral, A.:	Bone Changes in Leprosy: A Clinical and Roentgenologic Study of 505 Cases	Radiology **42:** 1-13 (Jan.) 1944.
Helfet, A. J.:	Acute Manifestations of Yaws of Bone and Joint	J. Bone & Joint Surg. **26:** 672 (Oct.) 1944.
Howorth, M. B.:	Echinococcosis of Bone	J. Bone & Joint Surg. **27:** 401 (July) 1945.
McMaster, P. E., and Gilfillan, C.:	Coccidioidal Osteomyelitis	J. A. M. A. **112:** 1233 (April 1) 1939.
Morton, J. J.:	Syphilis of Bone	Urol. & Cutan. Rev. **43:** 72 (Jan.) 1939.
Rhinehart, W. J., and Bauer, J. T.:	Disseminated Granuloma	Am. J. Roentgenol. **57:** 562-567 (May) 1947.
Sashin, O., Brown, G. N., Laffer, N. C., and McDowell, H. C.:	Disseminated Coccidioidomycosis Localized in Bone	Am. J. M. Sc. **212:** 565-573 (Nov.) 1946.
Steindler, A.:	Orthopedic Complications of Brucellosis	J. Iowa M. Soc. **30:** 256 (June) 1940.
Thomason, H. A., and Mayoral, A.:	Syphilitic Osteomyelitis	J. Bone & Joint Surg. **22:** 203 (Jan.) 1940.

Chapter VII

Infections of Joints (Exclusive of Tuberculosis)

Pyogenic Infections of Joints

Badgley, C. E., et al.:	Study of the End Results in 113 Cases of Septic Hips	J. Bone & Joint Surg. **18:** 1047 (Oct.) 1936.
Boger, W. P.:	Pneumococcic Arthritis	J. A. M. A. **126:** 1062-1065 (Dec. 23) 1944.
Carnett, J. B.:	Typhoid Spine	Ann. Surg. **61:** 456 (April) 1915.
Everidge, J.:	A New Method of Treatment for Suppurative Arthritis of the Knee-Joint	Brit. J. Surg. **6:** 566 (April) 1919.
Fox, M. J., and Gilbert, J.:	Meningococcus Infections With Articular Complications	Am. J. M. Sc. **208:** 63 (July) 1944.
Freiberg, J. A., and Perlman, R.:	Pelvic Abscesses Associated With Acute Purulent Infection of the Hip Joint	J. Bone & Joint Surg. **18:** 417 (April) 1936.

Hampton, O. P., Jr.:	The Management of Penetrating Wounds and Suppurative Arthritis of the Knee Joint in the Mediterranean Theatre of Operations	J. Bone & Joint Surg. **28**: 659 (Oct.) 1946.
Harmon, P. H., and Adams, C. O.:	Pyogenic Coxitis: End Results and Considerations of Diagnosis and Treatment	Am. J. Roentgenol. **51**: 707 (June) 1944.
Heberling, J. A.:	Review of Two Hundred and One Cases of Suppurative Arthritis	J. Bone & Joint Surg. **23**: 917 (Oct.) 1941.
Miller, O. L.:	Acute Transient Epiphysitis of the Hip Joint	J. A. M. A. **96**: 575 (Feb. 21) 1931.
Ober, F. R.:	Posterior Arthrotomy of the Hip Joint: Report of 5 Cases	J. A. M. A. **83**: 1500 (Nov. 8) 1924.
Phemister, D. B.:	Changes in Articular Surfaces in Tuberculous and in Pyogenic Infections of Joints	Am. J. Roentgenol. **12**: 1 (July) 1924.
Thomson, J. E. M.:	Pyogenic Infections of the Joints (Nontuberculous), in Cyclopedia of Medicine, Surgery, Specialties, Vol. 7, 581	Philadelphia, F. A. Davis Co., 1950.
Willems, C.:	Treatment of Purulent Arthritis by Wide Arthrotomy Followed by Immediate Active Mobilization	Surg., Gynec. & Obst. **28**: 546 (June) 1919.

Gonococcal Arthritis

Ginsberg, S.:	Roentgenographic Findings in Acute Gonococcal Synovitis of the Knee Treated by Pneumarthrosis: Report of 2 Cases With a Plea for Early Motion	J. Bone & Joint Surg. **15**: 615 (July) 1933.
Hench, P. S., Slocumb, C. H., and Popp, W. C.:	Fever Therapy	J. A. M. A. **104**: 1779 (May 18) 1935.
Kendall, H. W., Webb, W. W., and Simpson, W. M.:	Artificial Fever Therapy of Gonorrheal Arthritis: Report of 31 Cases.	Am. J. Surg. **29**: 428 (Sept.) 1935.
Spink, W. W., and Keefer, C. S.:	The Diagnosis, Treatment and End Results in Gonococcal Arthritis	New England J. Med. **218**: 453 (Mar. 17) 1938.

Syphilis of Joints

Klauder, J. V., and Robertson, H. F.:	Symmetrical Serous Synovitis (Clutton's Joints): Congenital Syphilis and Interstitial Keratitis	J. A. M. A. **103**: 236 (July 28) 1934.
Kling, D. H.:	Syphilitic Arthritis With Effusion	Am. J. M. Sc. **183**: 538 (April) 1932.

Ankylosis and Arthroplasty

Baer, W. S.:	Arthroplasty With the Aid of Animal Membrane	Am. J. Orthop. Surg. **16**: 1 (Jan.) 1918.
	Arthroplasty of the Hip	J. Bone & Joint Surg. **8**: 769 (Oct.) 1926.
Bennett, G. E.:	Lengthening of the Quadriceps Tendon	J. Bone & Joint Surg. **4**: 279 (April) 1922.
Campbell, W. C.:	Arthroplasty of the Hip: An Analysis of 48 Cases	Surg., Gynec. & Obst. **43**: 9 (July) 1926.
	Arthroplasty of the Knee	Surg., Gynec. & Obst. **47**: 89 (July) 1928.
	The Physiology of Arthroplasty	J. Bone & Joint Surg. **13**: 223 (April) 1931.
	Surgery of the Ankylosed Joint	Surg., Gynec. & Obst. **55**: 747 (Dec.) 1932.
Judet, J., and Judet, R.:	Use of Artificial Femoral Head for Arthroplasty of Hip Joint	J. Bone & Joint Surg. **32B**: 166-173 (May) 1950.
Kelikian, H.:	Method of Mobilizing Temporomandibular Joint	J. Bone & Joint Surg. **32A**: 113-131 (Jan.) 1950.
Knight, R. A.:	Arthroplasty, in Monographs on Surgery for 1952, 253-309	Baltimore, The Williams & Wilkins Co., 1952.
MacAusland, W. R.:	Knee Joint Arthroplasty	J. A. M. A. **101**: 1699 (Nov. 25) 1933.
Putti, V.:	Arthroplasty	J. Orthop. Surg. **3**: 421 (Sept.) 1921.
Schrock, R. D.:	Fixation Position for Optimum Joint Function	Nebraska M. J. **19**: 211 (June) 1934.
Smith-Petersen, M. N.:	Arthroplasty of the Hip —A New Method	J. Bone & Joint Surg. **21**: 269 (April) 1939.
	Evolution of Mould Arthroplasty of Hip Joint	J. Bone & Joint Surg. **30B**: 59-75 (Feb.) 1948.
Speed, J. S., and Trout, P. C.:	Arthroplasty of Knee, Follow-up Study	J. Bone & Joint Surg. **31B**: 53-60 (Feb.) 1949.
Stinchfield, F. E., and Carroll, R. E.:	Vitallum-Cup Arthroplasty of Hip Joint	J. Bone & Joint Surg. **31A**: 628-638 (July) 1949.
Thompson, T. C.:	Quadricepsplasty	Ann. Surg. **121**: 751-755 (May) 1945.

Chapter VIII

Tuberculosis of Bones and Joints: The Spine and Pelvis

General Considerations

Barr, J. S.: Heliotherapy in the Treatment of Surgical Tuberculosis — New England J. Med. **208:** 131 (Jan. 19) 1933.

Blair, J. E., and Hallmann, F. A.: Diagnosis of Surgical Tuberculosis; Comparison of Diagnosis by Inoculation of Guinea-Pigs and by Culture — Arch. Surg. **27:** 178 (July) 1933.

Bosworth, D.: Orthopaedic Problems in Tuberculosis — S. Clin. North America, Symposium on Orthopaedic Surgery (April) 1951.

Bosworth, D. M., and Wright, H. A.: Streptomycin in Bone and Joint Tuberculosis — J. Bone & Joint Surg. **34A:** 255-266 (April) 1952.

Brav, E. A., and Hench, P. S.: Tuberculous Rheumatism; A Résumé — J. Bone & Joint Surg. **16:** 839 (Oct.) 1934.

Brock, B. J.: Streptomycin in the Treatment of Draining Tuberculous Sinuses — J. A. M. A. **135:** 147-149 (Sept. 20) 1947.

Carrell, W. B., and Childress, H. M.: Tuberculosis of Large Long Bones of Extremities — J. Bone & Joint Surg. **22:** 569 (July) 1940.

Erlacher, P. J.: The Radical Operative Treatment of Bone and Joint Tuberculosis — J. Bone & Joint Surg. **17:** 536 (July) 1935.

Fraser, J.: Tuberculosis of the Bones and Joints in Children — London, A. & C. Black, 1914.

Ghormley, R. K.: Joint Disease; A Clinical-Pathological Study — J. Bone & Joint Surg. **8:** 858 (Oct.) 1926.

Girdlestone, G. R.: Tuberculosis of Bone and Joint — London, Oxford University Press, 1940.

Harris, R. I., and Coulthard, H. S.: Prognosis in Bone and Joint Tuberculosis: Analysis of Results of Treatment and Consideration of Factors Which Influence End Results — J. Bone & Joint Surg. **24:** 382 (April) 1942.

Harris, R. I., Coulthard, H. S., and Dewar, F. P.: Streptomycin in the Treatment of Bone & Joint Tuberculosis — J. Bone & Joint Surg. **34A:** 279-287 (April) 1952.

Hsieh, C. K., Miltner, L. J., and Chang, C. P.: Tuberculosis of the Shaft of the Large Long Bones of the Extremities — J. Bone & Joint Surg. **16:** 545 (July) 1934.

Kite, J. H.:	Tuberculosis of Bones and Joints, in Cyclopedia of Medicine, Surgery, Specialties, Vol. 7, 639	Philadelphia, F. A. Davis Co., 1950.
Peabody, C. W.:	Chronic Synovial Tuberculosis	Ann. Surg. **86**: 92 (July) 1927.
Phemister, D. B.:	Changes in the Articular Surfaces in Tuberculous Arthritis	J. Bone & Joint Surg. **7**: 835 (Oct.) 1925.
Pomeranz, M. M.:	Roentgen Diagnosis of Bone and Joint Tuberculosis	Am. J. Roentgenol. **29**: 753 (June) 1933.
Rollier, A.:	The Conservative Treatment in Surgical Tuberculosis of the Lower Extremity	J. Bone & Joint Surg. **12**: 733 (Oct.) 1930.
Rosencrantz, E., Piscitelli, A., and Bost, F. C.:	Analytical Study of Bone and Joint Lesions in Relation to Chronic Pulmonary Tuberculosis	J. Bone & Joint Surg. **23**: 628 (July) 1941.
Van Alstyne, G. S., and Gowen, G. H.:	Osteitis Tuberculosa Multiplex Cystica (Jüngling); Report of a Case Involving the Larger Long Bones With Complete Proof of Its Tuberculous Etiology; A Review of the Literature	J. Bone & Joint Surg. **15**: 193 (Jan.) 1933.

Spine and Pelvis

Albee, F. H.:	The Bone-Graft Operation for Tuberculosis of the Spine; Twenty Years' Experience	J. A. M. A. **94**: 1467 (May 10) 1930.
Auerbach, O., and Stemmerman, M. G.:	Roentgen Interpretation of Pathology in Pott's Disease	Am. J. Roentgenol. **52**: 57 (July) 1944.
Baker, L. D., and Hoyt, W. A.:	Arthrodesis of the Spine, in Monographs on Surgery for 1950, 465-490	New York, Thos. Nelson & Sons, 1950.
Bosworth, D. M., and Levine, J.:	Tuberculosis of Spine—Analysis of Cases Treated Surgically.	J. Bone & Joint Surg. **31A**: 267-274 (April) 1949.
Butler, R. W.:	Paraplegia in Pott's Disease, With Special Reference to Pathology and Etiology	Brit. J. Surg. **22**: 738 (April) 1935.
Campbell, W. C.:	An Operation for Extra-Articular Fusion of the Sacro-Iliac Joint	Surg., Gynec. & Obst. **45**: 218 (Aug.) 1927.

Cave, E. F.:	Tuberculosis of the Spine in Children	New England J. Med. **217**: 853 (Nov. 25) 1937.
Cleveland, M.:	Treatment of Tuberculosis of Spine	J. Bone & Joint Surg. **22**: 824 (July) 1940.
Cleveland, M., and Bosworth, D. M.:	Pathology of Tuberculosis of Spine	J. Bone & Joint Surg. **24**: 527 (July) 1942.
Cleveland, M., Bosworth, D. M., and Thompson, F. R.:	Pseudarthrosis in Lumbosacral Spine	J. Bone & Joint Surg. **30A**: 302-312 (April) 1948.
Dobson, J.:	Tuberculosis of Spine	J. Bone & Joint Surg. **33B**: 517-532 (Nov.) 1951.
Finkelstein, H., Greenberg, B. B., Jahss, S. A., and Mayer, L.:	Operative and Conservative Treatment of Tuberculosis of the Spine	J. A. M. A. **110**: 480 (Feb. 12) 1938.
Garceau, G. J., and Brady, T. A.:	Pott's Disease	J. Bone & Joint Surg. **32A**: 87-96 (Jan.) 1950.
Hibbs, R. A., and Risser, J. C.:	Treatment of Vertebral Tuberculosis by the Spine Fusion Operation; A Report of 286 Cases	J. Bone & Joint Surg. **10**: 805 (Oct.) 1928.
Kite, J. H.:	Non-Operative Versus Operative Treatment of Tuberculosis of the Spine in Children; A Review of 50 Consecutive Cases Treated by Each Method	South. M. J. **26**: 918 (Nov.) 1933.
	Tuberculosis of the Spine with Paraplegia	South, M. J. **29**: 883 (Sept.) 1936.
McKee, G. K.:	A Comparison of Results of Spinal Fixation Operations and Non-Operative Treatment in Pott's Disease in Adults	Brit. J. Surg. **24**: 456 (Jan.) 1937.
Seddon, H. J.:	Pott's Paraplegia: Prognosis and Treatment	Brit. J. Surg. **22**: 769 (April) 1935.
Swett, P. P., Bennett, G. E., and Street, D. M.:	Pott's Disease — Initial Lesion, Relative Infrequency of Extension by Contiguity, Nature and Type of Healing, Role of Abscess, and Merits of Operative and Non-Operative Treatment	J. Bone & Joint Surg. **22**: 878 (July) 1940.

Chapter IX

Tuberculosis of Bones and Joints: The Extremities

Badgley, C. E., and Hammond, G.: Tuberculosis of Hip: Review of Seventy-Six Patients With Proved Tuberculous Arthritis of Seventy-Seven Hips Treated by Arthrodesis J. Bone & Joint Surg. **24:** 135 (Jan.) 1942.

Bosworth, D. M.: Femoro-Ischial Transplantation J. Bone & Joint Surg. **24:** 38-46 (Jan.) 1942.

Brav, E. A.: Subchondral Granulation Tissue in Tuberculosis of the Knee Joint J. Bone & Joint Surg. **15:** 631 (July) 1933.

Brittain, H. A.: Architectural Principles in Arthrodesis Edinburgh, E. & S. Livingstone, Ltd., 1942.

Ischiofemoral Arthrodesis J. Bone & Joint Surg. **30B:** 642-650 (Nov.) 1948.

Charnley, J. C.: Positive Pressure in Arthrodesis of Knee Joint J. Bone & Joint Surg. **30B:** 478-486 (Aug.) 1948.

Dobson, J.: Prognosis in Tuberculosis of the Hip J. Bone & Joint Surg. **33B:** 149-159 (May) 1951.

Ghormley, R. K.: The Use of the Anterior Superior Spine and Crest of the Illium in Surgery of the Hip Joint J. Bone & Joint Surg. **13:** 784 (Oct.) 1931.

Ghormley, R. K., and Brav, E. A.: Resected Knee Joints Arch. Surg. **26:** 465 (Mar.) 1933.

Hallock, H., and Toumey, J. W., Jr.: Hip Joint Tuberculosis Treated by Fusion Operation; End-Result Study of 170 Unselected Cases J. A. M. A. **103:** 1836 (Dec. 15) 1934.

Hatcher, C. H., and Phemister, D. B.: The Primary Point of Infection in Tuberculosis of the Hip Joint Surg., Gynec. & Obst. **65:** 721 (Dec.) 1937.

Hibbs, R. A.: A Preliminary Report of Twenty Cases of Hip Joint Tuberculosis Treated by an Operation Devised to Eliminate Motion by Fusing the Joint J. Bone & Joint Surg. **8:** 522 (July) 1926.

Hibbs, R. A., and von Lackum, H. L.: End-Results in Treatment of Knee Joint Tuberculosis J. A. M. A. **85:** 1289 (Oct. 24) 1925.

Knight, R. A., and Bluhm, M. M.: Brittain Ischiofemoral Arthrodesis J. Bone & Joint Surg. **27:** 578 (Oct.) 1945.

Lo Grasso, H.: The Non-Operative Treatment of Tuberculous Joints of the Lower Extremities — J. Bone & Joint Surg. **12**: 755 (Oct.) 1930.

McCarroll, H. R., and Heath, R. D.: Tuberculosis of the Hip in Children — J. Bone & Joint Surg. **29**: 889-906 (Oct.) 1947.

Miltner, L. J., and Fang, H. C.: Prognosis and Treatment of Tuberculosis of the Bones of the Foot — J. Bone & Joint Surg. **18**: 287 (April) 1936.

Pease, C. N.: Fusion of the Hip in Children, The Chandler Method — J. Bone & Joint Surg. **29**: 874-888 (Oct.) 1947.

Soliolt, S.: Tuberculosis of Sacro-iliac Joint — J. Bone & Joint Surg. **33A**: 119-130 (Jan.) 1951.

Stinchfield, F. E., and Cavallaro, W. U.: Arthrodesis of Hip Joint, Follow-up Study — J. Bone & Joint Surg. **32A**: 48 - 58 (Jan.) 1950.

Toumey, J. W., Jr.: Knee Joint Tuberculosis; Two Hundred Twenty-Two Patients Treated by Operative Fusion — Surg., Gynec. & Obst. **68**: 1029 (June) 1939.

Van Gorder, G. W.: Trumble Operation for Fusion of Hip — J. Bone & Joint Surg. **31A**: 717-727 (Oct.) 1949.

Wilson, J. C.: Operative Fixation of Tuberculous Hips in Children; End-Result Study of 33 Patients from the Orthopaedic Department of the Children's Hospital — J. Bone & Joint Surg. **15**: 22 (Jan.) 1933.

Yu, H. I.: Tuberculosis of Hip — J. Bone & Joint Surg. **33A**: 131-143 (Jan.) 1951.

Chapter X

Chronic Arthritis

Adams, C. H., and Cecil, R. L.: Gold Therapy in Early Rheumatoid Arthritis — Ann. Int. Med. **33**: 163-173 (July) 1950.

Allison, N., and Ghormley, R. K.: Diagnosis in Joint Disease — New York, William Wood & Co., 1931.

American Rheumatism Association Committee: Primer on Rheumatic Diseases — J. A. M. A. **139**: 1068-1076, 1138-1146, 1268-1273 (April) 16, 23, 30, 1949.

Bach, F.: Dietetic Aspects of Rheumatism — Brit. J. Rheumatism **1**: 173 (Jan.) 1939.

Bauer, W., and Bennett, G. A.: Experimental and Pathological Studies in the Degenerative Type of Arthritis — J. Bone & Joint Surg. **18**: 1 (Jan.) 1936.

Bauer, W., and Short, C. L.: The Treatment of Degenerative Joint Disease — New England J. Med. **225**: 145 (July 24) 1941.

Cecil, R. L., Kammerer, W., and de Prume, F. J.: Gold Salts in Treatment of Rheumatoid Arthritis: Study of Two Hundred and Forty-Five Cases — Ann. Int. Med. **16**: 811 (May) 1942.

Collins, D. H.: The Pathology of Osteoarthritis — Brit. J. Rheumatism **1**: 248 (April) 1939.

Comroe, B. I.: Arthritis and Allied Conditions, Hollander, J. L., Editor, 4th Edition — Philadelphia, Lea & Febiger, 1949.

Common Mistakes in Handling of Patients With Arthritis and Allied Conditions — J. A. M. A. **127**: 392 (Feb. 17) 1945.

Dickson, F. D.: The Surgical Treatment of Arthritis — Ann. Surg. **113**: 869 (May) 1941.

Edmonds, E. P.: Psychosomatic Non-articular Rheumatism — Ann. Rheumat. Dis. **6**: 36-49 (March) 1947.

Fletcher, A. A.: The Nutritional Factor in Chronic Arthritis — J. Lab. & Clin. Med. **15**: 1140 (Aug.) 1930.

Fletcher, A. A., and Graham, D.: The Large Bowel in Chronic Arthritis — Am. J. M. Sc. **179**: 91 (Jan.) 1930.

Forkner, C. E., Shands, A. R., Jr., and Poston, M.: Synovial Fluid in Chronic Arthritis — Arch. Int. Med. **42**: 675 (Nov.) 1928.

Freyberg, R. H.: Symposium on Analysis and Interpretation of Symptoms: Joint Pain — Clinics **2**: 1586-1619 (April) 1944.

Goldberg, A. S.: Pathology of Osteoarthritis — Am. J. Clin. Path. **14**: 1 (Jan.) 1944.

Graham, J. W., and Fletcher, A. A.: Gold Therapy in Rheumatoid Arthritis — Canad. M. A. J. **49**: 483 (Dec.) 1943.

Hall, F. C.: Menopausal Arthralgia. A Study of Seventy-One Women at Artificial Menopause — New England J. Med. **219**: 1015 (Dec. 29) 1938.

Hall, F. C., and Monroe, R. T.: Thyroid Gland Deficiency in Chronic Arthritis — J. Lab. & Clin. Med. **18**: 439 (Feb.) 1933.

Hench, P. S., et al.: Rheumatism and Arthritis; Review of American and English Literature of Recent Years — Ann. Int. Med. **28**: 66-168 (Jan.), 309-451 (Feb.) 1948.

Hench, P. S.:   Reversibility of Certain   Ann. Int. Med. **36:** 1-38
                Rheumatic and Non-   (Jan.) 1952.
                rheumatic Conditions
                by Use of Cortisone or
                of Pituitary Adreno-
                corticotropic Hormone

Hench, P. S., and   Palindromic Rheumatism   Arch. Int. Med. **73:**
   Rosenberg, E. F.:   293-321 (April) 1944.

Horwitz, T.:   Bone and Cartilage De-   J. Bone & Joint Surg.
                bris in Synovial Mem-   **30A:** 579-588 (July)
                brane   1948.

Kling, D. H.:   The Synovial Membrane   Los Angeles, Medical
                and the Synovial Fluid   Press, 1938.
                With Special Reference
                to Arthritis and In-
                juries of the Joints

Kuhns, J. G.:   Surgery in Chronic Ar-   New England J. Med.
                thritis   **240:** 605-610 (April)
                                         1949.

                Orthopedic Aspects of   Philadelphia, F. A. Davis
                Chronic Arthritis, in   Co., 1950.
                Cyclopedia of Med-
                icine, Surgery, Special-
                ties, Vol. 1, 818-856

Nichols, E. H., and   Arthritis Deformans   J. Med. Research **21:** 149
   Richardson, F. L.:   (Sept.) 1909.

Polley, H. F., and Ma-   Rheumatoid Arthritis   J. A. M. A. **143:** 1474-
   son, H. L.:   1481 (Aug.) 1950.

Portis, R. B.:   Pathology of Chronic   Am. J. Dis. Child. **55:**
                Arthritis of Children   1000 (May) 1938.
                (Still's Disease)

Preiser, G.:   Static Joint Diseases,   Am. J. Orthop. Surg. **10:**
                Their Etiology and   100 (Aug.) 1912.
                Their Relation to
                Arthritis Deformans

Slocumb, C. H.:   Rheumatic Diseases   Philadelphia, W. B. Saun-
                              ders Co., 1952.

Small, J. C.:   Mechanics of Deformities   Ann. Int. Med. **32:**
                of Hands in Atrophic   1 0 8 7 - 1 0 9 4 (June)
                Arthritis, and Discus-   1950.
                sion of Their Preven-
                tion and Correction

Snow, W. B.:   Relation of Physical Ther-   New England J. Med.
                apy to Arthritis   **229:** 959 (Dec. 23)
                              1943.

Soeur, R.:   Synovial Membrane of   J. Bone & Joint Surg.
                Knee in Pathological   **31A:** 317-340 (April)
                Conditions   1949.

Steinbrocker, O. (With   Arthritis in Modern Prac-   Philadelphia, W. B.
   Supplemental Chapters   tice. The Diagnosis and   Saunders Co., 1941.
   by Kuhns, J. G.):   Management of Rheu-
                matic and Allied Con-
                ditions

Steindler, A.:   Arthritic Deformities of   J. Bone & Joint Surg.
                                  Wrist and Fingers   33A: 849-863 (Oct.)
                                                               1951.

Swaim, L. T., and   The Prevention of De-
Kuhns, J. G.:   formities in Chronic
                                  Arthritis

                                  (1) The Upper Extrem-   J. A. M. A. 93: 1853
                                      ity   (Dec. 14) 1929.

                                  (2) The Spine and Head   J. A. M. A. 94: 1123
                                                               (April 12) 1930.

                                  (3) The Lower Extrem-   J. A. M. A. 94: 1743
                                      ity   (May 31) 1930.

Swett, P. P.:   A Review of Synovectomy   J. Bone & Joint Surg. 20:
                                                               68 (Jan.) 1938.

Thorn, G. W., and   Medical Progress; Studies   New England J. Med.
others: on Relation of Pitui-   241: 529-537 (Oct.)
                                  tary-Adrenal Function   1949.
                                  to Rheumatic Disease

Chapter XI

Chronic Arthritis: Special Joints

Baker, L. D., Coonrad,   Marie-Strumpell Arthri-   J. Bone & Joint Surg.
R. W., Reeves, R. J.,   tis: Follow-up Study   32A: 848-855 (Oct.)
and Hoyt, W. A. Jr.:   of Roentgenographic,   1950.
                                  Physical, and Ortho-
                                  paedic Therapy

Bennett, G. A.,   Changes in the Knee Joint   New York, The Common-
Waine, H., and   at Various Ages, With   wealth Fund, 1942.
Bauer, W.:   Particular Reference to
                                  the Nature and De-
                                  velopment of Degener-
                                  ative Joint Disease

Boland, E. W., and   Rheumatoid Spondylitis: J. A. M. A. 129: 843
Present, A. J.:   A Study of One Hun-   (Nov. 24) 1945.
                                  dred Cases, With Spe-
                                  cial Reference to Di-
                                  agnostic Criteria

Boland, E. W., and   Rheumatoid Spondylitis: Radiology 47: 551
Shebesta, E. M.:   Correlation of Clinical   (Dec.) 1946.
                                  and Roentgenographic
                                  Features

Freyberg, R. H.:   Roentgen Therapy for   M. Clin. North America
                                  Rheumatic Diseases   30: 603-615 (May)
                                                               1946.

Ghormley, R. K., and   Surgical Treatment of   J. Bone & Joint Surg. 24:
Coventry, M. B.:   Painful Hips of Adults   424 (April) 1942.

Golding, F. C.:   Spondylitis Ankylopoi-   Brit. J. Surg. 23: 484
                                  etica   (Jan.) 1936.

Inge, G. A. L.:   Eighty-Six Cases of   J. A. M. A. **111**: 2451
                               Chronic Synovitis of   (Dec. 31) 1938.
                               Knee Joint Treated by
                               Synovectomy

Keefer, C. S.,   Relationship Between An-   Arch. Int. Med. **53**: 325
   Parker, F., Jr.,   atomic Changes in   (March) 1934.
   Myers, W. K., and   Knee Joint With Ad-
   Irwin, R. L.:   vancing Age and De-
                               generative Arthritis

Knaggs, R. L.:   A Report on the Strange-   Brit. J. Surg. **20**: 113,
                               way's Collection of   309 and 425, 1932-33.
                               Rheumatoid Joints in
                               Museum of the Royal
                               College of Surgeons

Kuhns, J. G.:   Orthopaedic Treatment   J. Bone & Joint Surg. **24**:
                               of Hypertrophic Arth-   547 (July) 1942.
                               ritis of the Hip

                               Treatment of Arthritic   New England J. Med.
                               Contractures of the   **227**: 975 (Dec. 24)
                               Knee   1942.

Law, W. A.:   Surgical Treatment of the J. Bone & Joint Surg.
                               Rheumatic Diseases   **34B**: 215-225 (May)
                                                          1952.

McMurray, T. P.:   Osteoarthritis of the Hip J. Bone & Joint Surg. **21**:
                               Joint   1 (Jan.) 1939.

Polley, H. F., and   Rheumatoid Spondylitis;   Ann. Int. Med. **26**: 240-
   Slocumb, C. H.:   Study of 1035 Cases   249 (Feb.) 1947.

Shands, A. R., Jr.,   Atrophic and Hyper-   South. M. J. **26**: 384
   and Oates, M. O.:   trophic Arthritis of the   (May) 1933.
                               Spine

Chapter XII

Neuromuscular Disabilities: Infantile Paralysis

Abbott, L. C.:   The Operative Lengthen-   J. Bone & Joint Surg. **9**:
                               ing of the Tibia and   128 (Jan.) 1927.
                               Fibula

Allan, F. G.:   Bone Lengthening   J. Bone & Joint Surg.
                                                          30B: 490-505 (Aug.)
                                                          1948.

American Orthopaedic   Infantile Paralysis, or   J. A. M. A. **131**: 1411-
   Association, Primer   Acute Poliomyelitis: A   1419 (Aug. 24) 1946.
   Committee on   Brief Primer of the Dis-
   Poliomyelitis: ease and Its Treatment

American Orthopaedic   Survey of End Results on   J. Bone & Joint Surg. **24**:
   Association, Research   Stabilization of Para-   699 (July) 1942.
   Committee: lytic Shoulder

Bennett, G. E.,   Molded Plaster Shells for J. A. M. A. **109**: 1120-
   Cobey, M. C., and   Rest and Protection   1121 (Oct. 2) 1937.
   Kendall, H. O.:   Treatment of Infantile
                               Paralysis

Blount, W. P., and Clarke, G. R.: Control of Bone Growth by Epiphyseal Stapling — J. Bone &. Joint Surg. **31A:** 464-478 (July) 1949.

Campbell, W. C.: Bone-Block Operation for Drop-Foot; Analysis of End Results — J. Bone & Joint Surg. **12:** 317 (April) 1930.

Cleveland, M.: Operative Fusion of the Unstable or Flail Knee Due to Anterior Poliomyelitis; A Study of the Late Results — J. Bone & Joint Surg. **14:** 525 (July) 1932.

Colonna, P. C., and vom Saal, F.: Study of Paralytic Scoliosis Based on Five Hundred Cases of Poliomyelitis — J. Bone & Joint Surg. **23:** 335 (April) 1941.

Crego, C. H., and McCarroll, H. R.: Recurrent Deformities in Stabilized Paralytic Feet — J. Bone & Joint Surg. **20:** 609 (July) 1938.

Davis, G. G.: The Treatment of Hollow Foot (Pes Cavus) — Am. J. Orthop. Surg. **11:** 231 (Oct.) 1913.

Dickson, F. D.: An Operation for Stabilizing Paralytic Hips; A Preliminary Report — J. Bone & Joint Surg. **9:** 1 (Jan.) 1927.

Drew, A. J.: Late Results of Arthrodesis of Foot — J. Bone & Joint Surg. **33B:** 496-503 (Nov.) 1951.

Dunn, N.: Stabilizing Operations in the Treatment of Paralytic Deformities of the Foot — Proc. Roy. Soc. Med. (Sect. Orthop.) **15:** 15 (Feb.) 1922.

Fitzgerald, F. P., and Seddon, H. J.: Lambrinudi's Operation for Drop-Foot — Brit. J. Surg. **25:** 283 (Oct.) 1937.

Ghormley, R. K., and others: Evaluation of the Kenny Treatment of Infantile Paralysis — J. A. M. A. **125:** 466 (June 17) 1944.

Gill, A. B.: Operation for Correction of Paralytic Genu Recurvatum — J. Bone & Joint Surg. **13:** 49 (Jan.) 1931.

New Operation for Arthrodesis of the Shoulder — J. Bone & Joint Surg. **13:** 287 (April) 1931.

An Operation to Make a Posterior Bone Block at the Ankle to Limit Foot-Drop — J. Bone & Joint Surg. **15:** 166 (Jan.) 1933.

The Kenny Concepts and Treatment of Infantile Paralysis — J. Bone & Joint Surg. **26:** 87-98 (Jan.) 1944.

Goldner, J. L., and Irwin, C. E.: Analysis of Paralytic Thumb Deformities — J. Bone & Joint Surg. **32A:** 627-639 (July) 1950.

Green, W. T., and Anderson, M.: Experiences With Epiphyseal Arrest in Correcting Discrepancies in Length of the Lower Extremities in Infantile Paralysis, A Method of Predicting the Effect — J. Bone & Joint Surg. **29**: 659-675 (July) 1947.

Hart, V. L.: Arthrodesis of the Foot in Infantile Paralysis — Surg., Gynec. & Obst. **64**: 794 (April) 1937.

Hellgrimsson, S.: Studies on Reconstructive and Stabilizing Operations on the Skeleton of the Foot With Special Reference to Subastragalar Arthrodesis in the Treatment of Foot Deformities Following Infantile Paralysis — Acta. Chir. Scandinav. 88, Suppl. 78, 1943.

Hoke, M.: An Operation for Stabilizing Paralytic Feet — J. Orthop. Surg. **3**: 494 (Oct.) 1921.

Hughes, R. E.: Knee-Flexion Deformity Following Poliomyelitis; Its Correction by Operative Procedures — J. Bone & Joint Surg. **17**: 627 (July) 1935.

Ingram, A. J., and Hundley, J. M.: Posterior Bone Block of Ankle for Paralytic Equinus: End - Result Study — J. Bone & Joint Surg. **33A**: 679-692 (July) 1951.

Irwin, C. E.: Transplants to Thumb to Restore Function of Opposition: End Results — South. M. J. **35**: 257 (March) 1942.

Genu Recurvatum Following Poliomyelitis; Controlled Method of Operative Correction — J. A. M. A. **120**: 277 (Sept. 26) 1942.

Iliotibial Band, Its Role in Producing Deformity in Poliomyelitis — J. Bone & Joint Surg. **31A**: 141-146 (Jan.) 1949.

The Calcaneus Foot — South, M. J. **44**: 191-197 (March) 1951.

Irwin, C. E., and Eyler, D. L.: Surgical Rehabilitation of Hand and Forearm Disabled by Poliomyelitis — J. Bone & Joint Surg. **33A**: 825-836 (Oct.) 1951.

Johnson, R. W., Jr.: Results of Modern Methods of Treatment of Poliomyelitis — J. Bone & Joint Surg. **27**: 223 (April) 1945.

Kendall, H. O., and Kendall, F. P.: Care During the Recovery Period in Paralytic Poliomyelitis — Public Health Bulletin 242, U. S. Treasury Department, Public Health Service (Revised) 1939.

Kendall, H. O., and Kendall, F. P.: | Muscles, Testing and Function | Baltimore, Williams & Wilkins Co., 1949.

Kleinberg, S.: | Paralytic Scoliosis: An Analysis of Fifty-One Cases | Am. J. Surg. 64: 301-312 (June) 1944.

Legg, A. T.: | Tensor Fasciae Femoris Transplantation in Cases of Weakened Gluteus Medius | New England J. Med. 209: 61 (July 13) 1933.

Prognosis in Poliomyelitis | J. Bone & Joint Surg. 25: 132 (Jan.) 1943.

Lenhard, R. E.: | Results of Poliomyelitis in Baltimore | J. Bone & Joint Surg. 32A: 71 - 79 (Jan.) 1950.

Levinthal, D. H.: | Tendon Transplantation in the Lower Extremity | S. Clin. North America 19: 79 (Feb.) 1939.

Lewin, P.: | Surgery in Infantile Paralysis | S. Clin. North America 19: 115 (Feb.) 1939.

Infantile Paralysis — Anterior Poliomyelitis | Philadelphia, W. B. Saunders Co., 1941.

Lovett, R. W.: | The Treatment of Infantile Paralysis, 2nd Edition | Philadelphia, P. Blakiston's Son & Co., 1917.

Lowman, C. L.: | Plastic Repair for Paralysis of Abdominal Musculature | New England J. Med. 205: 1187 (Dec. 17) 1931.

The Relation of the Abdominal Muscles to Paralytic Scoliosis | J. Bone & Joint Surg. 14: 763 (Oct.) 1932.

Mayer, L.: | Transplantation of the Trapezius for Paralysis of the Abductors of the Arm | J. Bone & Joint Surg. 9: 412 (July) 1927.

Further Studies of Fixed Paralytic Pelvic Obliquity | J. Bone & Joint Surg. 18: 87 (Jan.) 1936.

The Physiological Method of Tendon Transplantation in the Treatment of Paralytic Drop-Foot | J. Bone & Joint Surg. 19: 389 (April) 1937.

Operative Reconstruction of the Paralyzed Upper Extremity | J. Bone & Joint Surg. 21: 377 (April) 1939.

Surgery of Tendons, in Cyclopedia of Medicine, Surgery, Specialties, Vol. 13, 723-759 | Philadelphia, F. A. Davis Co., 1951.

Moldaver, J.: | Analysis of Neuromuscular Disorders in Poliomyelitis | J. Bone & Joint Surg. 26: 103 (Jan.) 1944.

Moore, B. H.: Critical Appraisal of Leg Lengthening Operation — Am. J. Surg. **52:** 415 (June) 1941.

Ober, F. R.: An Operation for the Relief of Paralysis of the Gluteus Maximus Muscle — J. A. M. A. **88:** 1063 (April 2) 1927.

Tendon Transplantation in the Lower Extremity — New England J. Med. **209:** 52 (July 13) 1933.

Patterson, R. L., Parrish, F. F., and Hathaway, E. N.: Stabilizing Operations of Foot, Study of Indications, Techniques Used, and End-Results — J. Bone & Joint Surg. **32A:** 1-26 (Jan.) 1950.

Petch, C. P.: Guillain-Barré Syndrome or Acute Infective Polyneuritis — Lancet **2:** 405-408 (Sept.) 1949.

Phemister, D. B.: Operative Arrestment of Longitudinal Growth of Bones in the Treatment of Deformities — J. Bone & Joint Surg. **15:** 1 (Jan.) 1933.

Russell, W. R.: Paralytic Poliomyelitis — Brit. M. J. **1:** 465-471 (March) 1949.

Ryerson, E. W.: Arthrodesing Operations on the Feet — J. Bone & Joint Surg. **5:** 453 (July) 1923.

Schwartz, R. P., Bouman, H. D., and Smith, W. K.: The Significance of Muscle Spasm — J. A. M. A. **126:** 695 (Nov. 11) 1944.

Schwartzmann, J. R., and Crego, C. H., Jr.: Hamstring Tendon Transplantation for Relief of Quadriceps Femoris Paralysis in Residual Poliomyelitis, Follow-up Study of 134 Cases. — J. Bone & Joint Surg. **30A:** 541-549 (July) 1948.

Smith, A. D.: Arthrodesis, in Monographs on Surgery for 1951, 471-496 — New York, Thos. Nelson & Sons, 1951.

Steindler, A.: Tendon Transplantation in the Upper Extremity — Am. J. Surg. **44:** 260 (April) 1939.

The Newer Pathological and Physiological Concepts of Anterior Poliomyelitis and Their Clinical Interpretation — J. Bone & Joint Surg. **29:** 59 (Jan.) 1947.

Stinchfield, A. J., Reidy, J. A., and Barr, J. S.: Prediction of Unequal Growth of Lower Extremities in Anterior Poliomyelitis — J. Bone & Joint Surg. **31A:** 478-484 (July) 1949.

Straub, L. R., Thompson, T. C., and Wilson, P. D.: The Results of Epiphyseodesis and Femoral Shortening in Relation to Equalization of Limb Length — J. Bone & Joint Surg. **27:** 254 (April) 1945.

Thompson, C. F.:	Fusion of Metacarpals of Thumb and Index Finger to Maintain Functional Position of Thumb	J. Bone & Joint Surg. 24: 907 (Oct.) 1942.
Thompson, T. C.:	Astragalectomy and the Treatment of Calcaneovalgus	J. Bone & Joint Surg. 21: 627 (July) 1939.
	Modified Operation for Opponens Paralysis	J. Bone & Joint Surg. 24: 632 (July) 1942.
Wagner, L. C.:	Ankle Bone Block for Paralytic Drop Foot	Ann. Surg. 101: 1091 (April) 1935.
Ward, R.:	The Epidemiology of Poliomyelitis	J. Bone & Joint Surg. 26: 829 (Oct.) 1944.
White, J. W.:	Femoral Shortening for Equalization of Leg Length	J. Bone & Joint Surg. 17: 597 (July) 1935.
Yount, C. C.:	The Rôle of the Tensor Fasciae Femoris in Certain Deformities of the Lower Extremities	J. Bone & Joint Surg. 8: 171 (Jan.) 1926.

Chapter XIII

Neuromuscular Disabilities (Exclusive of Infantile Paralysis) · Involvement of the Brain and Spinal Cord

Cerebral Palsy

Benda, C. E.:	Developmental Disorders of Mentation and Cerebral Palsies	New York, Grune & Stratton, Inc., 1952.
Chandler, F. A.:	Surgical Procedures Commonly Used in Correcting Deformities of Spastic Paralysis	Clinics 2: 992-1001 (Dec.) 1943.
Crothers, B., and Putnam, M. C.:	Obstetrical Injuries of the Spinal Cord	Medicine 6: 41 (Feb.) 1927.
Foerster, O.:	Resection of the Posterior Spinal Nerve Roots in the Treatment of Gastric Crises and Spastic Paralysis	Proc. Roy. Soc. Med. (Surg. Sect.) 4: 226 (June) 1911.
Gill, A. B.:	Stoffel's Operation for Spastic Paralysis	J. Orthop. Surg. 3: 52 (Feb.) 1921.
Green, W. T., and McDermott, R. J.:	Operative Treatment of Cerebral Palsy of Spastic Type	J. A. M. A. 118: 434 (Feb. 7) 1942.
Heyman, C. H.:	The Surgical Treatment of Spastic Paralysis	Surg., Gynec. & Obst. 68: 792 (April) 1939.
Irish, C. W.:	Cerebral Vascular Lesions in Newborn Infants and Young Children	J. Pediat. 15: 64 (July) 1939.

Phelps, W. M.:	Symposium on Orthopaedic Surgery: Treatment of Cerebral Palsies	Clinics **2**: 981-991 (Dec.) 1943.
	Recent Significant Trends in the Care of Cerebral Palsy	South, M. J. **39**: 132 (Feb.) 1946.
Pohl, J. F.:	Cerebral Palsy	St. Paul, Bruce Publishing Co., 1950.
Putnam, T. J.:	Results of Treatment of Athetosis by Section of the Extra - Pyramidal Tracts in the Spinal Cord	Arch. Neurol. & Psychiat. **39**: 258 (Feb.) 1938.
Royle, N. D.:	The Treatment of Spastic Paralysis by Sympathetic Ramisection	Surg., Gynec. & Obst. **39**: 701 (Dec.) 1924.
Stoffel, A.:	The Treatment of Spastic Contractures	Am. J. Orthop. Surg. **10**: 611 (May) 1913.

Progressive Muscular Atrophy

Aring, C. D., and Cobb, S.:	The Muscular Atrophies and Allied Disorders	Medicine **14**: 77 (Feb.) 1935.
Jacobs, J. E., and Carr, C. R.:	Progressive Muscular Atrophy of Peroneal Type (Charcot-Marie -Tooth Disease) Orthopaedic Management and End-Result Study	J. Bone & Joint Surg. **32A**: 27 - 38 (Jan.) 1950.

Neuropathic Disease of the Bones and Joints

Cleveland, M.:	Surgical Fusion of Unstable Joints Due to Neuropathic Disturbance	Am. J. Surg. **43**: 580 (Feb.) 1939.
Delano, P. J.:	The Pathogenesis of Charcot's Joint	Am. J. Roentgenol. **56**: 189 (Aug.) 1946.
Pomeranz, M. M., and Rothberg, A. S.:	Review of Fifty - Eight Cases of Tabetic Arthropathy	Am. J. Syph., Gonor., & Ven. Dis. **25**: 103 (Jan.) 1941.
Potts, W. J.:	The Pathology of Charcot Joints	Ann. Surg. **86**: 596 (Oct.) 1927.
Shands, A. R., Jr.:	Neuropathies of the Bones and Joints; Report of a Case of an Arthropathy of the Ankle Due to a Peripheral Nerve Lesion	Arch. Surg. **20**: 614 (April) 1930.
Shands, A. R., Jr., and Hakala, E. W.:	Neuropathic Affections of Bones and Joints, in Cyclopedia o f Medicine, Surgery, Specialties, Vol. 7, 733-738	Philadelphia, F. A. Davis Co., 1950.

Soto-Hall, R., and Haldeman, K. O.: — Diagnosis of Neuropathic Joint Disease (Charcot Joint): Analysis of Forty Cases — J. A. M. A. **114:** 2076 (May 25) 1940.

Steindler, A.: — The Tabetic Arthropathies — J. A. M. A. **96:** 250 (Jan. 24) 1931.

Joint Disabilities of Cerebral Origin

Luck, J. V.: — Psychosomatic Problems in Military Orthopaedic Surgery — J. Bone & Joint Surg. **28:** 213 (April) 1946.

Myerson, A.: — Hysterical Paralysis and Its Treatment — J. A. M. A. **105:** 1565 (Nov. 16) 1935.

Spina Bifida

Smith, R. S.: — Orthopaedic Considerations in the Treatment of Spina Bifida — Surg., Gynec. & Obst. **62:** 218-227 (Feb.) 1936.

Chapter XIV

Neuromuscular Disabilities (Exclusive of Infantile Paralysis): Involvement of Peripheral Nerves and of Muscles

Peripheral Nerve Injuries

Barnes, R.: — Traction Injuries to Brachial Plexus in Adults — J. Bone & Joint Surg. **31B:** 10 - 16 (Feb.) 1949.

Cobb, S., and Coggeshall, H. C.: — Neuritis — J. A. M. A. **103:** 1608 (Nov. 24) 1934.

Cullen, C. H.: — Causalgia, Diagnosis and Treatment — J. Bone & Joint Surg. **30B:** 467-477 (Aug.) 1948.

Davidson, A. J., and Horwitz, M. T.: — Late or Tardy Ulnar Nerve Paralysis — J. Bone & Joint Surg. **17:** 844 (Oct.) 1935.

Delageniere, H.: — A Contribution to the Study of the Surgical Repair of Peripheral Nerves — Surg. Gynec. & Obst. **39:** 543 (Nov.) 1924.

Forrester, C. R. G.: — Peripheral Nerve Injuries With Results of Early and Delayed Suture — Am. J. Surg. **47:** 555 (March) 1940.

Gay, J. R., and Love, J. G.: — Diagnosis and Treatment of Tardy Paralysis of the Ulnar Nerve — J. Bone & Joint Surg. **29:** 1087-1097 (Oct.) 1947.

Gurdjian, E. S., and Goetz, A. G.: — Radial Paralysis Complicating Fracture and Dislocation in the Upper Limb — Ann. Surg. **99:** 487 (Mar.) 1934.

Haymaker, W.: — Pathology of Peripheral Nerve Injuries — Mil. Surgeon **102:** 448-459 (June) 1948.

Haymaker, W., and Woodhall, B.:	Peripheral Nerve Injuries, Principles of Diagnosis	Philadelphia, W. B. Saunders Co., 1945.
Kolodny, A.:	Traction Paralysis of Brachial Plexus	Am. J. Surg. **51**: 620 (March) 1941.
Lewis, D., and Miller, E. M.:	Peripheral Nerve Injuries Associated With Fractures	Ann. Surg., **76**: 528 (Oct.) 1922.
Lyons, W. R., and Woodhall, B.:	Atlas of Peripheral Nerve Injuries	Philadelphia, W. B. Saunders Co., 1949.
McGowan, A. J.:	Results of Transposition of Ulnar Nerve for Traumatic Ulnar Neuritis	J. Bone & Joint Surg. **32B**: 293-301 (Aug.) 1950.
Mouat, T. B.:	Peripheral Nerve Injuries, Recent Progress in Treatment	Brit. M. J. **2**: 983 (Dec. 28) 1946.
Overpeck, D. O., and Ghormley, R. K.:	Paralysis of Serratus Magnus Muscle, Caused by Lesions of Long Thoracic Nerve	J. A. M. A. **114**: 1994 (May 18) 1940.
Pollock, L. J., and Davis, L.:	Peripheral Nerve Injuries	New York, Paul B. Hoeber, Inc., 1933.
Schnitker, M. T.:	Principles of Treatment in Peripheral Nerve Injuries	Northwest Med. **43**: 5 (Jan.) 1944.
Scuderi, C.:	Tendon Transplants for Irreparable Radial Nerve Paralysis	Surg., Gynec. & Abst. **88**: 643 - 651 (May) 1949.
Shallow, T. A.:	Traumatic Lesions of the Brachial Plexus	Ann. Surg. **92**: 182 (Aug.) 1930.
Shumacker, H. B., Jr., Speigel, I. J., and Upjohn, R. H.:	Causalgia, I, Role of Sympathetic Interruption in Treatment.	Surg., Gynec. & Obst. **86**: 76-86 (Jan.) 1948.
	Causalgia, II, Signs and Symptoms, With Particular Reference to Vasomotor Disturbances	Surg., Gynec & Obst. **86**: 452-640 (April) 1948.
Stookey, B.:	Meralgia Paraesthetica; Etiology and Surgical Treatment	J. A. M. A. **90**: 1705 (May 26) 1928.
Sunderland, S.:	Course and Rate of Regeneration of Motor Fibers Following Lesions of the Radial Nerve	Arch. Neurol. & Psychiat. **56**: 133 (Aug.) 1946.
Wilson, G., and Hadden, S. B.:	Neuritis and Multiple Neuritis Following Serum Therapy	J. A. M. A. **98**: 123 (Jan. 9) 1932.

Young, F.:   Peripheral Nerve Paral-   J. A. M. A. **98**: 1139
                            yses Following the Use   (April 2) 1932.
                            of Various Serums; Re-
                            port of a Case and
                            Review of the Liter-
                            ature

                            Obstetric Paralysis

Kleinberg, S.:   Reattachment of the   J. A. M. A. **98**: 294
                            Capsule and External   (Jan. 23) 1932.
                            Rotators of the Shoul-
                            der for Obstetric Pa-
                            ralysis

L'Episcopo, J. B.:   Tendon Transplantation   Am. J. Surg. **25**: 122
                            in Obstetrical Paralysis   (July) 1934.

Sever, J. W.:   Obstetric Paralysis; Its   Am. J. Dis. Child. **12**:
                            Etiology, Pathology,   541 (Dec.) 1916.
                            Clinical Aspects and
                            Treatment, With a Re-
                            port of 470 Cases

                            Obstetrical Paralysis   Surg., Gynec. & Obst.
                                                         44: 547 (April) 1927.

                            Progressive Muscular Dystrophy

Geschickter, C. F., and   Affections of Muscles   J. Bone & Joint Surg.
Maseritz, I. H.:   **21**: 576 (July) 1939.

Scheman, L., Lewin, P.,   Pseudohypertrophic Mus-   J. A. M. A. **111**: 2265
and Soskin, S.:   cular Dystrophy: An   (Dec. 17) 1938.
                            Evaluation of Recent
                            Studies

Voshell, A. F.:   Progressive Pseudohyper-   South. M. J. **26**: 156
                            trophic Muscular Dys-   (Feb.) 1933.
                            trophy

                            Amyotonia Congenita

Burdick, W. F., Whipple,   Amyotonia Congenita   Am. J. Dis. Child. **69**:
D. V., and   (Oppenheimer): Re-   295 (May) 1945.
Freeman, W.:   port of 5 Cases With
                            Necropsy

Chapter XV

Tumors

Tumors of Bone

Alldredge, R. H.:   Localized Fibrocystic Dis-   J. Bone & Joint Surg.
                            ease of Bone: Results   **24**: 795 (Oct.) 1942.
                            of Treatment in One
                            Hundred and Fifty-
                            Two Cases

Badgley, C. E., and Batts, M., Jr.: | Osteogenic Sarcoma: Analysis of Eighty Cases | Arch. Surg. **43**: 541 (Oct.) 1941.

Bayrd, E. D., and Heck, F. J.: | Multiple Myeloma, A Review of Eighty-three Proved Cases | J. A. M. A. **133**: 147-157 (Jan.) 1947.

Chandler, F. A., and Kaell, H. I.: | Osteoid-osteoma | Arch. Surg. **60**: 294-304 (Feb.) 1950.

Codman, E. A.: | Bone Sarcoma | New York, Paul B. Hoeber, Inc., 1925.

Coley, B. L.: | The Diagnosis of Neoplasms of Bone | S. Clin. North America **26**: 410-421 (April) 1946.

Neoplasms of Bone and Related Conditions, Their Etiology, Pathogenesis, Diagnosis and Treatment | New York, Paul B. Hoeber, Inc., 1949.

Coley, B. L., Bowdin, L., and Higinbotham, N. L.: | Endothelioma of Bone (Ewing's Sarcoma) | Ann. Surg. **128**: 533-560 (Sept.) 1948.

Coley, B. L., and Higinbotham, N. L.: | Giant-Cell Tumor of Bone | J. Bone & Joint Surg. **20**: 870 (Oct.) 1938.

Conservative Surgery in Tumors of Bone With Special Reference to Segmental Resection | Ann. Surg. **127**: 231-242 (Feb.) 1948.

Coley, B. L., and Lenson, N.: | Osteoid-Osteoma | Am. J. Surg. **77**: 3-9 (Jan.) 1949.

Coley, B. L., and Peterson, R. L.: | Primary Bone Tumors in Children | Am. J. Surg. **39**: 335 (Feb.) 1938.

Coley, B. L., and Stewart, F. W.: | Bone Sarcoma in Polyostotic Fibrous Dysplasia | Ann. Surg. **121**: 872-881 (June) 1945.

Copeland, M. M.: | Bone Tumors With Reference to Their Treatment | Surgery **11**: 436 (March) 1942.

Benign Tumors of Bone | Surg., Gynec. & Obst. **90**: 697-712 (June) 1950.

Copeland, M. M., and Geschickter, C. F.: | Bone Tumors and Their Treatment, in Monographs on Surgery for 1951, 392-442 | New York, Thos. Nelson & Sons, 1951.

Dunne, R. E.: | Primary Adamantinoma of the Tibia | New England J. Med. **218**: 634 (April 14) 1938.

Ellis, F., Russell, D. S., Willis, R. A., Prossor, T. M., Windeyer, B. W., and Woodyatt, P. B.: | Giant-Cell Tumor Symposium (five articles) | J. Bone & Joint Surg. **31B**: 236-290 (May) 1949.

Ewing, J.: | A Review of the Classification of Bone Tumors | Surg., Gynec. & Obst. **68**: 971 (May) 1939.

Ewing, J.:	Neoplastic Diseases, 4th Edition	Philadelphia, W. B. Saunders Co., 1940.
Ferguson, A. B.:	Treatment of Osteogenic Sarcoma	J. Bone & Joint Surg. 22: 916 (Oct.) 1940.
Freund, E., and Meffert, C. B.:	On the Different Forms of Non - Generalized Fibrous Osteodystrophy	Surg., Gynec. & Obst. 62: 541 (Mar.) 1936.
Galloway, J. D. B., Broders, A. C., and Ghormley, R. K.:	Xanthoma of Tendon Sheaths and Synovial Membranes: Clinical and Pathologic Study	Arch. Surg. 40: 485 (March) 1940.
Geschickter, C. F., and Copeland, M. M.:	Multiple Myeloma	Arch. Surg. 16: 807 (April) 1928.
	Tumors of Bone	New York, Am. J. Cancer, 3rd Edition, 1949.
	Parosteal Osteoma of Bone: A New Entity	Ann. Surg. 133: 790-807 (June) 1951.
Geschickter, C. F., and Maseritz, I. H.:	Ewing's Sarcoma	J. Bone & Joint Surg. 21: 26 (Jan.) 1939.
	Skeletal Metastasis in Cancer	J. Bone & Joint Surg. 21: 314 (April) 1939.
Ghormley, R. K., and Adson, A. W.:	Hemangioma of Vertebrae	J. Bone & Joint Surg. 23: 887 (Oct.) 1941.
Hamilton, J. F.:	Ewing's Sarcoma (Endothelial Myeloma)	Arch. Surg. 41: 29 (July) 1940.
Hill, R. M.:	Non - specific Granuloma of Bone (Eosinophilic)	Brit. J. Surg. 37: 69-76 (July) 1949.
Jaffe, H. L., and Lichtenstein, L.:	Osteoid Osteoma	J. Bone & Joint Surg. 22: 645 (July) 1940.
	Solitary Unicameral Bone Cyst With Emphasis on the Roentgen Picture, the Pathologic Appearance and the Pathogenesis	Arch. Surg. 44: 1004 (June) 1942.
	Solitary Benign Enchondroma of Bone	Arch. Surg. 46: 480 (April) 1943.
Kolodny, A.:	Bone Sarcoma: The Primary Malignant Tumors of Bone and the Giant-Cell Tumor	Chicago, Surgical Publishing Co., 1927.
Levinthal, D. H., and Kraft, G. L.:	Eradication of Benign Lytic Bone Tumors and Immediate Reconstructive Surgery With Emphasis on Benign Giant Cell Tumors.	Surg. Gynec. & Obst. 89: 735-747 (Dec.) 1949.
Lichtenstein, L.:	Bone Tumors	St. Louis, The C. V. Mosby Co., 1952.
Lichtenstein, L., and Jaffe, H. L.:	Chondrosarcoma of Bone	Am. J. Path. 19: 553 (July) 1943.

Lichtenstein, L., and Jaffe, H. L.: | Ewing's Sarcoma of Bone | Am. J. Path. **23**: 43-78 (Jan.) 1947.

Luck, J. V.: | A Correlation of Roentgenogram and Pathological Changes in Ossifying and Chondrifying Primary Osteogenic Neoplasms | Radiology **40**: 253 (March) 1943.

Lumb, G., and Prossor, T. M.: | Plasma Cell Tumours | J. Bone & Joint Surg. **30B**: 124-152 (Feb.) 1948.

Mabrey, R. E.: | Chordoma: A Study of 150 Cases | Am. J. Cancer **25**: 501 (Nov.) 1935.

Morton, J. J., and Mider, G. B.: | Chondrosarcoma | Ann. Surg. **126**: 895-931 (Dec.) 1947.

Prevo, S. R.: | Clinical Analysis of 205 Cases of Malignant Bone Tumor | J. Bone & Joint Surg. **32A**: 298-306 (April) 1950.

Rosh, R., and Raider, L.: | The Results of Treatment of Osteogenic Sarcoma | J. Bone & Joint Surg. **20**: 933 (Oct.) 1938.

| Primary Malignant Bone Tumors | Am. J. Roentgenol. **56**: 75 (July) 1946.

Sherman, M. S.: | Osteoid-Osteoma, Review of the Literature and Report of Thirty Cases | J. Bone & Joint Surg. **29**: 918-939 (Oct.) 1947.

Stewart, M. J., and Richardson, T. R.: | Giant-Cell Tumor of Bone | J. Bone & Joint Surg. **34A**: 372-386 (April) 1952.

Thomas, G. L.: | Metastasis to Bone in Gastrointestinal Malignancy | S. Clin. North America **26**: 692-694 (June) 1946.

Turner, J. W., and Jaffe, H. L.: | Metastatic Neoplasms: Clinical and Roentgenologic Study of Involvement of Skeleton and Lungs | Am. J. Roentgenol. **43**: 479 (April) 1940.

Upshaw, J. E., McDonald, J. R., and Ghormley, R. K.: | Extension of Primary Neoplasms of Bone to Bone Marrow | Surg., Gynec. & Obst. **89**: 704 - 714 (Dec.) 1949.

Woodard, H. Q.: | Role of the Chemical Laboratory in Diagnosis of Neoplastic Diseases of Bone | Arch. Surg. **47**: 368 (Oct.) 1943.

Tumors of Soft Tissues

Bennett, G. A.: | Malignant Neoplasms Originating in Synovial Tissues (Synoviomas) | J. Bone & Joint Surg. **29**: 259-291 (April) 1947.

Berger, L.: | Synovial Sarcomas in Serous Bursae and Tendon Sheaths | Am. J. Cancer **34**: 501 (Dec.) 1938.

Bick, E. M.: Fibrosarcoma of the Extremities — Ann. Surg. **101**: 759 (Feb.) 1935.

Brooks, B., and Lehman, E. P.: The Bone Changes in Recklinghausen's Neurofibromatosis — Surg., Gynec. & Obst. **38**: 587 (May) 1924.

Cobey, M. C.: Hemangioma of Joints — Arch. Surg. **46**: 465 (April) 1943.

De Santo, D. A., and Wilson, P. D.: Xanthomatous Tumors of Joints — J. Bone & Joint Surg. **21**: 531 (July) 1939.

Foster, L. N.: Benign Giant Cell Tumor of Tendon Sheaths — Am. J. Path. **23**: 567-583 (July) 1947.

Tumors of the Peripheral Nerves — Am. J. Cancer **25**: 377 (Oct.) 1935.

Geschickter, C. F., and Lewis, D.: Tumors of Tendon Sheaths, Joints and Bursae — Am. J. Cancer **22**: 96 (Sept.) 1934.

Gross, P., and Cameron, D. W.: Synovialoma — Arch. Path. **33**: 687 (May) 1942.

Haagensen, C. D., and Stout, A. P.: Synovial Sarcoma — Ann. Surg. **120**: 826 (Dec.) 1944.

King, E. S. J.: Concerning the Pathology of Tumors of Tendon-Sheaths — Brit. J. Surg. **18**: 594 (April) 1931.

Tissue Differentiation in Malignant Synovial Tumors — J. Bone & Joint Surg. **34B**: 97-115 (Feb.) 1952.

Knox, L. C.: Synovial Sarcoma — Am. J. Cancer **28**: 461 (Nov.) 1936.

Lewis, D., and Hart, D.: Tumors of Peripheral Nerves — Ann. Surg. **92**: 961 (Dec.) 1930.

Mason, M. L., and Woolston, W. H.: Isolated Giant Cell Xanthomatic Tumors of the Fingers and Hand — Arch. Surg. **15**: 499 (Oct.) 1927.

McCarroll, H. R.: Clinical Manifestations of Congenital Neurofibromatosis — J. Bone & Joint Surg. **32A**: 601-617 (July) 1950.

Minear, W. L.: Xanthomatous Joint Tumors — J. Bone & Joint Surg. **33A**: 451-459 (April) 1951.

Morton, J. J.: Tumors of the Tendon Sheaths; Their Close Biological Relationship to Tumors of the Joints and Bursae — Surg., Gynec. & Obst. **59**: 441 (Sept.) 1934.

Shallow, T. A., Eger, S. A., and Wagner, F. B., Jr.: Primary Hemangiomatous Tumors of Skeletal Muscle — Ann. Surg. **119**: 700 (May) 1944.

Sharpe, J. C., and Young, R. H.: Recklinghausen's Neurofibromatosis: Clinical Manifestations in 31 Cases — Arch. Int. Med. **59**: 298 (Feb.) 1937.

Stewart, F. W., and Copeland, M. M.:   Neurogenic Sarcoma   Am. J. Cancer **15**: 1235 (July) 1931.

Tillotson, J. F.. McDonald, J. R., and Janes, J. M.:   Synovial Sarcomata   J. Bone & Joint Surg. **33A**: 459-473 (April) 1951.

Wagner, L. C.:   Intraarticular Endothelial Tumors Arising From Synovial Membrane   Ann. Surg. **92**: 421 (Sept.) 1930.

Chapter XVI

Fracture Deformities

General Problems of Bone Formation and Repair

Blum, G.:   Phosphatase and the Repair of Fractures   Lancet **2**: 75-78 (July 15) 1944.

Eggers, G. W. N.:   Internal Contact Splint   J. Bone & Joint Surg. **30A**: 40 - 52 (Jan.) 1948.

Eggers, G. W. N., Shindler, T. O., and Pomerat, C. M.:   Influence of Contact Compression Factor on Osteogenesis in Surgical Fractures   J. Bone & Joint Surg. **31A**: 693-716 (Oct.) 1949.

Fitts, W. T.:   The Healing of Fractures   S. Clin. North America **26**: 1470 (Dec.) 1946.

Franseen, C. C., Simmons, C. C., and McLean, R.:   The Phosphatase Determination in the Differential Diagnosis of Bone Lesions   Surg., Gynec. & Obst. **68**: 1038 (June) 1939.

Gallie, W. E., and Robertson, D. E.:   The Repair of Bone   Brit. J. Surg. **7**: 211 (Oct.) 1919.

Haldeman, K. O.:   Factors Determining Deposition and Demineralization of Bone   J. Bone & Joint Surg. **32A**: 596-600 (July) 1950.

Howard, J. E.:   Some Current Concepts on Mechanism of Calcification   J. Bone & Joint Surg. **33A**: 801-807 (July) 1951.

Johnson, R. W., Jr.:   A Physiological Study of the Blood Supply of the Diaphysis   J. Bone & Joint Surg. **9**: 153 (Jan.) 1927.

   A Study of the Healing Processes in Injuries to the Carpal Scaphoid   J. Bone & Joint Surg. **9**: 482 (July) 1927.

Jones, R. W., and Roberts, R. E.:   Calcification, Decalcification, and Ossification   Brit. J. Surg. **21**: 461 (Jan.) 1934.

Kay, H. D.:   Phosphatase in Growth and Disease of Bone   Physiol. Rev. **12**: 384 (July) 1932.

Leriche, R., and Policard, A.:   The Normal and Pathological Physiology of Bone   St. Louis, The C. V. Mosby Co., 1928.

Lord, I. J.:	Alkaline Phosphatase and Mechanism of Ossification	J. Bone & Joint Surg. **31B:** 94 - 99 (Feb.) 1949.
Martland, M., and Robison, R.:	The Possible Significance of Hexose-Phosphoric Esters in Ossification; The Bone Phosphatase	Biochem. J. **21:** 665, (Mar.) 1927.
May, H.:	The Regeneration of Bone Transplants	Ann. Surg. **106:** 441 (Sept.) 1937.
Pearse, H. E., Jr., and Morton, J. J.:	The Influence of Alterations in the Circulation on the Repair of Bone	J. Bone & Joint Surg. **13:** 68 (Jan.) 1931.
Petersen, H. A.:	A Clinical Study of Ununited Fractures With Special Reference to the Inorganic Bone-Forming Elements in the Blood Serum	J. Bone & Joint Surg. **6:** 885 (Oct.) 1924.
Phemister, D. B.:	Repair of Bone in Presence of Aseptic Necrosis Resulting From Fractures, Transplantations, and Vascular Obstruction	J. Bone & Joint Surg. **12:** 769 (Oct.) 1930.
Robinson, W. H.:	The Rôle of the Circulation in the Healing of Fractures	Arch. Surg. **17:** 420 (Sept.) 1928.
Todd, T. W., and Iler, D. H.:	Phenomena of the Early Stages in Bone Repair	Ann. Surg. **86:** 715 (Nov.) 1927.

Delayed Union, Malunion, and Nonunion

Abbott, L. C., Schottstaedt, E. R., Saunders, J. B. deC. M., and Bost, F. C.:	Evaluation of Cortical and Cancellous Bone as Grafting Material	J. Bone & Joint Surg. **29:** 381-414 (April) 1947.
Bennett, G. E.:	Fractures of the Humerus With Particular Reference to Non-Union and Its Treatment	Ann. Surg., **103:** 994 (June) 1936.
Bickel, W. H.:	Bone Repair, Delayed Union, Nonunion, and Malunion, Cyclopedia of Medicine, Surgery, Specialties, Vol. 5, 843	Philadelphia, F. A. Davis Co., 1950.
Bishop, W. A., Stauffer, R. C., and Swenson, A. L.:	Bone Grafts, An End-Result Study of the Healing Time	J. Bone & Joint Surg. **29:** 961-972 (Oct.) 1947.
Blair, H. C.:	Diamond - Shaped Graft From Ilium for Non-Union of Tibia.	J. Bone & Joint Surg. **33A:** 362-371 (April) 1951.
Boyd, H. B.:	Congenital Pseudarthrosis: Treatment by Dual Bone Grafts	J. Bone & Joint Surg. **23:** 497 (July) 1941.

Boyd, H. B., and Fox, K. W.:   Congenital Pseudarthrosis   J. Bone & Joint Surg. **30A**: 274-283 (April) 1948.

Brackett, E. G.:   Fractured Neck of the Femur: Operation of Transplantation of Femoral Head to Trochanter   Boston M. & S. J. **192**: 1118 (June 4) 1925.

Bush, L. F., and Garber, C. Z.:   The Bone Bank, in Monographs on Surgery for 1950, 383-410   New York, Thos. Nelson & Sons, 1950.

Campbell, W. C.:   Malunited Fractures and Unreduced Dislocations About the Elbow   J. A. M. A. **92**: 122 (Jan. 12) 1929.

    Malunited Colles Fractures   J. A. M. A. **109**: 1105 (Oct. 2) 1937.

    Onlay Bone Graft for Ununited Fractures   Arch. Surg. **38**: 313 (Feb.) 1939.

Cleveland, M., and Bailey, W. L.:   End Result Study of Intracapsular Fracture of Neck of Femur   Surg., Gynec. & Obst. **90**: 393 - 405 (April) 1950.

Colonna, P. C.:   A New Type of Reconstruction Operation for Old Ununited Fracture of the Neck of the Femur   J. Bone & Joint Surg. **17**: 110 (Jan.) 1935.

Cooper, W.:   Aseptic (Avascular) Necrosis of the Femoral Head in Adults, in Monographs on Surgery for 1952, 214-252   Baltimore, The Williams & Wilkins Co., 1952.

Davis, A. G.:   Fibular Substitution for Tibial Defects   J. Bone & Joint Surg. **26**: 229 (April) 1944.

Dehne, E., and Immermann, E. W.:   Dislocation of Hip Combined With Fracture of Shaft of Femur on Same Side   J. Bone & Joint Surg. **33A**: 731-746 (July) 1951.

Dickson, J. A.:   The High Geometric Osteotomy, With Rotation and Bone Graft for Ununited Fractures of the Neck of the Femur   J. Bone & Joint Surg. **29**: 1005-1018 (Oct.) 1947.

Durman, D. C.:   An Operation for Correction of Deformities of the Wrist Following Fracture   J. Bone & Joint Surg. **17**: 1014 (Oct.) 1935.

Eggers, G. W. N.:   The Internal Fixation of Fractures of the Shafts of Long Bones, in Monographs on Surgery for 1952, 130-178   Baltimore, The Williams & Wilkins Co., 1952.

Farkas, A., Wilson, M. J., and Hayner, J. C.: — An Anatomical Study of the M e c h a n i c s, Pathology and Healing of Fracture of the Femoral Neck — J. Bone & Joint Surg. **30:** 53-69 (Jan.) 1948.

Flanagan, J. J. and Burem, H. S.: — Reconstruction of Defects of the Tibia and Femur With Apposing Massive Grafts From the Affected Bone — J. Bone & Joint Surg. **29:** 5 8 7 - 5 9 7 (July) 1947.

Ghormley, R. K.: — Choice of Bone Graft Methods in Bone and Joint Surgery — Ann. Surg. **115:** 427 (Mar.) 1942.

Gibson, A., and Loadman, B.: — Bridging of Bone Defects — J. Bone & Joint Surg. **30A:** 381-396 (April) 1948.

Green, W. T., and Rudo, N.: — Pseudoarthrosis and Neurofibromatosis — Arch. Surg. **46:** 639 (May) 1943.

Hallock, H.: — The Use of Multiple Small Bone Transplants in the Treatment of Pseudoarthosis of the Tibia of Congenital Origin or **Following** Osteotomy for the Correction of Congenital Deformity — J. Bone & Joint Surg. **20:** 648 (July) 1938.

Arthrodesis of the Ankle Joint for Old Painful Fracture — J. Bone & Joint Surg. **27:** 49 (Jan.) 1945.

Henderson, M. S.: — Bone Grafts in Ununited Fractures — J. Bone & Joint Surg. **20:** 635 (July) 1938.

Henderson, M. S., and Stuck, W. G.: — Fractures of the Ankle: Recent and Old — J. Bone & Joint Surg. **15:** 882 (Oct.) 1933.

Higgs, S. L.: — The Use of Cancellous Chips in Bone-Grafting — J. Bone & Joint Surg. **28:** 15 (Jan.) 1946.

Horwitz, T.: — Behavior of Bone Grafts — Surg., Gynec. & Obst. **91:** 310-316 (Dec.) 1950.

Horwitz, T., and Lambert, R. G.: — M a s s i v e I l i a c Bone Grafts in the Treatment of U n u n i t e d Fractures and L a r g e Defects of Long Bones. The Combined Bone Graft — Metallic Plate Technique — Surg., Gynec. & Obst. **84:** 435-450, 1947.

Kimberley, A. G.: — Malunited Fractures Affecting the Ankle Joint — Surg., Gynec. & Obst. **62:** 79 (Jan.) 1936.

King, D., and Secor, C.: — Bow Elbow (Cubitus Varus) — J. Bone & Joint Surg. **33A:** 572-576 (July) 1951.

King, T.:

The Closed Operation for Intracapsular Fracture of the Neck of the Femur; Final Results in Recent and Old Cases

Brit. J. Surg. **26:** 721 (April) 1939.

Lauge-Hausen, N.:

Fractures of Ankle, I, Analytic Historic Survey as Basis of New Experimental Roentgenologic and Clinical Investigations

Arch. Surg. **56:** 259-317 (March) 1948.

Fractures of Ankle, II, Combined Experimental - Surgical and Experimental - Roentgenologic Investigations

Arch. Surg. **60:** 957-985 (May) 1950.

Leadbetter, G. W.:

A Treatment for Fracture of the Neck of the Femur

J. Bone & Joint Surg. **15:** 931 (Oct.) 1933.

Cervical-Axial Osteotomy of the Femur: A Preliminary Report

J. Bone & Joint Surg. **26:** 713 (Oct.) 1944.

Luckey, C. A., and Adams, C. O.:

The Use of Iliac Bone in Bone-Grafting and Arthrodesis

J. Bone & Joint Surg. **28:** 521 (July) 1946.

McFarland, B.:

Pseudarthrosis of Tibia in Childhood

J. Bone & Joint Surg. **33B:** 36 - 46 (Feb.) 1951.

McKeever, F. M.:

Fractures of Tarsal and Metatarsal Bones

Surg., Gynec. & Obst. **90:** 735-745 (June) 1950.

Moore, J. R.:

Cartilaginous Cup Arthroplasty in Ununited Fractures of Neck of Femur

J. Bone & Joint Surg. **30A:** 313-330 (April) 1948.

Delayed Autogenous Bone Graft in Treatment of Congenital Pseudarthrosis

J. Bone & Joint Surg. **31A:** 23-39 (Jan.) and 586-598 (July) 1949.

Murray, C. R.:

Basic Problems in Bone Grafting for Ununited Compound Fractures

J. Bone & Joint Surg. **26:** 437 (July) 1944.

Murray, G.:

End Results of Bone-Grafting for Non-Union of the Carpal Navicular

J. Bone & Joint Surg. **28:** 749 (Oct.) 1946.

Peterson, L. T.:

Fixation of Bones by Plates and Screws

J. Bone & Joint Surg. **29:** 335-347 (April) 1947.

Pusitz, M. E., and Davis, E. V.:

Bone-Drilling in Delayed Union of Fractures

J. Bone & Joint Surg. **26:** 560 (July) 1944.

Reich, R. S.:	The Present Status of Treatment of Fractures of the Calcaneus	Surg., Gynec. & Obst. **68**: 302 (March) 1939.
Reynolds, F. C., and Oliver, D. R.:	Experimental Evaluation of Homogenous Bone Grafts	J. Bone & Joint Surg. **32A**: 283-297 (April) 1950.
Schottstaedt, E. R., Larsen, L. J., and Bost, F. C.:	Intracapsular Fractures of the Femoral Neck, Their Care and Complications, in Monographs on Surgery for 1952, 179-213	Baltimore, The Williams & Wilkins Co., 1952.
Schumm, H. C.:	The Schanz Osteotomy for Fractures of the Neck of the Femur	J. Bone & Joint Surg. **19**: 955 (Oct.) 1937.
Sever, J. W.:	Nonunion in Fracture of the Shaft of the Humerus; Report of 5 Cases	J. A. M. A. **104**: 382 (Feb. 2) 1935.
Shands, A. R., Jr.:	Malunited Fractures of Lower End of Humerus	Am. J. Surg., **37**: 679 (June) 1937.
Sherman, M. S., and Phemister, D. B.:	The Pathology of Ununited Fractures of the Neck of the Femur	J. Bone & Joint Surg. **29**: 19 (Jan.) 1947.
Smith-Petersen, M. N.:	Treatment of Fractures of the Neck of the Femur by Internal Fixation	Surg., Gynec. & Obst. **64**: 287 (Feb. 15) 1937.
Snedecor, S. T., and Coffey, F. L.:	Bone Grafts in Non-Union of War Fractures	Am. J. Surg. **71**: 577-586 (May) 1946.
Speed, J. S., and Boyd, H. B.:	Operative Reconstruction of Malunited Fractures About the Ankle Joint	J. Bone & Joint Surg. **18**: 270 (April) 1936.
Speed, J. S., and Knight, R. A.:	The Treatment of Malunited Colles's Fractures	J. Bone & Joint Surg. **27**: 361 (July) 1945.
Speed, J. S., and Macey, H. B.:	Fractures of the Humeral Condyles in Children	J. Bone & Joint Surg. **15**: 903 (Oct.) 1933.
Speed, J. S., and Smith, H.:	Trochanteric Osteotomy for Ununited Fractures of Neck of Femur	South. M. J. **34**: 798 (Aug.) 1941.
Speed, K.:	A Discussion of Pott's Fracture With Complications; Based on a Series of 208 Cases	Surg., Gynec. & Obst. **19**: 73 (July) 1914.
Street, D. M.:	Medullary Nailing of Femur: Comparative Study of Skeletal Traction, Dual Plating and Medullary Nailing	J. A. M. A., **143**: 709-714 (June 24) 1950.

Thompson, V. P., and Epstein, H. C.:	Traumatic Dislocation of Hip: Survey of 204 Cases Covering Period of 21 Years	J. Bone & Joint Surg. **33A:** 731-745 (July) 1951.
Trethowan, W. H.:	Fractures in the Neighborhood of the Ankle-Joint	Lancet **1:** 90 (Jan. 9) 1926.
Venable, C. S., and Stuck, W. G.:	Electrolysis Controlling Factor in the Use of Metals in Treating Fractures	J. A. M. A. **111:** 1349 (Oct. 8) 1938.
	The Internal Fixation of Fractures	Springfield, Ill., Charles C. Thomas, 1947.
Watson-Jones, R., and Coltart, W. D.:	Slow Union of Fractures With Study of 804 Fractures of Shafts of Tibia and Femur	Brit. J. Surg. **30:** 260 (Jan.) 1943.
Whitman, R.:	The Reconstruction Operation for Ununited Fracture of the Neck of the Femur	Surg., Gynec. & Obst. **32:** 479 (June) 1921.
Williams, E. R.:	Two Congenital Deformities of the Tibia: Congenital Angulation and Congenital Pseudarthrosis	Brit. J. Radiol. **16:** 371 (Dec.) 1943.
Wilson, P. D.:	Fracture of the Lateral Condyle of the Humerus in Childhood	J. Bone & Joint Surg. **18:** 301 (April) 1936.
	Experiences With a Bone Bank	Ann. Surg. **126:** 932-946 (Dec.) 1947.
	Experience With Use of Refrigerated Homogenous Bone	J. Bone & Joint Surg., **33B:** 301-315 (Aug.) 1951.

Chapter XVII

Body Mechanics and Physical Therapy

American Academy of Orthopaedic Surgeons: Report of Posture Committee	Posture and Its Relationship to Orthopaedic Disabilities	Chicago, American Academy of Orthopaedic Surgeons, 1947.
Bierman, W.:	Physical Medicine in General Practice	New York, Paul B. Hoeber, Inc., 1944.
Covalt, N. K.:	Bed Exercises	Arch. Phys. Med. **28:** 18 (Jan.) 1947.
DeLorme, T. L.:	Restoration of Muscle Power by Heavy Resistance Exercises	J. Bone & Joint Surg. **27:** 645 (Oct.) 1945.
DeLorme, T. L., and Watkins, A. L.:	Progressive Resistance Exercise: Technic and Medical Application	New York, Appleton-Century-Crofts, 1951.

Ewerhardt, F. H.:	Exercise in Medicine	South. M. J. **38:** 662 (Oct.) 1945.
Goldthwait, J. E.:	The Backgrounds and Foregrounds of Orthopaedics	J. Bone & Joint Surg. **15:** 279 (April) 1933.
Goldthwait, J. E., Brown, L. T., Swaim, L. T., and Kuhns, J. G.:	Essentials of Body Mechanics in Health and Disease, 4th Edition	Philadelphia, J. B. Lippincott Co., 1945.
Hart, V. L.:	Physiological Rest and the Preservation of Locomotion	Surg., Gynec. & Obst. **56:** 687 (March) 1933.
Hellebrandt, F. A., and Franseen, E. B.:	Physiological Study of the Vertical Stance of Man	Physiol. Rev. **23:** 220 (July) 1943.
Howorth, B.:	Dynamic Posture	J. A. M. A. **131:** 1398 (Aug. 24) 1946.
Keith, A.:	Man's Posture; Its Evolution and Disorders	Brit. M. J. **1:** 451 (March 17) 1923.
Kendall, H. O., and Kendall, F. P.:	Posture and Pain	Baltimore, The Williams & Wilkins Co., 1951.
Kovacs, R.:	Electrotherapy and Light Therapy With the Essentials of Hydrotherapy and Mechanotherapy, 6th Edition	Philadelphia, Lea and Febiger, 1949.
Krusen, F. H.:	Light Therapy, 2nd Edition	New York, Paul B. Hoeber, Inc., 1937.
Lowman, C. L.:	Technique of Underwater Gymnastics	Los Angeles, American Publications Corp., 1937.
	Underwater Gymnastics	J. A. M. A. **97:** 1074 (Oct. 10) 1931.
Mennell, J. B.:	Physical Treatment of Movement, Manipulation and Massage, 5th Edition	Philadelphia, The Blakiston Co., 1945.
Mortimer, B., and Osborne, S. L.:	Tissue Heating by Short Wave Diathermy; Some Biologic Observations	J. A. M. A. **104:** 1413 (April 20) 1935.
Murray, C. R.:	The Exact Rôle of Physical Therapy in the Treatment of Fractures	Surg., Gynec. & Obst. **56:** 479 (Feb. 15) 1933.
Osborne, S. L., and Holmquest, H. J.:	Technic of Electrotherapy and Its Physical and Physiological Basis	Springfield, Ill., and Baltimore, Charles C. Thomas, 1944.
Osgood, R. B.:	Body Mechanics and Posture	J. A. M. A. **96:** 2032 (June 13) 1931.
Phelps, W. M., and Kiphuth, R. J. H.:	The Diagnosis and Treatment of Postural Defects	Springfield, Ill., Charles C. Thomas, 1932.

Plastridge, A. L.: | Gaits | Physiotherapy Rev. **21**: 24 (Jan.-Feb.) 1941.

| Principles and Practices of Physical Therapy | Hagerstown, Md., W. F. Prior Co., 1932.

Schwartz, R. P.: | Kinetics of Human Gait | J. Bone & Joint Surg. **16**: 343 (April) 1934.

Schwartz, R. P., and Heath, A. L.: | The Definition of Human Locomotion on t h e Basis of Measurement | J. Bone & Joint Surg. **29**: 203 (Jan.) 1947.

Smith, O. F. G.: | Rehabilitation, Re-Education and Remedial Exercises | Baltimore, William Wood & Co., 1943.

Stafford, G. T., DeCook, H. B., and Picard, J. L.: | Individual Exercises: Selected Exercises for Individual Conditions | New York, A. S. Barnes & Co., 1935.

Steindler, A.: | Biomechanics | J. Bone & Joint Surg. **15**: 567 (July) 1933.

| Mechanics of Normal and Pathological Locomotion in Man | Springfield, Ill., Charles C. Thomas, 1935.

Chapter XVIII
Affections of the Spine and Thorax

Abbott, E. G.: | Scoliosis | Am. J. Orthop. Surg. **15**: 26, 108, 172, 243, **and** 362, 1917.

American Orthopaedic Association, Research Committee | End - Result Study of Treatment of Idiopathic Scoliosis | J. Bone & Joint Surg. **23**: 963 (Oct.) 1941.

Buchman, J.: | Vertebral Epiphysitis: A Cause of Spinal Deformity | J. Bone & Joint Surg. **7**: 814 (Oct.) 1925.

| Osteochondritis of the Vertebral Body | J. Bone & Joint Surg. **9**: 55 (Jan.) 1927.

| A Résumé of the Osteochondritides | Surg., Gynec. & Obst. **49**: 447 (Oct.) 1929.

Calvé, J.: | A Localized Affection of the Spine Suggesting Osteochondritis of the Vertebral Body, With the Clinical Aspect of Pott's Disease | J. Bone & Joint Surg. **7**: 41 (Jan.) 1925.

Cardis, J., Walker, G. F., and Olver, R. H.: | Kümmell's Disease | Brit. J. Surg. **15**: 616-625 (April) 1928.

Cobb, J. R.: | Treatment of Scoliosis | Connecticut M. J. **7**: 467 (July) 1943.

| Technique, After-Treatment and Results of Spine Fusion for Scoliosis | Am. Acad. Orthopaedic S u r g. Instructional C o u r s e Lectures, **9**: 65-70, 1952.

Edelstein, J. M.: | Adolescent Kyphosis | Brit. J. Surg. **22**: 119 (July) 1934.

Ellis, J. D.:	Compression Fractures of Vertebral Bodies and Other Changes Mistaken for Them	J. Bone & Joint Surg. **26:** 139-145 (Jan.) 1944.
Frejka, B.:	Kyphosis Adolescentium	J. Bone & Joint Surg. **14:** 545 (July) 1932.
Galeazzi, R.:	The Treatment of Scoliosis	J. Bone & Joint Surg. **11:** 81 (Jan.) 1929.
Hibbs, R. A., Risser, J. C., and Ferguson, A. B.:	Scoliosis Treated by the Fusion Operation; An End-Result Study of 360 Cases	J. Bone & Joint Surg. **13:** 91 (Jan.) 1931.
Hodgen, J. T., and Frantz, C. H.:	Juvenile Kyphosis	Surg., Gynec., & Obst. **72:** 798 (April) 1941.
Kleinberg, S.:	Scoliosis, 2nd Edition	New York, Paul B. Hoeber, Inc., 1951.
Lovett, R. W.:	Lateral Curvature of the Spine and Round Shoulders	Philadelphia, P. Blakiston's Son & Co., 1931.
Lovett, R. W., and Brewster, A. H.:	The Treatment of Scoliosis by a Different Method From That Usually Employed	J. Bone & Joint Surg. **6:** 847 (Oct.) 1924.
MacGowan, T. J. B. A.:	Adolescent Kyphosis	Lancet **1:** 211-214 (Feb. 12) 1944.
McElvenny, R. T.:	Principles Underlying Treatment of Scoliosis by Wedging Jacket	Surg., Gynec., & Obst. **72:** 228 (Feb.) 1941.
McKenzie, K. G., and Dewar, F. P.:	Scoliosis With Paraplegia	J. Bone & Joint Surg. **31B:** 162-174 (May) 1949.
Mitchell, J. I.:	Vertebral Osteochondritis	Arch. Surg. **25:** 544 (Sept.) 1932.
Nathan L., and Kuhns, J. G.:	Epiphysitis of the Spine	J. Bone & Joint Surg. **22:** 55 (Jan.) 1940.
O'Brien, F. W.:	Kümmell's Disease	New England J. Med. **204:** 641 (March 26) 1931.
Ponseti, I. V., and Friedman, B.:	Prognosis in Idiopathic Scoliosis	J. Bone & Joint Surg. **32A:** 381-401 (April) 1950.
	Changes in Scoliotic Spine After Fusion	J. Bone & Joint Surg. **32A:** 751-766 (Oct.) 1950.
Rogers, S. P.:	Mechanics of Scoliosis	Arch. Surg. **26:** 962 (June) 1933.
Smith, A. DeF., Butte, F. L., and Ferguson, A. B.:	Treatment of Scoliosis by the Wedging Jacket and Spine Fusion	J. Bone & Joint Surg. **20:** 825 (Oct.) 1938.
Steindler, A.:	Diseases and Deformities of the Spine and Thorax	St. Louis, The C. V. Mosby Co., 1929.

Steindler, A.:	Conservative Compensation-Derotation Treatment of Scoliosis	J. Bone & Joint Surg. **23**: 67 (Jan.) 1941.
Truesdale, P. E., and Hyatt, G. T.:	Funnel Chest	New England J. Med. **215**: 101 (July 16) 1936.
Ullrich, H. F.:	The Operative Treatment of Scoliosis	Am. J. Surg. **45**: 235 (Aug.) 1939.
Willis, T. A.:	Structure and Development of the Spine	J. A. M. A. **125**: 407-412 (June 10) 1944.

Chapter XIX

Affections of the Low Back

Adams, J. D., and Coonse, G. K.:	Back Injuries in Industry	Am. J. Surg. **74**: 258-269 (Sept.) 1947.
Aitken, A. P., and Bradford, C. H.:	End-Results of Ruptured Intervertebral Disks in Industry	Am. J. Surg. **73**: 365-380 (March) 1947.
Baer, W. S.:	Sacro-Iliac Strain	Bull. Johns Hopkins Hosp. **28**: 159 (May) 1917.
Barr, J. S.:	Ruptured Intervertebral Disk and Sciatic Pain	J. Bone & Joint Surg. **29**: 429-437 (April) 1947.
	Low-back and Sciatic Pain — Results of Treatment	J. Bone & Joint Surg. **33A**: 633-649 (July) 1951.
Barr, J. S., Hampton, A. O., and Mixter, W. J.:	Pain Low in the Back and "Sciatica" Due to Lesions of the Intervertebral Disks	J. A. M. A. **109**: 1265 (Oct. 16) 1937.
Barr, J. S., and Mixter, W. J.:	Posterior Protrusions of the Lumbar Intervertebral Discs	J. Bone & Joint Surg. **23**: 444-456, 1941.
Bennett, G. E.:	Tumors of Cauda Equina and Spinal Cord; Report of 4 Cases in Which Marked Spasm of Erector Spinae and Hamstring Muscles Was Outstanding Sign	J. A. M. A. **89**: 1480 (Oct. 29) 1927.
Billington, R. W., Willis, T. A., and O'Reilly, A.:	Backache; Report for the Clinical Orthopaedic Society	J. Bone & Joint Surg. **10**: 290 (April) 1928.
Brahdy, L.:	Mechanics of the Physical Signs in Lower Trunk Injuries	Surg., Gynec. & Obst. **60**: 802 (April) 1935.
Brailsford, J. F.:	Deformities of the Lumbosacral Region of the Spine	Brit. J. Surg. **16**: 562 (April) 1929.

Caldwell, G. A.:	Spondylolisthesis. Analysis of Fifty-Nine Consecutive Cases	Ann. Surg. **119:** 485 (April) 1944.
Camp, J. D.:	Contrast Myelography, Past and Present	Radiology 54:477-506 (April) 1950.
Capener, N.:	Spondylolisthesis	Brit. J. Surg. **19:** 374 (Jan.) 1932.
Chandler, F. A.:	Spinal Fusion Operations in the Treatment of Low Back and Sciatic Pain	J. A. M. A. **93:** 1447 (Nov. 9) 1929.
	Lesions of the "Isthmus" (Pars Inter - Articularis) of the Laminae of the Lower Lumbar Vertebrae and Their Relation to Spondylolisthesis	Surg., Gynec. & Obst. **53:** 273 (Sept.) 1931.
Colonna, P. C., and Friedenberg, Z. B.:	Disc Syndrome, Results of Conservative Care of Patients With Positive Myelograms	J. Bone & Joint Surg. **31A:** 614-618 (July) 1949.
Coventry, M. B., Ghormley, R. K., and Kernohan, J. W.:	The Intervertebral Disc. Its Microscopic Anatomy and Pathology	J. Bone & Joint Surg. **27:** 105 (Jan.) 1945; **27:** 233 (April) 1945; and **27:** 460 (July) 1945.
Danforth, M. S., and Wilson, P. D.:	The Anatomy of the Lumbo-Sacral Region in Relation to Sciatic Pain	J. Bone & Joint Surg. **7:** 109 (Jan.) 1925.
Davis, A. G., and Contributors:	Symposium on the Intervertebral Disc at Meeting of American Orthopaedic Association in June, 1946	J. Bone & Joint Surg. **29:** 424-475 (April) 1947.
Dittrich, R. J.:	Lumbosacral Spina Bifida Occulta	Surg., Gynec. & Obst. **53:** 378 (Sept.) 1931.
	Coccygodynia as Referred Pain	J. Bone & Joint Surg. **33A:** 715-719 (July) 1951.
Duncan, G. A.:	Painful Coccyx	Arch. Surg. **34:** 1088 (June) 1937.
Duncan, W. S.:	The Relation of the Prostate Gland to Orthopaedic Problems	J. Bone & Joint Surg. **18:** 101 (Jan.) 1936.
Ellis, J. D., Editor:	The Injured Back and Its Treatment	Springfield, Ill., Charles C. Thomas, 1940.
Ferguson, A. B.:	The Clinical and Roentgenographic Interpretation of Lumbosacral Anomalies	Radiology **22:** 548 (May) 1934.
Fisher, A. G. T.:	Treatment by Manipulation	New York, The Macmillan Co., 1947.

Ford, L. T., and Key, J. A.: — Evaluation of Myelography in Diagnosis of Intervertebral Disc Lesions of Low Back — J. Bone & Joint Surg. **32A:** 257-266 (April) 1950.

Freiberg, A. H., and Vinke, T. H.: — Sciatica and the Sacro-Iliac Joint — J. Bone & Joint Surg. **16:** 126 (Jan.) 1934.

Friberg, S.: — Studies on Spondylolisthesis — Stockholm, P. A. Norstedt & Son, 1939; supplement to vol. 82, Acta chir. Scandinav.

Ghormley, R. K.: — Low Back Pain, With Special Reference to the Articular Facets, With Presentation of an Operative Procedure — J. A. M. A. **101:** 1773 (Dec. 2) 1933.

Haynes, W. G.: — Problem of Herniated Nucleus Pulposus in the Military Service — War Med. **3:** 585-595 (June) 1943.

Heyman, C. H.: — Posterior Fasciotomy in the Treatment of Back Pain — J. Bone & Joint Surg. **21:** 397 (April) 1939.

Hibbs, R. A., and Swift, W. E.: — Developmental Abnormalities at the Lumbosacral Juncture Causing Pain and Disability; A Report of 147 Patients Treated by the Spine Fusion Operation — Surg., Gynec. & Obst. **48:** 604 (May) 1929.

Hitchcock, H. H.: — Spondylolisthesis: Observations on Its Development, Progression and Genesis — J. Bone & Joint Surg. **22:** 1 (Jan.) 1940.

Jostes, F. A.: — Place of Manipulative Procedures in the Overall Treatment Rationale for Painful Back Conditions — Arch. Phys. Therapy **25:** 716-720 (Dec.) 1944.

Kendall, H. O., and Kendall, F. P.: — Study and Treatment of Muscle Imbalance in Cases of Low Back and Sciatic Pain — Privately printed, Baltimore, Feb., 1936.

Key, J. A.: — Operative Treatment of Coccygodynia — J. Bone & Joint Surg. **19:** 759 (July) 1937.

Kleinberg, S.: — Sciatic Scoliosis — Am. J. Surg. **37:** 418 (Sept.) 1937.

Kreuscher, P. H.: — The Orthopedic Aspect of Low Back Pain in Connection With Pelvic Disorders — Surg., Gynec. & Obst. **45:** 482 (Oct.) 1927.

Le Cocq, E.: — Anomalies of the Lumbosacral Spine — Am. J. Surg. **22:** 118 (Oct.) 1933.

Lennon, M. B.:	The Traumatic Neurosis	J. A. M. A. **83**: 738 (Sept. 6) 1924.
Lewin, P.:	Backache and Sciatic Neuritis; Back Injuries, Deformities, Diseases, Disabilities, With Notes on the Pelvis, Neck, and Brachial Neuritis	Philadelphia, Lea & Febiger, 1943.
Love, J. G.:	Protruded Intervertebral Disk	S. Clin. North America **26**: 997-1006 (Aug.) 1946.
Lowman, C. L.:	Rôle of Iliolumbar Ligaments in Low Back Strains	J. A. M. A. **87**: 1002 (Sept. 25) 1926.
Magnuson, P. B.:	Intervertebral Disks	Am. J. Surg. **67**: 228-236 (Feb.) 1945.
Meyerding, H. W.:	Spondylolisthesis: Surgical Treatment and Results	J. Bone & Joint Surg. **25**: 65 (Jan.) 1943.
Mitchell, G. A. G.:	The Lumbosacral Junction	J. Bone & Joint Surg. **16**: 233 (April) 1934.
	The Significance of Lumbosacral Transitional Vertebrae	Brit. J. Surg. **24**: 147 (July) 1936.
Moore, B. H.:	Sacralization of the Fifth Lumbar Vertebra	J. Bone & Joint Surg. **7**: 271 (April) 1925.
Naffziger, H. C., Inman, V. T., and Saunders, J. B. deC. M.	Lesions of the Intervertebral Discs and Ligamenta Flava	Surg., Gynec. & Obst. **66**: 288 (Feb.) 1938.
Newman, P. H.:	Sprung Back	J. Bone & Joint Surg. **34B**: 30-37 (Feb.) 1952.
Ober, F. R.:	Back Strain and Sciatica	J. A. M. A. **104**: 1580 (May 4) 1935.
O'Connell, J. E. A.:	Protrusion of Lumbar Intervertebral Discs	J. Bone & Joint Surg. **33B**: 8-30 (Feb.) 1951.
Osgood, R. B.:	Etiologic Factors in Certain Cases of So-Called Sciatic Scoliosis	J. Bone & Joint Surg. **9**: 667 (Oct.) 1927.
Pitkin, H. C., and Pheasant, H. C.:	Sacrarthrogenetic Telalgia	J. Bone & Joint Surg. **18**: 111 (Jan.), 365 (April), 706 (July), 1008 (Oct.) 1936, and **19**: 169 (Jan.) 1937.
Poppen, J. L.:	The Herniated Intervertebral Disc; An Analysis of 400 Verified Cases	New England J. Med. **232**: 211-215 (Feb. 22) 1945.
Raney, R. B.:	Isthmus Defects of the Fifth Lumbar Vertebra	South. M. J. **38**: 166 (March) 1945.
Rhodes, M. P., and Colangelo, C.:	Spondylolysis and Its Relation to Spondylolisthesis	Am. J. Surg. **72**: 20-25 (July) 1946.

Schumacher, F. L.: Evaluation of Disability in Low Back Injuries Radiology **41**: 18 (July) 1943.

Smith-Petersen, M. N., and Rogers, W. A.: End-Result Study of Arthrodesis of the Sacro-Iliac Joint for Arthritis, Traumatic and Non-Traumatic J. Bone & Joint Surg. **8**: 118 (Jan.) 1926.

Steindler, A.: Diseases and Deformities of the Spine and Thorax St. Louis, The C. V. Mosby Co., 1929.

Thiele, G. H.: Coccygodynia, Mechanisms of Its Production and Its Relationship to Anorectal Disease Am. J. Surg. **79**: 110-116 (Jan.) 1950.

Toumey, J. W., Poppen, J. L., and Hurley, M. T.: Cauda Equina Tumors as Cause of Low Back Syndrome J. Bone & Joint Surg. **32A**: 249-256 (April) 1950.

Williams, P. C.: Lesions of the Lumbosacral Spine. Part I: Acute Traumatic Destruction of the Lumbosacral Intervertebral Disc J. Bone & Joint Surg. **19**: 343 (April) 1937.

Part II: Chronic Traumatic (Postural) Destruction of the Lumbosacral Intervertebral Disc J. Bone & Joint Surg. **19**: 690 (July) 1937.

Willis, T. A.: An Analysis of Vertebral Anomalies Am. J. Surg. **6**: 163 (Feb.) 1929.

Chapter XX

Affections of the Hip

Coxa Plana

Buchman, J.: A Résumé of the Osteochondritides Surg., Gynec. & Obst. **49**: 447 (Oct.) 1929.

Calvé, J.: Osteochondritis of the Upper Extremity of Femur J. Orthop. Surg. **3**: 489 (Oct.) 1921.

Cole, W. H.: The Clinical Diagnosis, Treatment, and Prognosis of Epiphyseal Disturbances in Childhood J. A. M. A. **127**: 318-320 (Feb. 10) 1945.

Danforth, M. S.: The Treatment of Legg-Calvé-Perthes' Disease Without Weight-Bearing J. Bone & Joint Surg. **16**: 516 (July) 1934.

Doub, H. P.:	Aseptic Necrosis of the Epiphyses and Short Bones: Roentgen Studies	J. A. M. A. **127**: 311 (Feb. 10) 1945.
Ferguson, A. B., and Howorth, M. B.:	Coxa Plana and Related Conditions at the Hip	J. Bone & Joint Surg. **16**: 781 (Oct.) 1934.
Gill, A. B.:	Legg-Perthes Disease of Hip: Its Early Roentgenographic Manifestations and Its Cyclical Course	J. Bone & Joint Surg. **22**: 1013 (Oct.) 1940.
Heyman, C. H., and Herndon, C. H.:	Legg-Perthes Disease, Method of Measuring Roentgenographic Result	J. Bone & Joint Surg. **32A**: 767-778 (Oct.) 1950.
Howorth, M. B.:	Coxa Plana	J. Bone & Joint Surg. **30A**: 601-620 (July) 1948.
Kreuz, F. P., and Shands, A. R., Jr.:	Some Congenital and Developmental Problems of Hip Joint in Infancy and Childhood	New York, Monographs of Surg. p. 327-392, Thomas Nelson & Sons, 1951.
Legg, A. T.:	An Obscure Affection of the Hip-Joint	Boston M. & S. J. **162**: 202 (Feb. 17) 1910.
	The End Results of Coxa Plana	J. Bone & Joint Surg. **9**: 26 (Jan.) 1927.
Mundell, E. R., and Sherman, M. S.:	Late Results in Legg-Perthes Disease	J. Bone & Joint Surg. **33A**: 1-23 (Jan.) 1951.
Pedersen, H. E., and McCarroll, H. R.:	Treatment of Legg-Perthes Disease	J. Bone & Joint Surg. **33A**: 591-600 (July) 1951.
Pike, M. M.:	Legg-Perthes Disease, Method of Conservative Treatment	J. Bone & Joint Surg. **32A**: 663-670 (July) 1950.
Snyder, C. H.:	Sling for Use in Legg-Perthes Disease	J. Bone & Joint Surg. **29**: 524-526 (April) 1947.
Waldenstrom, H.:	First Stages of Coxa Plana	J. Bone & Joint Surg. **20**: 559 (July) 1938.
Zemansky, A. P., Jr.:	The Pathology and Pathogenesis of Legg-Calvé-Perthes' Disease (Osteochondritis Juvenilis Deformans Coxae)	Am. J. Surg. **4**: 169 (Feb.) 1928.

Coxa Vara

Babb, F. S., Ghormley, R. K., and Chatterton, C. C.:	Congenital Coxa Vara	J. Bone & Joint Surg. **31A**: 115-131 (Jan.) 1949.
Duncan, G. A.:	Congenital Developmental Coxa Vara	Surgery **3**: 741 (May) 1937.

LeMesurier, A. B.:	Developmental Coxa Vara	J. Bone & Joint Surg. **30B**: 595-605 (Nov.) 1948.
Ollerenshaw, R.:	The Femoral Neck in Childhood	Proc. Roy. Soc. Med. London **32**: 113 (Dec.) 1938.
Zadek, I.:	Congenital Coxa Vara	Arch. Surg. **30**: 62 (Jan.) 1935.

Slipping of the Upper Femoral Epiphysis

Badgley, C. E., Isaacson, A. S., Wolgamot, J. C., and Miller, J. W.:	Operative Therapy for Slipped Upper Femoral Epiphysis, an End-Result Study	J. Bone & Joint Surg. **30**: 19-30 (Jan.) 1948.
Cleveland, M., Bosworth, D. M., Naly, J. N., and Hess, W. E.:	Study of Displaced Capital Femoral Epiphyses	J. Bone & Joint Surg. **33A**: 955-967 (Oct.) 1951.
Compere, C. L.:	Correction of Deformity and Prevention of Aseptic Necrosis in Late Cases of Slipped Femoral Epiphysis	J. Bone & Joint Surg. **32A**: 351-362 (April) 1950.
Ghormley, R. K., and Fairchild, R. D.:	Diagnosis and Treatment of Slipped Epiphyses	J. A. M. A. **114**: 229 (Jan. 20) 1940.
Harris, W. R.:	Endocrine Basis for Slipping of Upper Femoral Epiphysis: Experimental Study	J. Bone & Joint Surg. **32B**: 5-11 (Feb.) 1950.
Heyman, C. H.:	Treatment of Slipping of Upper Femoral Epiphysis: Study of Results of 42 Cases	Surg., Gynec. & Obst. **89**: 559-565 (Nov.) 1949.
Howorth, M. B.:	Slipping of Upper Femoral Epiphysis	J. Bone & Joint Surg. **31A**: 734-747 (Oct.) 1949.
Klein, A., Joplin, R. J., and Reidy, J. A.:	Treatment of Slipped Capital Femoral Epiphysis	J. A. M. A. **136**: 445-451 (Feb. 14) 1948.
Klein, A., Joplin, R. J., Reidy, J. A., and Hanelin, J.:	Roentgeno-graphic Changes in Nailed Slipped Capital Femoral Epiphysis	J. Bone & Joint Surg. **31A**: 1-22 (Jan.) 1949.
Lacroix, P.:	Slipping of Upper Femoral Epiphysis: Pathological Study	J. Bone & Joint Surg. **33A**: 371-382 (April) 1951.
Martin, P. H.:	Slipped Epiphysis in Adolescent Hip; a Reconsideration of Open Reduction	J. Bone & Joint Surg. **30A**: 9-19 (Jan.) 1948.
Milch, H.:	Epiphysiolysis or Epiphyseal Coxa Anteverta	J. Bone & Joint Surg. **19**: 97 (Jan.) 1937.

Pomeranz, M. M.:   Epiphyseolysis or Separa-   Am. J. Roentgenol. **40:**
                        tion of the Capital   581 (Oct.) 1938.
                        Epiphysis of the Femur
                        in Adolescence

Sever, J. W.:   Slipping Epiphysis of the   New England J. Med.
                        Head of the Femur   **211:** 1179 (Dec. 27)
                                                     1934.

Wilson, P. D.:   The Treatment of Slip-   J. Bone & Joint Surg.
                        ping of the Upper Fe-   **20:** 379 (April) 1938.
                        moral Epiphysis With
                        Minimal Displacement

                        Pathologic Dislocation

Bryson, A. F.:   Treatment of Pathologi-   J. Bone & Joint Surg.
                        cal Dislocation of Hip   **30B:** 449-453 (Aug.)
                        Joint After Suppura-   1948.
                        tive Arthritis in In-
                        fants

Elzinga, E. R., and Key, Paralytic Dislocation at   J. Bone & Joint Surg.
J. A.:   the Hip in Poliomye-   **14:** 867 (Oct.) 1932.
                        litis

Gill, A. B.:   Pathological Dislocations   South. M. J. **22:** 207
                        of the Hip   (March) 1929.

Hart, V. L.:   Spontaneous Dislocations   Arch. Surg. **17:** 587
                        of the Hip Joint Dur-   (Oct.) 1928.
                        ing Early Life

Milch, H., and Green,   Pathological Dislocation   Arch. Surg. **32:** 880
H. H.:   of the Hip   (May) 1936.

                        Other Conditions

Albee, F. H.:   Injuries and Diseases of   New York, Paul B. Hoe-
                        the Hip   ber, Inc., 1937.

Dickinson, A. M.:   Bilateral Snapping Hip   Am. J. Surg. **6:** 97
                                                     (Jan.) 1929.

Ferguson, A. B., and   Coxa Magna: A Condi-   J. A. M. A. **104:** 808
Howorth, M. B.:   tion of the Hip Related   (March 9) 1935.
                        to Coxa Plana

Finder, J. G.:   Iliopectineal Bursitis   Arch. Surg., **36:** 519
                                                     (March) 1938.

Gellman, M.:   Arthrokatadysis of the   South. M. J. **27:** 215
                        Hip Joint   (March) 1934.

Gibson, A.:   Posterior Exposure of   J. Bone & Joint Surg.
                        Hip Joint   **32B:** 183-186 (May)
                                                     1950.

Gilmour, J.:   Adolescent Deformities of   Brit. J. Surg. **26:** 670
                        the Acetabulum: An   (April) 1939.
                        Investigation Into the
                        Nature of Protrusio
                        Acetabuli

Golding, F. C.:   Protrusio Acetabuli (Cen-   Brit. J. Surg. **22:** 56
                        tral Luxation)   (July) 1934.

Jansen, M.:	Flattened Hip Socket and Its Sequelae (Coxa Plana, Valga, Vara, and Malum Coxae)	J. Bone & Joint Surg. **5**: 528 (July) 1923.
Jones, F. W.:	The Anatomy of Snapping Hip	J. Orthop. Surg. **2**: 1 (Jan.) 1920.
Rechtman, A. M.:	Etiology of Deep Acetabulum and Intrapelvic Protrusion	Arch. Surg. **33**: 122 (July) 1936.
Smith-Petersen, M. N.:	A New Supra-Articular Subperiosteal Approach to the Hip Joint	Am. J. Orthop. Surg. **15**: 592 (Aug.) 1917.
	Treatment of Malum Coxae Senilis, Old Slipped Upper Femoral Epiphysis, Intrapelvic Protrusion of the Acetabulum, and Coxa Plana by Means of Acetabuloplasty	J. Bone & Joint Surg. **18**: 869 (Oct.) 1936.
Tucker, F. R.:	Arterial Supply to Femoral Head and Its Clinical Importance	J. Bone & Joint Surg. **31B**: 82-93 (Feb.) 1949.

Chapter XXI

Affections of the Knee

Internal Derangements

Abbott, L. C., Saunders, J. B. DeC. M., Bost, F. C., and Anderson, C. E.:	Injuries to the Ligaments of the Knee Joint	J. Bone & Joint Surg. **26**: 503 (July) 1944.
Bennett, G. E.:	The Use of Fascia for the Reinforcement of Relaxed Joints	Arch. Surg. **13**: 655 (Nov.) 1926.
	Relaxed Knees and Torn Ligaments	Proc. Internat. Assem., Interstate Postgrad. M. A. North America **6**: 351, 1931.
	Internal Derangement of the Knee Joint	Am. J. Surg. **42**: 670 (Dec.) 1938.
Bennett, G. E., and Shaw, M. B.:	Cysts of the Semilunar Cartilages	Arch. Surg. **33**: 92 (July) 1936.
Brantigan, O. C., and Voshell, A. F.:	Mechanics of Ligaments and Menisci of the Knee Joint	J. Bone & Joint Surg. **23**: 44 (Jan.) 1941.
Bristow, W. R.:	Internal Derangement of the Knee Joint	J. Bone & Joint Surg. **17**: 605 (July) 1935.
Bronitsky, J.:	Chondromalacia Patellae	J. Bone & Joint Surg. **29**: 931-945 (Oct.) 1947.

Burman, M. S., and Sutro, C. J.:	A Study of the Degenerative Changes of the Menisci of the Knee Joint and the Clinical Significance Thereof	J. Bone & Joint Surg. **15:** 835 (Oct.) 1933.
Carrell, W. B.:	Use of Fascia Lata in Knee-Joint Instability	J. Bone & Joint Surg. **19:** 1018 (Oct.) 1937.
Cave, E. F.:	Internal Derangements of the Knee, in Monographs on Surgery for 1951, 443-470	New York, Thos. Nelson & Sons, 1951.
Cave, E. F., Rowe, C. R., and Yee, L. B. K.:	Selection of Cases for Arthrotomy of the Knee in an Overseas General Hospital	J. Bone & Joint Surg. **27:** 603 (Oct.) 1945.
Colonna, P. C.:	Osteochondromatosis of the Knee Joint	Surg., Gynec. & Obst. **53:** 698 (Nov.) 1931.
Dickson, F. D.:	Injuries of the Knee Joint	J. A. M. A. **110:** 122 (Jan. 8) 1938.
Dunn, N.:	Observations on Some Injuries of the Knee-Joint	Lancet **1:** 1267 (June 16) 1934.
Fairbank, H. A. T.:	Osteo-chondritis Dissecans	Brit. J. Surg. **21:** 67 (July) 1933.
Finder, J. G.:	Discoid External Semilunar Cartilage; A Cause of Internal Derangement of the Knee Joint	J. Bone & Joint Surg. **16:** 804 (Oct.) 1934.
Fisher, A. G. T.:	Internal Derangements of the Knee Joint, 2nd Edition	New York, The Macmillan Co., 1933.
Ghormley, R. K., and Clegg, R. S.:	Bone and Joint Changes in Hemophilia With Report of Cases of So-Called Hemophilic Pseudotumor	J. Bone & Joint Surg. **30A:** 589 (July) 1948.
Henderson, M. S.:	Bucket-Handle Fractures of the Semilunar Cartilages	J. A. M. A. **90:** 1359 (April 28) 1928.
	Injuries to the Semilunar Cartilages of the Knee Joint	Surg., Gynec. & Obst. **51:** 720 (Nov.) 1930.
Horwitz, M. T., and Davidson, A. J.:	Newer Concepts in the Treatment of Injuries to the Ligaments of the Knee Joint: An Evaluation of the Mauck Operation	Surgery **3:** 407 (March) 1938.
Jones, H. T.:	Loose Body Formation in Synovial Osteochondromatosis With Special Reference to the Etiology and Pathology	J. Bone & Joint Surg. **6:** 407 (April) 1924.

King, D.:	The Healing of Semilunar Cartilages	J. Bone & Joint Surg. **18**: 333 (April) 1936.
	The Function of Semilunar Cartilages	J. Bone & Joint Surg. **18**: 1069 (Oct.) 1936.
Krida, A.:	Instability of the Knee Joint Due to Injury of the Anterior Crucial Ligament; A Report of Eleven Operated Cases	J. Bone & Joint Surg. **15**: 897 (Oct.) 1933.
Lipscomb, P. R., and Henderson, M. S.:	Internal Derangements of the Knee	J. A. M. A. **135**: 827 (Nov. 29) 1947.
MacAusland, W. R.:	A Study of Derangement of Semilunar Cartilage Based on 850 Cases	Surg., Gynec. & Obst. **77**: 141 (Aug.) 1943.
Mauck, H. P.:	A New Operative Procedure for Instability of the Knee	J. Bone & Joint Surg. **18**: 984 (Oct.) 1936.
	Severe Acute Injuries of the Knee	Am. J. Surg. **56**: 54 (April) 1942.
Middleton, D. S.:	Congenital Disc-Shaped Lateral Meniscus With Snapping Knee	Brit. J. Surg. **24**: 246 (Oct.) 1936.
Moulonguet, P.:	Foreign Bodies in Joints	J. Bone & Joint Surg. **11**: 353 (Apr.) 1929.
Mussey, R. D., and Henderson, M. S.:	Osteochondromatosis	J. Bone & Joint Surg. **31A**: 619-627 (July) 1949.
O'Donoghue, D. H.:	Surgical Treatment of Fresh Injuries to Major Ligaments of Knee	J. Bone & Joint Surg. **32A**: 721-738 (Oct.) 1950.
Peabody, C. W., and Walsh, F. P.:	Lesions of Patellar Cartilage as Cause of Internal Derangements of Knee	Arch. Surg. **57**: 589-598 (Oct.) 1949.
Phemister, D. B.:	The Causes of and Changes in Loose Bodies Arising From the Articular Surface of the Joint	J. Bone & Joint Surg. **6**: 278 (April) 1924.
Shands, A. R., Jr., Hutchison, J. L., and Ziv, L.:	Derangements of the Semilunar Cartilages of the Knee; A Clinical and Experimental Study	South. M. J. **29**: 1045 (Nov.) 1936.
Smillie, I. S.:	Observations on the Regeneration of the Semilunar Cartilages in Man	Brit. J. Surg. **31**: 398-401 (April) 1944.
	Congenital Discoid Meniscus	J. Bone & Joint Surg. **30B**: 671-682 (Nov.) 1948.

Smillie, I. S.:   Injuries of Knee Joint   Edinburgh, E. & S. Liv-
                                                        ingstone, Ltd., 1951.

Stein, B. H., Ikins, R. G., Osteochondritis Dissecans   Am. J. Surg. **64:** 328-
  and Lowry, F. C.:   337 (June) 1944.

Steindler, A.:   Synovectomy a n d F a t   J. A. M. A. **84:** 16
                             Pad Removal in the   (Jan. 3) 1925.
                             Knee

Wilmoth, C. L.:   Osteochondromatosis   J. Bone & Joint Surg.
                                                        23: 367 (April) 1941.

                          Other Affections

Bierring, W. L.:   Intermittent Hydrarthro-   J. A. M. A. **77:** 785
                            sis   (Sept. 3) 1921.

Bosworth, D. M.:   Autogenous Bone Pegging   J. Bone & Joint Surg.
                            for Epiphysitis of the   **16:** 829 (Oct.) 1934.
                            Tibial Tubercle

Cave, E. F., and   Patella, Its Importance   J. Bone & Joint Surg.
  Rowe, C. R.:   in Derangements of   **32A:** 542-553 (July)
                            Knee   1950.

Cole, J. P.:   A Study of Osgood-   Surg., Gynec. & Obst.
                            Schlatter's Disease   **65:** 55 (July) 1937.

Conway, F. M.:   Rupture of the Quadri-   Am. J. Surg. **50:** 3
                            ceps Tendon With Re-   (Oct.) 1940.
                            port of Three Cases

Goldthwait, J. E.:   Slipping or Recurrent   Boston M. & S. J. **150:**
                            Dislocation of the Pa-   169 (Feb.) 1904.
                            tella

Haggart, G. E.:   Synovial Cysts of the   Ann. Surg. **118:** 438
                            Popliteal Space: Clin-   (Sept.) 1943.
                            ical Significance and
                            Treatment

Hauser, E. D. W.:   Total Tendon Transplant   Surg., Gynec. & Obst.
                            for Slipping Patella.   **66:** 199 (Feb.) 1938.
                            A New Operation for
                            Recurrent Dislocation
                            of the Patella

Hedrick, D. W., and   Pellegrini - Stieda's Dis-   Radiology **23:** 180-188
  Jones, H. C.:   ease: Clinical and   (Aug.) 1934.
                            Roentgenologic Con-
                            sideration

Hughes, E. S. R.:   Osgood - Schlatter's Dis-   Surg., Gynec. & Obst.
                            ease   **86:** 323-328 (March)
                                                         1948.

Keefer, C. S., and   Hemophilic Arthritis   New England J. Med.
  Myers, W. K.:   **208:** 1183 (June 8)
                                                         1933.

Key, J. A.:   Hemophilic Arthritis   Ann. Surg. **95:** 198
                            (Bleeder's Joints)   (Feb.) 1932.

Kulowski, J.:   Chondromalacia of the   J. A. M. A. **100:** 1837
                            Patella   (June 10) 1933.

Kulowski, J.: Post-Traumatic Para-Articular Ossification of Knee Joint (Pellegrini-Stieda's Disease) — Am. J. Roentgenol. **47:** 392 (March) 1942.

McCarroll, H. R., and Schwartzmann, J. R.: Lateral Dislocation of the Patella, Correction by Simultaneous Transplantation of the Tibial Tubercle and Semitendinosus Tendon — J. Bone & Joint Surg. **27:** 446 (July) 1945.

Morris, H. D., and Mosiman, R. S.: Arthrodesis of Knee: Comparison of Compression Method With Non-Compression Method — J. Bone & Joint Surg. **33A:** 982-988 (Oct.) 1951.

Newcomber, N. B.: The Joint Changes in Hemophilia — Radiology **32:** 573 (May) 1939.

Osgood, R. B.: Lesions of the Tibial Tubercle Occurring During Adolescence — Boston M. & S. J. **148:** 114 (Jan. 29) 1903.

Thomas, H. B.: Some Orthopaedic Findings in 98 Cases of Hemophilia — J. Bone & Joint Surg. **18:** 140 (Jan.) 1936.

Uhry, E., Jr.: Osgood-Schlatter Disease — Arch. Surg. **48:** 406-414 (May) 1944.

Voshell, A. F., and Brantigan, O. C.: Bursitis in the Region of the Tibial Collateral Ligament — J. Bone & Joint Surg. **26:** 793-798 (Oct.) 1944.

Wilson, P. D.: Posterior Capsuloplasty in Certain Flexion Contractures of the Knee — J. Bone & Joint Surg. **11:** 40 (Jan.) 1929.

Wilson, P. D., Eyre-Brook, A. L., and Francis, J. D.: A Clinical and Anatomical Study of the Semimembranosus Bursa in Relation to Popliteal Cyst — J. Bone & Joint Surg. **20:** 963 (Oct.) 1938.

Chapter XXII

Affections of the Ankle and Foot

Bernstein, A., and Stone, J. R.: March Fracture: A Report of Three Hundred and Seven Cases and a New Method of Treatment — J. Bone & Joint Surg. **26:** 743-750 (Oct.) 1944.

Bingold, A. C., and Collins, D. H.: Hallux Rigidus — J. Bone & Joint Surg. **32B:** 214-222 (May) 1950.

Butte, F. L.: Navicular-Cuneiform Arthrodesis for Flat-Foot — J. Bone & Joint Surg. **19:** 496 (April) 1937.

Chandler, F. A.:	Children's Feet, Normal and Presenting Common Abnormalities	Am. J. Dis. Child. **63:** 1136 (June) 1942.
Chang, C. C., and Miltner, L. J.:	Periostitis of the Os Calcis	J. Bone & Joint Surg. **16:** 355 (April) 1934.
Cleveland, M.:	End-Result Study of Keller Operation	J. Bone & Joint Surg. **32A:** 163-175 (Jan.) 1950.
Cole, W. H.:	Treatment of Clawfoot	J. Bone & Joint Surg. **22:** 895 (Oct.) 1940.
Crego, C. H., and Ford, I. T.:	End-Result Study of Various Operative Procedures for Correcting Flat Feet in Children	J. Bone & Joint Surg. **34A:** 183-196 (Jan.) 1952.
Dickson, F. D., and Diveley, R. L.:	Functional Disorders of the Foot. Their Diagnosis and Treatment, 2nd Edition	Philadelphia, J. B. Lippincott Co., 1944.
Dwight, T.:	Clinical Atlas: Variations of the Bones of the Hands and Feet	Philadelphia, J. B. Lippincott Co., 1907.
Fraser, J.:	Minor Orthopaedics of the Feet in General Practice	Brit. M. J. **1:** 383 (March 2) 1929.
Freiberg, A. H.:	The So-Called Infraction of the Second Metatarsal Bone	J. Bone & Joint Surg. **8:** 257 (April) 1926.
Graham, J.:	Weak Foot: Pathogenesis and Treatment	Am. J. Surg. **35:** 486 (March) 1937.
Haglund, P.:	Concerning some Rare but Important Surgical Injuries Brought on by Violent Exercise	Lancet **2:** 12 (July 4) 1908.
Harbin, M., and Zollinger, R.:	Osteochondritis of the Growth Centres	Surg., Gynec. & Obst. **51:** 145 (Aug.) 1930.
Hardy, R. H., and Clapham, J. R. C.:	Observations on Hallux Valgus	J. Bone & Joint Surg. **33B:** 376-391 (Aug.) 1951.
Harris, R. I., and Beath, T.:	Army Foot Survey	Ottawa, Canada National Research Council, 1947.
	Hypermobile Flat-foot With Short Tendo Achillis	J. Bone & Joint Surg. **30:** 116 - 140 (Jan.) 1948.
	Etiology of Peroneal Spastic Flat Foot	J. Bone & Joint Surg. **30B:** 624-634 (Nov.) 1948.
	Short First Metatarsal— Its Incidence and Clinical Significance	J. Bone & Joint Surg. **31A:** 553-565 (July) 1949.
Hartley, J. B.:	"Stress" or "Fatigue" Fractures of Bone	Brit. J. Radiol. **16:** 225 (Sept.) 1943.

Hauser, E. D. W.: Diseases of the Foot — Philadelphia, W. B. Saunders Co., 1950.

Hertzler, A. E.: Bursitides of the Plantar Surface of the Foot — Am. J. Surg 1: 117 (Sept.) 1926.

Hoke, M.: An Operation for the Correction of Extremely Relaxed Flat Feet — J. Bone & Joint Surg. 13: 773 (Oct.) 1931.

Holland, C. T.: The Accessory Bones of the Foot With Notes on a Few Other Conditions — The Robert Jones Birthday Volume, p. 157; London, Oxford University Press, 1928.

Hughes, E. S. R.: Painful Heels in Children — Surg., Gynec. & Obst. 86: 64-68 (Jan.) 1948.

Inge, G. A. L., and Ferguson, A. B.: Surgery of the Sesamoid Bones of the Great Toe; An Anatomic and Clinical Study, With a Report of 41 Cases — Arch. Surg. 27: 466 (Sept.) 1933.

Jones, E.: Operative Treatment of Chronic Dislocation of the Peroneal Tendons — J. Bone & Joint Surg. 14: 574 (July) 1932.

Jones, F. W.: Structure and Function as Seen in the Foot — Baltimore, William Wood & Co., 1944.

Karp, M. G.: Köhler's Disease of the Tarsal Scaphoid: An End-Result Study — J. Bone & Joint Surg. 19: 84 (Jan.) 1937.

Keith, A.: The History of the Human Foot and Its Bearing on Orthopaedic Practice — J. Bone & Joint Surg. 11: 10 (Jan.) 1929.

Keller, W. L.: Further Observations on the Surgical Treatment of Hallux Valgus and Bunions — New York M. J. 95: 696 (April 6) 1912.

Kernodle, H. B., and Jacobs, J. E.: Metatarsal March Fractures — South. M. J. 37: 579 (Oct.) 1944.

Kidner, F. C.: The Prehallux (Accessory Scaphoid) in Its Relation to Flat-Foot — J. Bone & Joint Surg. 11: 831 (Oct.) 1929.

Köhler, A.: Typical Disease of the Second Metatarsophalangeal Joint — Am. J. Roentgenol. 10: 705 (Sept.) 1923.

Lake, N. C.: The Foot, 4th Edition — Baltimore, The Williams & Wilkins Co., 1951.

Lapidus, P. W.: Spastic Flat-Foot — J. Bone & Joint Surg. 28: 126 (Jan.) 1946.

Leavitt, D. G., and Woodward, H. W.: March Fracture: A Statistical Study of Forty-Seven Patients — J. Bone & Joint Surg. 26: 733 (Oct.) 1944.

Lewin, P.: The Foot and Ankle. Their Injuries, Diseases, Deformities and Disabilities, 3rd Edition — Philadelphia, Lea & Febiger, 1947.

Mayo, C. H.: The Surgical Treatment of Bunion — Ann. Surg. 48: 300 (Aug.) 1908.

McElvenny, R. T.: The Etiology and Surgical Treatment of Intractable Pain About the Fourth Metatarsophalangeal Joint (Morton's Toe) — J. Bone & Joint Surg. 25: 675 (July) 1943.

Meyerding, H. W., and Stuck, W. G.: Painful Heels Among Children (Apophysitis) — J. A. M. A. 102: 1658 (May 19) 1934.

Morton, D. J.: Mechanism of the Normal Foot and of Flat Foot — J. Bone & Joint Surg. 6: 368 (April) 1924.

Metatarsus Atavicus; The Identification of a Distinctive Type of Foot Disorder — J. Bone & Joint Surg. 9: 531 (July) 1927.

The Human Foot — New York, Columbia University Press, 1935.

Myers, E. E.: The Management of Postural Deformities of the Lower Extremities — Am. J. Surg. 44: 232 (April) 1939.

Nissen, K. I.: Plantar Digital Neuritis, Morton's Metatarsalgia — J. Bone & Joint Surg. 30B: 84-94 (Feb.) 1948.

Perkins, G.: Removal of the Metatarsal Head for Hallux Valgus and Hallux Rigidus — Lancet 1: 540 (Mar. 12) 1927.

Roberts, P. W.: Fifty Cases of Bursitis of the Foot — J. Bone & Joint Surg. 11: 338 (April) 1929.

Saunders, J. T.: Etiology and Treatment of Clawfoot — Arch. Surg. 30: 179 (Feb.) 1935.

Shands, A. R., Jr.: The Accessory Bones of the Foot — South. Med. & Surg. 93: 326 (May) 1931.

Silver, D.: The Operative Treatment of Hallux Valgus — J. Bone & Joint Surg. 5: 225 (April) 1923.

Spitzy, H.: Operative Correction of Claw-Foot — Surg., Gynec. & Obst. 45: 813 (Dec.) 1927.

Steindler, A.: Stripping of the Os Calcis — J. Orthop. Surg. 2: 8 (Jan.) 1920.

Webster, F. S., and Roberts, W. M.: Tarsal Anomalies and Peroneal Spastic Flatfoot — J. A. M. A. 146: 1099-1104 (July 21) 1951.

Whitman, R.:	The Importance of Positive Support in the Curative Treatment of Weak Feet and a Comparison of the Means Employed to Assure It	Am. J. Orthop. Surg. **11**: 215 (Oct.) 1913.
Williams, A. A.:	Tenosynovitis of Tendo Achillis	Brit. M. J. **2**: 377 (Sept. 13) 1941.
Zadek, I.:	Transverse - Wedge Arthrodesis for the Relief of Pain in Rigid Flat-Foot	J. Bone & Joint Surg. **17**: 453 (April) 1935.
	Accessory Tarsal Scaphoid	J. Bone & Joint Surg. **30A**: 957-968 (July) 1948.

Chapter XXIII

Affections of the Neck and Shoulder

Torticollis

Adson, A. W., Young, H. H., and Ghormley, R. K.:	Spasmodic Torticollis	J. Bone & Joint Surg. **28**: 299 (April) 1946.
Chandler, F. A., and Altenberg, A.:	"Congenital" Muscular Torticollis	J. A. M. A. **125**: 476-483 (June 17) 1944.
Dickson, J. A.:	The Treatment of Torticollis	S. Clin. North America **17**: 1349 (Oct.) 1937.
Hulbert, K. F.:	Congenital Torticollis	J. Bone & Joint Surg. **32B**: 50-59 (Feb.) 1950.
Middleton, D. S.:	The Pathology of Congenital Torticollis	Brit. J. Surg. **18**: 188 (Oct.) 1930.
Rugh, J. T.:	Spasmodic Torticollis: Its Cause and Treatment	Am. J. Surg. **49**: 490 (Sept.) 1940.

Cervical Rib, Scalenus Anticus Syndrome, and Cervical Spine Lesions

Adson, A. W.:	Surgical Treatment for Symptoms Produced by Cervical Rib and the Scalenus Anticus Muscle	Surg., Gynec. & Obst. **85**: 687 - 700 (Dec.) 1947.
Adson, A. W., and Coffey, J. R.:	Cervical Rib	Ann. Surg. **85**: 839 (June) 1927.
Cohn, B. N. E.:	Painful Shoulder Due to Lesions of Cervical Spine	Am. J. Surg. **66**: 269 (Nov.) 1944.
Gage, M., and Parnell, H.:	Scalenus Anticus Syndrome	Am. J. Surg. **73**: 252-268 (Feb.) 1947.

McGowan, J. M.:   Cervical Rib: The Role   Ann. Surg. **124:** 71-89
                                of the Clavicle in Oc-   (July) 1946.
                                clusion of the Subcla-
                                vian Artery

Michelsen, J. J., and   Pain and Disability of   New   England J. Med.
  Mixter, W. J.:   Shoulder and Arm Due   **231:** 279 (Aug. 24)
                                to Herniation of the   1944.
                                Nucleus Pulposus of
                                Cervical Intervertebral
                                Disks

Patterson, R. H.:   Cervical Ribs and Scale-   Ann. Surg. **111:** 531
                                nus Muscle Syndrome   (April) 1940.

Reichert, F. L.:   Compression of Brachial   J. A. M. A. **118:** 294
                                Plexus; Scalenus An-   (Jan. 24) 1942.
                                ticus Syndrome

Swank, R. L., and   Scalenus Anticus Syn-   Arch. Neurol. & Psychiat.
  Simeone, F. A.:   drome: Types; Their   **51:** 432-445 (May)
                                Characterization, Diag-   1944.
                                nosis and Treatment

Telford, E. D., and   P r e s s u r e at Cervico- J. Bone & Joint Surg.
  Mothershead, S.:   brachial Junction, Op-   **30B:** 249-265 (May)
                                erative and Anatomi-   1948.
                                cal Study

Telford, E. D., and   The Vascular Complica-   Brit. J. Surg. **18:** 557
  Stopford, J. S. B.:   tions of Cervical Rib   (April) 1931.

                                     The Shoulder

Abbott, L. C.,   Surgical Approaches to   J. Bone & Joint Surg.
  Saunders, J. B. deC.   Shoulder Joint   **31A:** 235-255 (April)
  M., Hagey, H., and   1949.
  Jones, E. W., Jr.:

Adams, J. C.:   Recurrent Dislocation of   J. Bone & Joint Surg.
                                Shoulder   **30B:** 26-38 (Feb.)
                                                             1948.

Armstrong, J. R.,   Painful Shoulder Sym-   J. Bone & Joint Surg.
  Brown, J. T.,   posium (six articles)   **31B:** 414-442 (Aug.)
  Harrison, S. H.,   1949.
  Jones, G. B.,
  Simmonds, F. A., and
  Withers, R. J. W.:

Bankart, A. S. B.:   An Operation for Recur-   Brit. J. Surg. **26:** 320
                                rent Dislocation (Sub-   (Oct.) 1938.
                                luxation) of the Stern-
                                oclavicular Joint

                                The Pathology and Treat-   Brit. J. Surg. **26:** 23
                                ment of Recurrent Dis-   (July) 1938.
                                location of the Shoul-
                                der Joint

Bennett, G. E.:   The Use of Fascia for   Arch. Surg. **13:** 655
                                the Reenforcement of   (Nov.) 1926.
                                Relaxed Joints

Bennett, G. E.:   Recurrent Dislocation of the Shoulder   Internat. S. Digest **5:** 67 (Feb.) 1928.

Old Dislocations of the Shoulder   J. Bone & Joint Surg. **18:** 594 (July) 1936.

Bishop, W. A.:   Calcification of the Supraspinatus Tendon   Arch. Surg. **39:** 231 (Aug.) 1939.

Bost, F. C., and Inman, V. T.:   Pathological Changes in Recurrent Dislocation of the Shoulder: Report of Bankart's Operative Procedure   J. Bone & Joint Surg. **24:** 595 (July) 1942.

Bosworth, B. M.:   C a l c i u m Deposits in Shoulder a n d Subacromial Bursitis: Survey of 12,122 Shoulders   J. A. M. A. **116:** 2477 (May 31) 1941.

Bosworth, D. M.:   Supraspinatus Syndrome: Symptomatology, Pathology and Repair   J. A. M. A. **117:** 422 (Aug. 9) 1941.

Brewer, A. A., and Zink, D. C.:   R a d i a t i o n Therapy of Acute Subdeltoid Bursitis   J. A. M. A. **122:** 800-801 (July 17) 1943.

Caldwell, G. A., Broderick, T. F., Jr., and Rose, R. M.:   Sympathetic Block of the Stellate Ganglion. Its Application in Orthopedic Conditions   J. Bone & Joint Surg. **28:** 513 (July) 1946.

Caldwell, G. A., and Unkauf, B. M.:   Results of Treatment of Subacromial Bursitis in 340 Cases   Ann. Surg. **132:** 432-442 (Sept.) 1950.

Codman, E. A.:   The Shoulder: Rupture of t h e Supraspinatus Tendon and Other Lesions in or About the Subacromial Bursa   Boston, Thomas Todd Co., 1934.

Rupture of the Supraspinatus   Am. J. Surg. **42:** 603 (Dec.) 1938.

Conwell, H. E.:   Subcutaneous Rupture of the Biceps Flexor Cubiti; Report of One Case   J. Bone & Joint Surg. **10:** 788 (Oct.) 1928.

Cubbins, W. R., Callahan, J. J., and Scuderi, C. S.:   The Reduction of Old or Irreducible Dislocations of the Shoulder Joint   Surg., Gynec. & Obst. **58:** 129 (Feb.) 1934.

DePalma, A. F.:   Surgery of the Shoulder   Philadelphia, J. B. Lippincott Co., 1950.

Dickson, J. A., and Crosby, E. H.:   Periarthritis of the Shoulder   J. A. M. A. **99:** 2252 (Dec. 31) 1932.

Gilcreest, E. L.:   Rupture of Muscles and Tendons, Particularly Subcutaneous Rupture of the Biceps Flexor Cubiti   J. A. M. A. **84:** 1819 (June 13) 1925.

Gilcreest, E. L.: The Common Syndrome of Rupture, Dislocation and Elongation of the Long Head of the Biceps Brachii; An Analysis of 100 Cases — Surg., Gynec. & Obst. **58**: 322 (Feb. 15) 1934.

Dislocation and Elongation of the Long Head of the Biceps Brachii — Ann. Surg. **104**: 118 (July) 1936.

Gilcreest, E. L., and Albi, P.: Unusual Lesions of Muscles and Tendons of the Shoulder Girdle and Upper Arm — Surg., Gynec. & Obst. **68**: 903 (May) 1939.

Henderson, M. S.: Results Following Tenosuspension Operations for Habitual Dislocation of the Shoulder — J. Bone & Joint Surg. **17**: 978 (Oct.) 1935.

Henry, M. O.: Acromio-Clavicular Dislocations — Minnesota Med. **12**: 431 (July) 1929.

Hitchcock, H. H., and Bechtol, C. O.: Painful Shoulder; Observations on Role of Tendon of Long Head of Biceps Brachii in Its Causation — J. Bone & Joint Surg. **30A**: 263-273 (April) 1948.

Hitzrot, J. M.: Surgical Diseases of the Shoulder Bursae — Ann. Surg. **98**: 273 (Aug.) 1933.

Howorth, M. B.: Calcification of the Tendon Cuff of the Shoulder — Surg., Gynec. & Obst. **80**: 337-345 (April) 1945.

Inman, V. T., Saunders, J. B. deC. M., and Abbott, L. C.: Observations on the Function of the Shoulder Joint — J. Bone & Joint Surg. **26**: 1 (Jan.) 1944.

Keyes, E. L.: Observations on Rupture of the Supraspinatus Tendon, Based Upon the Study of 73 Cadavers — Ann. Surg. **97**: 849 (June) 1933.

King, J. M., Jr., and Holmes, G. W.: Diagnosis and Treatment of 450 Painful Shoulders — J. A. M. A. **89**: 1956 (Dec. 3) 1927.

Klein, I.: Treatment of Peritendinitis Calcarea of the Shoulder Joint by Roentgen Irradiation — Am. J. Roentgenol. **56**: 366 (Sept.) 1946.

Mayo Clinic Number: Symposium on Pain in the Shoulder and Arm — S. Clin. North America **26**: 799-840 (Aug.) 1946.

McLaughlin, H. L.: Lesions of the Musculotendinous Cuff of the Shoulder: I. The Exposure and Treatment of Tears With Retraction — J. Bone & Joint. Surg. **26**: 31 (Jan.) 1944.

McLaughlin, H. L.:   Lesions of the Musculo-   J. A. M. A. **128**: 563
                            tendinous Cuff of the   (June 23) 1945.
                            Shoulder: II. Differ-
                            ential Diagnosis of
                            Rupture

                            Lesions of the Musculo-   Ann. Surg. **124**: 354-362
                            tendinous Cuff of the   (Aug.) 1946.
                            Shoulder: III. Obser-
                            vations on the Path-
                            ology, Course and
                            Treatment of Calcified
                            Deposits

McLaughlin, H. L., and   Lesions of Musculotendi-   J. Bone & Joint Surg.
Asherman, E. G.:   nous Cuff of Shoulder   **33A**: 76-86 (Jan.)
                                                           1951.

McMaster, P. E.:   Tendon and Muscle Rup-   J. Bone & Joint Surg.
                            tures; Clinical and Ex-   **15**: 705 (July) 1933.
                            perimental Studies on
                            the Causes and Loca-
                            tions of Subcutaneous
                            Ruptures

Meyer, A. W.:   Spontaneous Dislocation   Arch. Surg. **17**: 493
                            and Destruction of   (Sept.) 1928.
                            Tendon of Long Head
                            of Biceps Brachii

Meyerding, H. W., and   Chronic Functional Le-   Arch. Surg. **35**: 646
Ivins, J. C.:   sions of the Shoulder   (Oct.) 1937.

                            Causation and Treatment   Arch. Surg. **56**: 693-708
                            of Painful Stiff Shoul-   (June) 1948.
                            der

Moseley, H. F.:   Shoulder Lesions   Springfield, Ill., Charles
                                                           C. Thomas, 1945.

Nicola, T.:   Recurrent Anterior Dis-   J. Bone & Joint Surg.
                            location of the Shoul-   **11**: 128 (Jan.) 1929.
                            der: A New Operation

                            Recurrent Dislocation of   J. Bone & Joint Surg.
                            the Shoulder   **16**: 663 (July) 1934.

Norwich, I.:   Calcification of Supra-   Surg., Gynec. & Obst.
                            spinatus Tendon: In-   **86**: 183-191 (Feb.)
                            filtration Therapy   1948.
                            With Local Anesthesia
                            and Multiple Needling

Osmond-Clarke, H.:   Habitual Dislocation of   J. Bone & Joint Surg.
                            Shoulder, Putti-Platt   **30B**: 19-25 (Feb.)
                            Operation   1948.

Patterson, R. L., and   Treatment of Acute Bur-   J. Bone & Joint. Surg.
Darrach, W.:   sitis by Needle Irriga-   **19**: 993 (Oct.) 1937.
                            tion

Schneider, C. C.:   Acromioclavicular Dislo-   J. Bone & Joint. Surg.
                            cation; Autoplastic Re-   **15**: 957 (Oct.) 1933.
                            construction

Skinner, H. A.:	Anatomical Considerations Relative to Rupture of the Supraspinatus Tendon	J. Bone & Joint. Surg. **19:** 137 (Jan.) 1937.
Steindler, A.:	Reconstructive Surgery of the Upper Extremity	New York, D. Appleton & Co., 1923.
	The Traumatic Deformities and Disabilities of the Upper Extremity	Springfield, Ill., Charles C. Thomas, 1946.
Urist, M. R.:	Complete Dislocations of the Acromioclavicular Joint	J. Bone & Joint Surg. **68:** 813 (Oct.) 1946.
Wilson, C. L.:	Lesions of Supraspinatus Tendon: Degeneration, Rupture and Calcification	Arch. Surg. **46:** 307 (March) 1943.
Young, B. R.:	The Roentgen Treatment of Bursitis of the Shoulder	Am. J. Roentgenol. **56:** 626 (Nov.) 1946.

Chapter XXIV

Affections of the Elbow, Wrist, Hand, and Jaw

The Elbow

Bristow, W. R.:	Myositis Ossificans and Volkmann's Paralysis	Brit. J. Surg. **10:** 475 (April) 1923.
Brooks, B.:	Pathologic Changes in Muscle as a Result of Disturbances of Circulation; An Experimental Study of Volkmann's Ischemic Paralysis	Arch. Surg. **5:** 188 (July) 1922.
Campbell, W. C.:	Malunited Fractures and Unreduced Dislocations About the Elbow	J. A. M. A. **92:** 122 (Jan. 12) 1929.
Carp, L.:	Tennis Elbow (Epicondylitis) Caused by Radiohumeral Bursitis; Anatomic, Clinical Roentgenologic, and Pathologic Aspects, With Suggestions as to Treatment	Arch. Surg. **24:** 905 (June) 1932.
Cyriax, J. H.:	The Pathology and Treatment of Tennis Elbow	J. Bone & Joint Surg. **18:** 921 (Oct.) 1936.
Dobbie, R. P.:	Avulsion of Lower Biceps Brachii Tendon: Analysis of Fifty-One Previously Unreported Cases	Am. J. Surg. **51:** 662 (March) 1941.

Foisie, P. S.:	Volkmann's Ischemic Contracture: Analysis of Its Proximate Mechanism	New England J. Med. **226:** 671 (April 23) 1942.
Geschickter, C. F., and Maseritz, I. H.:	Myositis Ossificans	J. Bone & Joint Surg. **20:** 661 (July) 1938.
Griffiths, D. L.:	Volkmann's Ischaemic Contracture (Hunterian Lecture)	Brit. J. Surg. **28:** 239 (Oct.) 1940.
Jones, R.:	Volkmann's Ischaemic Contracture, With Special Reference to Treatment	Brit. M. J. **2:** 639 (Oct. 13) 1928.
March, H. C.:	Osteochondritis of the Capitellum (Panner's Disease)	Am. J. Roentgenol. **51:** 682-684 (June) 1944.
Osgood, R. B.:	Radiohumeral Bursitis, Epicondylitis, Epicondylalgia (Tennis Elbow)	Arch. Surg. **4:** 420 (March) 1922.
Speed, J. S.:	An Operation for Unreduced Posterior Dislocation of the Elbow	South. M. J. **18:** 193 (March) 1925.
VanGorder, G. W.:	Surgical Approach in Old Posterior Dislocation of the Elbow	J. Bone & Joint Surg. **14:** 127 (Jan.) 1932.

The Wrist and Hand

Anton, J. I., Reitz, G. B., and Spiegel, M. B.:	Madelung's Deformity	Ann. Surg. **108:** 411 (Sept.) 1938.
Blair, H. C.:	Carpal Osteitis	Ann. Surg. **89:** 748 (May) 1929.
Buchman, J.:	Traumatic Osteoporosis of the Carpal Bones	Ann. Surg. **87:** 892 (June) 1928.
Bunnell, S.:	Surgery of the Hand, 2nd Edition	Philadelphia, J. B. Lippincott Co., 1949.
Cutler, C. W., Jr.:	The Hand. Its Disabilities and Diseases	Philadelphia, W. B. Saunders Co., 1942.
Davis, A. A.:	The Treatment of Dupuytren's Contracture	Brit. J. Surg. **19:** 539 (April) 1932.
Destot, E.:	Injuries of the Wrist: A Radiological Study	London, Ernest Benn Ltd., 1925.
Dwight, T.:	Clinical Atlas: Variations of the Bones of the Hands and Feet	Philadelphia, J. B. Lippincott Co., 1907.
Evans, J. A.:	Reflex Sympathetic Dystrophy; Report on 57 Cases	Ann. Int. Med. **26:** 417-426 (March) 1947.

Goldsmith, R.: | Kienböch's Disease of the Semilunar Bone | Ann. Surg. **81:** 857 (April) 1925.

Gurd, F. B.: | Post-Traumatic Acute Bone Atrophy (Sudeck's Atrophy) | Ann. Surg. **99:** 449 (March) 1934, and Arch. Surg. **32:** 271 (Feb.) 1936.

Hanlon, C. R.: | DeQuervain's Disease | Am. J. Surg. **77:** 491-498 (April) 1949.

Horwitz, T.: | Dupuytren's Contracture: Consideration of Anatomy of Fibrous Structures of Hand in Relation to This Condition With Interpretation of Histology | Arch. Surg. **44:** 687 (April) 1942.

Jones, R. W.: | Carpal Semilunar Dislocations and Other Wrist Dislocations With Associated Nerve Lesions | Proc. Roy. Soc. Med. (Sect. Orthop.) **22:** 43 (June) 1929.

Kanavel, A. B.: | Splinting and Physiotherapy in Infections of the Hand | J. A. M. A. **83:** 1984 (Dec. 20) 1924.

 | Infections of the Hand, 5th Ed. | Philadelphia, Lea & Febiger, 1925.

Koch, S. L.: | Acquired Contractures of the Hand | Am. J. Surg. **9:** 413 (Sept.) 1930.
 | Dupuytren's Contraction | J. A. M. A. **100:** 878 (March 25) 1933.

Loomis, L. K.: | Variations of Stenosing Tenosynovitis at Radial Styloid Process | J. Bone & Joint Surg. **33A:** 340-347 (April) 1951.

Meyerding, H. W., Black, J. R., and Broders, A. C.: | Etiology and Pathology of Dupuytren's Contracture | Surg., Gynec. & Obst. **72:** 582 (March) 1941.

Patterson, D. C., and Jones, E. K.: | DeQuervain's Disease: Stenosing Tendovaginitis at the Radial Styloid | Am. J. Surg. **67:** 296-301 (Feb.) 1945.

Rhoades, R. L.: | Tenosynovitis of the Forearm | Am. J. Surg. **73:** 248 (Feb.) 1947.

Smillie, I. S.: | Mallet Finger | Brit. J. Surg. **24:** 439 (Jan.) 1937.

Smith, F. M.: | Late Rupture of Extensor Pollicis Longus Tendon Following Colles's Fracture | J. Bone & Joint Surg. **28:** 49 (Jan.) 1946.

Thompson, C. F., and Kalayjian, B.: | Madelung's Deformity and Associated Deformity at Elbow | Surg., Gynec. & Obst. **69:** 221 (Aug.) 1939.

The Jaw

Burman, M., and
  Sinberg, S. W.:

Condylar Movement in
  the Study of Internal
  Derangement of the
  Temporomandibular
  Joint

J. Bone & Joint Surg.
  28: 351 (April) 1946.

Kazanjian, V. H.:

Ankylosis of the Tempo-
  romandibular Joint

Surg., Gynec. & Obst.
  67: 333 (Sept.) 1938.

Wakeley, C. P. G.:

The Surgery of the Tem-
  poromandibular Joint

Surgery **5**: 697 (May)
  1939.

INDEX

A

Abbott treatment of scoliosis, 386
Abnormalities of fingers and toes, congenital, 48
Abscess, Brodie's, 132
  cold, 160, 163
  psoas, 169, 175
  tuberculous, 160
Absence, congenital, of individual bones, 43
Accessory, bones of foot, 494
  of hand, 537
  scaphoid (tarsal), 494
Acetabulum, dysplasia of, 58
  intrapelvic protrusion of, 438
  wandering, 180
Achilles bursa, posterior, 491
  tendon, rupture of, 492
    shortening of, 478
    tenosynovitis of, 491
Achondroplasia, 92, 98
Aclasis, diaphyseal or metaphyseal, 99
Acromegaly, 121
Acromioclavicular dislocation, old, 517
ACTH (adrenocorticotrophic hormone), 202, 210, 217, 219
Actinomycosis, 135
Adamantinoma, extramaxillary, 307
Adolescent coxa vara, 431
  kyphosis, 388
  rickets, 85
Adult round back, 392
Albee bone peg operation, 347
  inlay bone graft, 341
  reconstruction of hip, 349
  technic of spinal fusion, 175
Albers-Schönberg disease, 105
Albright's syndrome, 113
Albuminuria, Bence-Jones, in multiple myeloma, 323
Amputation in neuropathic arthropathy, 275
  in old injury of sciatic nerve, 300
  in osteogenic sarcoma, 319
  in tuberculosis of ankle and foot, 193
    of knee, 192
    of wrist, 199
  in tuberculous dactylitis, 199
  intrauterine, 50
Amyoplasia congenita, 51
Amyotonia congenita, 305
Amyotrophic lateral sclerosis, 270
Anatomy of bones and joints, 19-21

Andry's *L'Orthopédie,* 17, 367
Anemia, bone changes in, 95
Aneurysm, bone, 319
Angioma, of bone, 307
  of muscle or fascia, 330
Angle, lumbosacral, 410
Ankle, ankylosis of, optimum position for, 153
  arthrodesis of, after old injury, 358
    in infantile paralysis, 254
    in tuberculosis, 193
  dislocation of, congenital, 74
  excision of, in tuberculosis, 193
  incision for drainage of, 144
  malunion of fracture in region of, 356
  reconstruction of, after old injury, 357
  swelling in region of, 496
  tuberculosis of, 192
Ankylosing arthritis, 201
Ankylosis, 148-151
  in atrophic arthritis, 203
  in pyogenic arthritis, 142
  of jaw, 542
  optimum positions for, 151
Annulus fibrosus, 392
Anomaly, developmental (*see* Deformity, congenital)
Anserina bursa, 466
Anterior bowleg, 86
  heel, Cook, 483
  metatarsalgia, 481
  poliomyelitis (*see* Infantile paralysis)
Apophysitis of os calcis, 492
  of tibial tuberosity, 459
Arachnodactyly, 49
Aran-Duchenne type of paralysis, 270
Arborescent lipomas, 458
Arch supports, 473, 475, 484
Arches of foot, 469
  pads for, 473, 484
Arthralgia, syphilitic, 148
Arthrectomy (*see* Excision of joint)
Arthritis, ankylosing, 201
  atrophic, 201
  chronic, 200-235
  classification of, 201
  climacteric, 213
  deformans, 201
  degenerative, 201
  gonococcal, 145
  gouty, 218
  gummatous, 148

T